EMOTIONAL CARE OF
HOSPITALIZED CHILDREN

EMOTIONAL CARE OF
HOSPITALIZED CHILDREN

An Environmental Approach
Second Edition

MADELINE PETRILLO, R.N., M.Ed.

Director of Pediatric Nursing
Memorial Sloan-Kettering
Cancer Center, New York

and

SIRGAY SANGER, M.D.

Director, Parent-Child Program
St. Luke's Hospital, New York

J. B. LIPPINCOTT COMPANY
PHILADELPHIA • TORONTO

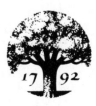

Dedicated to
The Association for the
Care of Children in Hospitals

and

Lilen, Terry and Vicky

Second Edition

COPYRIGHT © 1980 BY J. B. LIPPINCOTT COMPANY

6   5   4

Library of Congress Cataloging in Publication Data

Petrillo, Madeline
    Emotional care of hospitalized children.

    Includes bibliographies and index.
    1. Children—Hospital care.   2. Sick children
—Psychology.   3. Children—Preparation for medical care.   I. Sanger, Sirgay, 1935–   joint author.   II. Title. [DNLM: 1. Child, Hospi-talized—Psychology.   2. Mental health services—In infancy and childhood.   WS105 P495e]
RJ242.P47   1980   610.73′62   79-27462
ISBN 0-397-54343-3

Preface to the Second Edition

Since the first edition of this book, the care of children in hospitals has come to occupy a special niche in nursing and liaison psychiatry. Though the comprehensive program we evolved through pioneering efforts in the 1960s remains as a core curriculum in this edition, recent developments in neonatology, thanatology, ambulatory care, chronic disease, child abuse, consumerism in the general public, consciousness-raising of nursing, cumulative effects of television and inner-city life had to be integrated with the earlier text.

The need for this in-depth practical exposition of the facts, theories and techniques of humanizing the hospital experience for children and adolescents is greater than ever. If anything, life is more complicated for families, costs are much higher, medical science more arcane.

Clinical vignettes graphically illustrate the joys and challenges of working in this exciting field—one that occupies a nexus for many professionals and an in-vivo frontier of the best efforts caring people make as they combine expertise with humanitarian wishes to promote health in the newest members of our community. Our clinical vignettes are realistic and real: all the illustrations do not have happy endings.

It is not the purpose of this book to consider such issues as the placement of comprehensive pediatric care services in general and in children's hospitals, the separation of pediatric specialties in different community hospitals, the usefulness of separate facilities for long-term illness and acute illness, gathering community support for the cost of health care, the presence of child advocates, the communication and the architectural design of pediatric units.

Each of these is worthy of detailed consideration. However, they are parallel to the scope of what we have written—for example, though rooms should be provided for parent and family use during visits and rooming-in, we focus on the interpersonal events that would hold true whether a mother has a luxurious suite for rooming-in or sleeps on a cot next to her young child. In another example, hospitalized teenagers require their own kitchens, recreation areas and privacy, but without the staff's knowing how to control and use their feelings when the teenagers inevitably provoke and challenge authority, such facilities lack meaning.

The essence of what follows, therefore, transcends the community, the type of hospital, the arrangement of physical plant and organization of services. It is the basic understanding of everyone involved with comprehensive care that the child and family under the stress of illness can be effectively encouraged and supported toward emotional as well as physical health.

This book offers an essential, practical knowledge and its direct application without sacrificing the subtlety and sophistication that have been acquired over the past 30 years by many individual workers in these disciplines.

This book is intended for all those who have a part in the clinical management of children and for those professionals who see in the instance of a child's hospitalization an opportunity for promotion of growth, health and maturity. Specifically, it should prove to be beneficial to medical students, house officers, pediatricians, nurses, nursing students, physical and occupational therapists, psychiatric liaison, child psychiatry residents, hospital administrators, psychologists, clinical psychology students, dietitians, child life personnel, recreation workers, hospital teachers, chaplains, social workers and students of social work. Some sections should be useful as manuals for the technique of communicating with children; other sections, for the instruction of parents.

We hope to offer a beacon of light in the rough seas of hospitalization experiences that thousands of children must undergo. As more and more children are cared for on an ambulatory basis or via home care and hospice programs, we must remember to apply preventive and interventive practices for those children who are not so fortunate. The hospital—no matter how bright, how kind its people or how numerous its toys—remains a fearsome place.

MADELINE PETRILLO
SIRGAY SANGER

Preface to the
First Edition

In our work with children, parents and staff, we have evolved, through trial and error, a comprehensive program that applies theory to improving the lot of children who become hospitalized.

In seeing the effects of hospitalization on children, we thought there was a need for an explicit guide-in-depth of just how to deal with the common problems: (a) of the effects of severe stress, and (b) of everyday coping abilities of children and parents. This exposition is divided into major areas that coalesce into a health-promoting milieu. These areas are: a general knowledge of growth and development, the forces of family and culture, human reactions to stress, loss and separation. Also, preventive approaches that have the effect of minimizing trauma to children and their families are given in the form of our actual protocols.

Rationale for this presentation is to bridge the gap between understanding and action. This book offers a practical, essential knowledge and its direct application without sacrificing the subtlety and sophistication that have been acquired over the past 30 years by many individual workers in these disciplines.

This book is intended for all those who have a part in the clinical management of children, and for those professionals who see in the instance of a child's hospitalization, an opportunity for promotion of growth, health and maturity. Specifically, it should prove to be beneficial to medical students, house officers, pediatricians, nurses, student nurses, psychiatric liaison, child psychiatry residents, hospital administrators, clinical psychology students, dietitians, recreation workers, hospital teachers, social workers and student social workers. Sections should be useful as manuals for the technique of communicating with children, other sections for the instruction of parents. Finally, the book supports a systems theory approach to helping children that is implied throughout by the emphasis on the interplay of dynamisms, individually and collectively. Clinical vignettes graphically illustrate the success and failures of the work.

MADELINE PETRILLO
SIRGAY SANGER

Acknowledgments

The authors are grateful for the support of all who made possible the implementation of their ideas. Special appreciation is given to Page Brenner, Sally Everson and Joan Sheehan, assistants in the mental health program, for their outstanding contributions to the mental health of children.

The liaison work described herein took place first in The Children's Hospital and The Massachusetts General Hospital in Boston in the early 1960s, later in The New York Hospital–Cornell Medical Center. Inspirational teachers and colleagues at these hospitals whom we also wish to remember are: Gregory Rochlin, Richard Peebles, John Lamont, John Nemiah and Suzanne T. van Amerongen.

Contents

Introduction

Despite our present sophistication regarding the psychological responses of children to illness and hospitalization, and the impressive body of knowledge in child development, it is striking to note the discrepancies between what we know and what we do in the hospital environment.

With few exceptions, the policies and routines of the majority of pediatric departments in this country are little different from those of the pediatric departments of several decades ago. Research findings in human development and family dynamics have not been well integrated into practice, even though they are basic to the care of children. Indeed, we need to know more, and we need to encourage more relevant research. But at this time it is our belief that the most compelling need is for the application of existing knowledge by those most intimately involved in patient care. Application has been too long in coming.

Considering this current state of pediatric care, it may be surprising to learn that knowledge and practice were not initially at variance. Prior to 1900 and around the turn of the century, in the prescientific era, the literature overflowed with information on child-rearing practices and on socioeconomic conditions of the family and their consequences for child development, demonstrating that these areas were definitely within the purview of the new discipline of pediatrics.[1, 2]

The scientific era, however, worked against this philosophy. From 1920 to 1950, new advances in microbiology, immunology, biochemistry, physiology, pathology and pharmacology overshadowed child development and totally revamped medical education. As a result, interest shifted to the application of biological research. Although a number of child research institutes were organized simultaneously—some within universities divorced from medical centers and others under medical auspices—they had little influence. Publications in developmental research were for the most part neglected as the clinically oriented disciplines focused on the disease process.

Concern for child welfare in general was not evident again until the late '40s, once it was clear that more dramatic declines in infant morbidity and mortality could not be expected. Interest in psychosocial development and children's adaptation to a changing society was revived. But there were factors that discouraged progress: the academic community resisted this trend, and those in favor of it lacked direction. They therefore sought the assistance of child psychiatry. But this young discipline had a different frame of reference. Early studies in child behavior were oriented toward sickness, and their conclusions, presented in the language of pathology rather than in terms of adaptation, had little relevance for normal children. Theories expressed in psychiatric jargon were clear to only a select few. And so they failed to reach a wide audience. The child psychiatry of the period was not equipped to teach developmental theory and concepts of preventive psychiatry, and pediatrics itself was not, for the most part, motivated to research child development.

The new interest was reflected, nevertheless, in the creation of a section on child development of the Academy of Pediatrics for the purpose of stimulating child development research and incorporating the study of growth and development into pediatric education. While the objectives were clear, once again they had little impact on clinical practice.

In the literature of the period, there appeared a number of studies on the psychological significance of illness for children during various stages of development, conducted by both pediatricians and child psychiatrists: as early as 1936 by Beverly;[3] in 1942 by Jackson[4] and Bakwin;[5] in 1945 by Senn[6] and in 1948 by Langford.[7] During the same years, Levy,[8] Jessner and Kaplan,[9] Pearson[10] and Deutch[11] focused on children's emotional reactions to surgical procedures, thus enriching our understanding in this area. Investigators such as A. Freud,[12] Freud and Burlingham,[13] Spitz,[14] Goldfarb[15] and others studied the distortion of personality as the consequence of institutionalization or separation from parents. The works of

Bowlby,[16] Robertson[17] and A. Freud were most rewarding. In the hospitals of Great Britain, they brought about urgently needed reforms that served to humanize the hospital experience. In the late 1950s Parliament supported these research findings by passing a law permitting mothers of hospitalized children to room-in at government expense.

In the United States at this time, "A Study of the Emotional Reactions of Children and Families to Hospitalization and Illness" was carried out at Children's Medical Center in Boston by Dane Prugh and others and was published in the *American Journal of Orthopsychiatry* in January 1953. It revealed much of what we needed to know about hospital trauma in parents and children and recommended prophylactic measures. Regrettably, the conclusions drawn from this work did not generate similar responses as did those in Great Britain on the part of administrators of American institutions.

As the normal child increasingly became a subject of study, the situation appeared more hopeful. Other health professional personnel—nurses, social workers, physical and recreational therapists—were more frequently exposed to courses in the behavioral sciences. Still, this exposure was not reflected in actual child care practices. Theories were not yet translated into practical techniques applicable to hospitalized children. Little in the behavior of professionals indicated their having had special education in human development.

Skilled mental health personnel from various disciplines, working independently, have attempted to promote a comprehensive approach to child management, but they have found it difficult to effect permanent change without the wide support of colleagues. Others, such as volunteers or students, have succeeded in working creatively with individual children, but have been able to make only fleeting impressions on the field.

The climate was not suitable. The '50s were characterized by rigidity and conservatism and were thus unaccepting of innovations. Consequently, progress remained lopsided. Research findings brought about drastic changes in physical treatment over the decades but had minimal influence on the total care of patients.

Not until the '60s did we see a loosening of the old rigidity. The climate was right. We entered an era that emphasized the characteristics of feelings, emotions, imagination and creativity as desirable components of the human psyche. The mood was conducive to the expansion of knowledge and humanitarian reform. So it was not surprising to find signs of shifting attitudes that continue to the present.

A decade or so ago most progressive workers in the field of child development and child care would have been satisfied with limited goals in the emotional care of hospitalized children, knowing full well that the majority of pediatric facilities did not subscribe to child care practices leading to good hospital adjustment. The highest expectation was for minimal psychological damage. Today, however, in most enlightened areas we are no longer thinking small, in terms of minimal negative results, but rather in the more ambitious terms of the beneficial, constructive uses of the hospital experience for children and their families. It is our overall philosophy that only by being prepared to utilize all available knowledge in the many aspects of child development can we be of greatest service to children who, by the occasion of illness, present us with an extraordinary opportunity to look beyond their immediate sickness to their general adaptation and health.

To accomplish this goal, a change in the basic philosophy of most pediatric departments to affect the total environment for hospitalized children must occur. This change can be accomplished only with administrative support.

A change in the environment requires that the permanent pediatric staff of all disciplines be educated in the application of theory; that they become sensitive to the meaning of hospitalization and treatment to children; that they develop communication skills and techniques for working constructively with children and their families; and that they utilize their understanding of growth and development to identify problems that are present before hospitalization, as well as those induced by illness. Specifically, they need to know how to work with particular age groups and how to interpret medical/surgical conditions and treatment. They need to know how to help children master the stresses of hospitalization and how to recognize obstacles to optimal health. Our thesis is that professionals in child care ought to know as much about the mind as the body.

With this background, pediatric personnel become the role models who are able to indicate to new personnel how to intervene in certain situations. They point to the kind of approach that is valued and rewarded. In short, they demonstrate how to translate mental health concepts into skills that can be applied in tangible ways to child care. Until this occurs consistently, we shall see a continuation of existing practices, that is, the arbitrary, crisis-oriented and disease-oriented management of patients.

How can the lag between our understanding and our actions be overcome if not by focusing directly on the problem? This book is an attempt to do just this by describing programs designed to create a therapeutic environment for the care of hospitalized children and their families.

REFERENCES

1. Richmond, J. B.: Child development: a basic science for pediatrics. Pediatrics 39:649–58, 1967.
2. Sears, R. R.: Your ancients revisited: a history of child development. *In* Hetherington, M. E. (ed.): Review of Child Development Research. pp. 1–69. Chicago, University of Chicago Press, 1975.
3. Beverly, B. I.: Effect of illness upon emotional development. J. Pediat. 8:533, 1936.
4. Jackson, E. B.: Treatment of the young child in the hospital. Amer. J. Orthopsychiat. 12:56, 1942.
5. Bakwin, H.: Loneliness in infants. Amer. J. Dis. Child. 63:30, 1942.
6. Senn, M. J. E.: Emotional aspects of convalescence; fulfillment of child's emotional needs is factor in physical as well as psychological recovery. Child. 10:24, 1945.
7. Langford, W. S.: Physical illness and convalescence: their meanings to the child. J. Pediat. 33:242, 1948.
8. Levy, D. M.: Psychic traumas of operations in children. Amer. J. Dis. Child. 69:7, 1945.
9. Jessner, L., and Kaplan, S.: Observations on the emotional reactions of children to tonsillectomy and adenoidectomy. *In* Senn, M.

J. E. (ed.): Problems of Infancy and Early Childhood. New York, Macy Foundation, 1948.
10. Pearson, G. H. J.: Effect of operative procedures on emotional life of children. Amer. J. Dis. Child. 62:716, 1941.
11. Deutch, H.: Some psychoanalytic observations in surgery. Psychosom. Med. 4:105, 1942.
12. Freud, A.: The role of bodily illness in the mental life of children. *In* Eissler, R., *et al.* (eds.): The Psychoanalytic Study of the Child, vol. 7. New York, International Universities Press, 1952.
13. Freud, A., and Burlingham, D. T.: Infants Without Families. New York, International Universities Press, 1944.
14. Spitz, R. A.: Hospitalism. The Psychoanalytic Study of the Child 1:33, 1945.
15. Goldfarb, W.: Psychological privation in infancy and subsequent adjustment. Amer. J. Orthopsychiat. 15:247, 1945.
16. Bowlby, J.: The nature of the child's tie to his mother. Int'l. J. Psychoanalysis 39:350, 1958.
17. Robertson, J.: Young Children in Hospitals. London, Tavistock 1958.

Origins

The authors' initial work in the application of growth and development theory and concepts of preventive psychiatry to the care of hospitalized children evolved from the collaboration of two classic disciplines—nursing and psychiatry. Gradually it developed into an entity distinctly its own while retaining basic characteristics of each profession and expanding to include other disciplines.

The following account of beginning experiences in the organization of a pediatric mental health program is presented in the hope of encouraging and guiding others in similar work.

FROM THE PERSONAL POINT OF VIEW OF THE NURSING MENTAL HEALTH CONSULTANT

My interest in total child care began with my experience as an instructor in pediatric nursing. During this period, I was impressed with the ease of communicating to young students the essential needs —both physical and emotional—of hospitalized children. In the clinical area, students demonstrated eagerness and ability to apply classroom instruction. However, it was obvious that with their departure, clinical practice returned to the usual emphasis on physical treatment rather than on the care of the whole child.

I was disappointed to note that many of the same students returning to pediatrics as new graduates no longer functioned on the same level. In their initial encounters with sick children, they received the guidance and support of their instructors. At that time, teachers' values were most influential. Students also received grades for their ability to meet course objectives. In the roles of new staff members, however, they encountered a different set of values—all indisputably important. Priorities were efficiency in carrying out procedures, along with managerial and organizational skills.

Rewards for perpetuating the system and imitating established role models were made tangible by professional advancement and social acceptance. In this setting a child-centered approach to medical care failed to flourish—not because it was overtly discouraged, but simply because it was not highly regarded, and so not promoted.

It became increasingly apparent that a change in child care practices would not be brought about merely by preparing enthusiastic, well-equipped personnel. Change would entail the creation of a new clinical environment through the development of the permanent pediatric staff on all levels. This would ensure the maintenance of an atmosphere favoring comprehensive care, while at the same time supplying the role models for the teaching of all new and transient personnel.

Although it occurred to me how to effect this change, I did not imagine myself as the agent of change. This came later during the summer of 1966 when I worked for a time as a clinical supervisor in the pediatric department of a large medical center, expecting to return to a teaching-consultant position in the fall. Graduate education in mental health and psychiatric nursing led to my being called on frequently during those months to assist in the management of children whose behavior was disruptive. Within a few weeks the number of referrals so increased that I was devoting my time exclusively to working with this group of patients. As the months passed, the staff came to depend on this new service for dealing with patients and parents whom they found burdensome. Later I was asked to join the staff as the mental health consultant for pediatric nursing. In this capacity, I became an insider with the possibility of creating change from within.

The nursing staff made it clear that their need was not so much for consultation on the management of children, but rather for relief from the aggravation that "problem" patients imposed. In their estimation some children required attention beyond their capacity to supply, and my role was to supply it.

Thus, certain children were singled out for special care by the mental health consultant, while the nursing staff assumed responsibility for their physical welfare. Acting on the principle that one begins wherever permitted, I accepted this direction and worked independently for several months with the patients referred to me.

I could have tolerated this arrangement indefinitely for two reasons. First, the deep gratification derived from working in this manner was almost satisfying enough to deter me from the more important goal of motivating active staff involvement in a wider program. Second, I anticipated that a change from a role in which I was accepted conditionally to a more comprehensive one would precipitate greater resistance to the work being done.

Indeed, difficulties began when the focus shifted from a crisis orientation approach to a preventive one. The shift was a subtle and painstaking one. It started with keeping the staff informed on patients' progress, even when little interest was demonstrated. In this way, they were introduced to the basic concepts of working with each child. Gradually, a few nurses began to incorporate similar approaches and to parrot behavioral observations and management techniques without recalling the source. This indicated that the process of identification with a new role model had begun. But it was just a start—a long way from true integration of new attitudes and independent functioning. Chapter 1 describes the reeducation of one group that led subsequently to an environmental approach to child care and influenced the management of children in other pediatric hospitals as well.

FROM THE PERSONAL POINT OF VIEW OF THE LIAISON CHILD PSYCHIATRIST

As part of my residency training in child psychiatry, I spent a significant time during and subsequent to 1962 in Boston's Children's Hospital. In doing some routine pediatric consultations, I quickly became interested in innovative liaison programs. The flaws in the usual pediatric–psychiatric relationship were revealing. Calls for consultation from pediatric personnel were mainly for the relief from troublemaking children. Only those psychiatric problems accompanied by gross behavioral manifestations were being noticed.

There was usually an emergency atmosphere surrounding the referral, with an obvious potential for friction between members of the respective departments. In particular, working in the burn unit at Massachusetts General Hospital 1965–67 (reported in the Journal of American Academy of Child Psychiatry*), I found the weeklong crisis of survival and the emotional trauma of fear and guilt highlighting professional dichotomies. There was a difference in orientation between the two disciplines, in that pediatric time is in terms of hours, shifts, days and weeks while psychiatric time is in weeks, months and years. Further, the psychiatrist working in depth will respond to an immediate situation by thinking about the past, about the individual's unique and characteristic ways of responding and about how a personality is altered when it undergoes stress. The pediatrician is more inclined to limit the issue, deal with it in the present, and assume that a return to good health will assuage the rough spots in getting there. Later, while working in a large New York teaching hospital, I found the application of preventive mental health methods limited to a pilot program in nursing that had been evolving for a year but that was unrecognized by other staff. For the most part, only crises were managed; problems were not anticipated or modified before they were out of control.

Because they perceived their schedules as being overloaded, house officers and attending pediatricians wanted the child assigned to the psychiatrist and a report made. They were not motivated to acquire any diagnostic and therapeutic skills in the area. Therefore, at that time the most interested and motivated groups in the area of preventive mental health were those personnel who were most often with the children and who were confronted frequently with the subtle and gross personality characteristics of their charges. These personnel were nurses, play staff, teachers, occupational and physical therapists, and social workers.

It was apparent, however, that to work individually with these groups would not necessarily result in a team approach to the management of children in that the physicians were conspicuously missing. Although they carried the responsibility for the diagnostic and

*Bernstein, N. R., Sanger, S., Fras, I.: The Functions of the Child Psychiatrist in the Management of Severely Burned Children. J. Amer. Acad. Child Psychiat. 8 (4) 1969, pp. 620–36. Reprinted in Chess, S., and Thomas, A. (eds.): Annual Progress in Child Psychiatry and Child Development, New York, Brunner/Mazel, 1970.

treatment program, they were not motivated to participate in discussions of preventive mental health.

Though nursing and psychiatry were applying preventive methods, they were not truly environmental. The latter requires commitment to a total program on the part of each and every discipline that impinges on the child's awareness.

Representing the largest group and most pivotally situated between the doctors and the other professionals was the nursing mental health consultant. Discussions with her led rapidly to the use of environmental concepts: we were convinced that the child in a hospital was in a new environment and that all the people having a relationship to that child in giving care needed to know and apply emotional care. The opportunity for learning about a given young person and having an impact on him was not to be lost. The inclusion of all people in the hospital who had any relationship to, and responsibility for, the care of the children was necessary.

The subsequent large and small conferences that were held on every pediatric floor were open to everyone except parents; and occasionally, as professionals relaxed more about their prerogatives, parents were also included.

There were many surprises evolving from these "democratic" meetings. Some doctors were reluctant to accept information and formulations from nondoctors. The "psychopathology" of everyday life was a foreign notion, as was the application of family and cultural factors to the understanding of individual children. That psychiatry could concern itself with "normal" people was welcomed by some, feared by others. These meetings were the only nonstructured, nonstratified conferences in which persons of different disciplines could speak to each other as equals. This exchange had frequent repercussions; often it was difficult to stay with the topic of one particular child when there were pressing staff conflicts about diagnosis and management, and personal feelings evoked by the patient that needed resolution.

There were obvious built-in strains within pediatric hospital practice. Young doctors who were eager to apply their scientific acumen, and who enjoyed their authoritarian position, would often conflict with nurses who had to cope with personal needs in learning to live with the great responsibility of pediatric nursing and in exercising their maternal ideals. Doctors seemed overidentified with a "magic-bullet" remedy, cure-justifying-any-means attitude. Nurses were identified with the child as victim of illness and of curative procedures in which they often had to inflict pain without the doctors' ancillary rewards. Resentment was felt among both professions. Play staff, teachers, nursing aides and attendants were unaccustomed, by years of disregard, to contributing their valuable observations and innovations to the professionals higher on the "status ladder." Thus, some of the people working with children needed "deflation" in their role concept; others needed "inflation" in self-respect and job respect. It was a mixed surprise that no one could claim exclusive credit for the improvement of the children.

The ferment created by the environmental approach pointed out the need for integration of this approach in the education and orientation of all people working with children. Finally, the aim of this philosophy was to go beyond the most advanced prevention methods to so manage the hospitalization experience that it promoted and augmented growth.

1

The Dynamics of Change in Reeducation of the Staff for an Environmental Approach

The environment of a pediatric hospital is seldom defined as an emotionally therapeutic setting for the care of children and the interaction of families, visitors and staff. To qualify, an altered approach to pediatric care is required—going beyond the provision for adequate medical services to an approach that promotes the general adaptation of the family (its ability to cope during the crisis of illness) and that serves to bolster the family's emotional state to a level where it can perform as a stable unit and its members can function as stable individuals. In effect, the therapeutic environment supports the continuation of the normal functions of the family for the socialization of the child and the organization of the personality.

How well these functions can be maintained in the hospital depends on the staff's readiness to assume these family responsibilities in the event that parental involvement is absent or inappropriate under the stress of illness. The ability of the staff to "step in", as and when necessary, helps to reduce substantially the degree of regression in both children and parents and, in many instances, actually contributes to the growth of the entire family.

Effective participation and satisfaction from such a program is determined by the kind of education and support available to the caretakers—education and assistance in the clinical area that make it possible for them to supply the children and their families with basic needs for information, caring, belonging and gratification of dependency.

Although we now have an overabundance of knowledge to effect environmental change, we find that the majority of pediatric units are still organized around staff convenience, institutional routines and finances. Developmental needs, family stability and staff morale are not the usual priorities for most hospitals.

This failure in the application of knowledge, according to Schowalter, is attributed to several areas of interlocking conflict in adults that obstruct progress: (1) basic disregard for children who have no political–social impact, and low prestige for the caretakers of hospitalized children; (2) condescending or fearful attitudes toward the sick or troubled, resulting in withdrawal from patients; and (3) competition among adults—self-serving behavior that detracts from child/family-centered care.[1]

Experience confirms that these conflicts do, in fact, exist, though they are often difficult to identify, since they are largely unconscious phenomena. But remedial action cannot be taken to counter their negative effects unless the conflicts are uncovered and consciously resolved.

The following history of one pediatric department reveals many of these same basic conflicts in each phase of its struggle to promote a mental health program leading to environmental change. Four definite developmental phases were identified. One can see from this example just how difficult it is to initiate and maintain a therapeutic environment for hospitalized children even in the present day with all the research and accumulated supportive literature that proves the need for it.

PHASE 1: SETTING THE STAGE FOR INVOLVEMENT

An environmental approach was not in operation during the early months of the mental health program. The only children who received concentrated attention were those in apparent distress— those who obviously had regressed* or had caused difficulty for the staff. In pediatric literature hospitalization is repeatedly described as stressful for everyone, and experience has taught that even seemingly well-adjusted children and families are distressed when one

---

*Regression is a return to an earlier developmental state, such as recurrence of bed-wetting, baby talk, thumb-sucking, rocking, whining. The regression can be intractable or easily reversible.

looks beyond the facade. But because the number of patients who could be managed by the nurse mental health consultant working alone was limited, only the most disruptive situations were approached.

Expansion of the mental health program to include a greater number of children, and to shift the focus to a preventive approach, required the involvement of all the nurses. They held the key positions for determining the environment and experiences to which the children were exposed. In addition, they provided the greatest number of personnel on a 24-hour basis. In an effort to gain their assistance in caring for difficult children, a course in growth and development and in the management of problems most frequently observed in hospitalized children was offered. As a result, their ability to detect patients requiring special help increased appreciably, but the situation was only aggravated by the ensuing flood of referrals.

Obviously, other avenues for routine staff involvement had to be found. The nurses' willingness to use a consultant was a first step. However, in order to reach the numbers of children and families needing help and to influence the philosophy of child care in a lasting way, it was essential to have direct nursing participation. Also, in an environment where the care of patients is the responsibility of many professionals, it was important to plan for eventual widespread acceptance among the various members of the pediatric health care team.

Change in environment is accomplished neither by one person nor by one discipline. For significant change to occur, attention must be directed to influencing the total staff's attitudes on the needs of hospitalized children and on the policies that determine child care practices.

PHASE 2: THE BEGINNINGS OF SUCCESS

Opportunity for expansion of the program to include all patients on a preventive basis came through an incident involving Paul, a 5-year-old who had experienced several previous encounters with hospitalization and surgery, on each occasion becoming more difficult to manage. His reputation preceded him, and anticipation of his arrival caused some consternation. On his last admission for the correction of a bladder-neck obstruction and reimplantation of a ureter, his postoperative behavior was characteristic. He managed to pull out intravenous infusions, tugged at his urinary drainage tubes, regurgitated medications and resorted to frequent tantrums. The separation anxiety he demonstrated was typical of a toddler. Soon after his mother decided that she could safely leave him for a short time, there was a request for help in managing him. His reaction was chaotic; he lashed out at the harassed nurse who tried to distract him, and he banged at the elevator door. The staff was eager to abdicate responsibility for him.

Initially, the approach used to gain this boy's cooperation was commiseration rather than distraction. We encouraged him to re-count his problem, to express his feelings regarding his mother's "abandonment" of him (agreeing that it was difficult for him to bear), to talk about his mother—why she left, where she was and how long she would be there; we offered to stay with him in her place until she returned. Our efforts were geared to assuring him that his feelings were understood and were important to us. He became calm and talked about his family, home, friends and interests not connected with hospitalization. Before long, he appeared content with his newly found relationships.

The fact that Paul was beginning to respond to this approach was evident soon after when he announced the need to urinate. First, we tried to get his impression of what had happened to him, but he remained silent. The importance of helping the child to express his fantasies of his experiences was repeatedly expressed to the staff. This gives the child an opportunity to gain ego mastery over a problem area by putting words to thoughts and provides the occasion to clarify reality. In Paul's case the confusion was apparent, although he was not able to speak about it directly. He had been told on other occasions the purpose of the drainage tubes, but it did not seem to affect his understanding. This time an explanation was delivered visually. A body outline including the genitourinary system was sketched. This was followed by a simple interpretation of the anatomy and physiology, the congenital defects, surgical correction and the placement and purpose of the tubes; and, most significantly in his case, we dealt with the mutilation and castration fantasies common to Paul's period of development. "In the phallic phase . . . whatever part of the body is operated on will take over by displacement the role of the injured genital part.''[2] This was done by playful repetition to clarify his understanding in this way: ''This is where your operation is, right here on your belly. No other part of your body was operated on.'' (Then, pointing to body parts in a playful manner), ''Not your head, not your ears, not your eyes, nor your nose and mouth, not your arms and chest, not your 'peepee,' nor your legs, feet or toes.''

In conjunction with this explanation, Paul was given a stuffed doll on which he was helped to place tubes and bandages in the appropriate areas for his type of surgery. Subsequently, with this doll he was helped to pretend administering medication (oral and intramuscular) and to perform the other procedures that were a part of his treatment.

Paul's reaction was striking; he became cooperative with treatments, accepted the staff and was interested in play. This behavioral change became the subject of a nursing team conference the following day. The consensus was that some of Paul's difficulties had been the result of previous hospital trauma and that much of his turmoil could have been prevented had the new approach been introduced at his first admission. Then the nurses suggested that every patient could profit from similar management by the nursing staff—that is, of rationalizing treatment to a child, providing human closeness and talking to him about experiences as a way of coping with fear. This was the natural opening that promoted active staff involvement and marked the beginning of change in child care activities on a large scale throughout the department.

Once the nurses themselves suggested how they could contribute, and interest was high, it was important to initiate a program quickly. A series of conferences was held to determine how to proceed. At first because of their experience with Paul, attention was directed primarily to preparing children for urologic surgery, focusing on the special needs and considerations for teaching a specific age group—the child's intellectual and emotional development, the child's fantasies and preoccupations and the kinds of explanations needed for a particular medical or surgical problem. Initially, the number of patients and the type of problems considered were deliberately limited to order to allow time for the development of expertise and gratification.

Each newly admitted patient became the responsibility of one nurse whose work schedule permitted her to care for him on several consecutive days and to become well acquainted with him. In preparation for this assignment, each participant witnessed the procedure the child was to undergo and made an outline of the routine. She then received assistance in introducing and interpreting the material to the child.

The direct supervision and support of nurses during their initial efforts proved effective in diminishing the anxiety they experienced in dealing with negative feelings and fantasy material (related to abandonment, mutilation and death). The meaning of illness to children and their various responses to threats of hospitalization were the topics of numerous group and individual conferences. Understanding in these areas increased the staff's tolerance for difficult behavior, helped them to maintain objectivity and taught them not to assume that children easily accepted treatment.

After the nurses felt comfortable with this approach, they allowed parents to witness and to participate in the actual sessions. As the staff became more accomplished and satisfied with their progress, they extended their program to include a variety of genitourinary problems. Within a month, news of the work traveled, and requests were received from a few attending physicians and nurses on other units for help in preparing children for many different surgical procedures.

It was easier at this point to conduct continuous orientation classes for the entire department. Included in these sessions were personnel from the x-ray department, intensive care unit, operating and recovery rooms—areas where we needed support and cooperation in order to continue our close relationships with children. Close clinical supervision of new participants was still feasible because it was possible to draw from the more experienced staff for assistance. On occasion the teaching was carried out with medical students, pediatricians, surgeons and recreational therapists who expressed interest. However, because the nursing group was in the best position to offer this aspect of the program consistently, it remained in their purview.

Initially, the program was underplayed. There was never an intent to include experiences that children did not actually witness; for example, no details of the operating room and of the operative procedure were included. Quite often, information on suctioning, endotracheal tubes and monitoring equipment was excluded because the staff believed that the material was too provocative. Unfortunately, the subjects deleted became the preoccupations of our patients. When children were asked to tell, write or draw about their experiences, the themes frequently concerned the unexplained areas and their fears, confusion or anger over being deceived. Clearly, we were not helping children by protecting them from the inevitable. Any omission of information meant leaving them to bear the complete burden. This indicated that the events needed to be presented in an attenuated form so that they could be viewed with less anxiety, imminence and surprise.

Some of the children were so frightened that they either could not respond immediately to teaching or rejected it altogether. This was primarily true for those who had not received advance preparation by their parents for admission. The prospect of remaining in the hospital was already sufficiently alarming. For them, a more successful approach was to depersonalize the events—that is, to talk about the many other children who were also in the hospital—their reasons for admission, their treatment and the equipment used in their care. Thus, it was possible to touch on the relevant areas indirectly. In addition, much of the essential information was given through playing out procedures on dolls, by allowing the children to take the roles of physicians and nurses—becoming caretakers instead of victims.

One of the major difficulties was in finding the time for work with the child prior to the scheduled procedure. For minor treatment (from a medical, not the child's point of view), the essential aspects of the procedure could be covered even when a child was admitted the afternoon before the event. There was not adequate time, however, for adjustment to the hospital or for thinking through and asking questions about the information given. In complicated procedures, such as cardiac surgery, the material could not be delivered in a condensed fashion because too much, too quickly would be overwhelming for the patients. Because the children also required intensive physical preparation, competition from physicians and technicians from various departments—x-ray, hematology and cardiology—was great. Therefore, it was necessary to interpret to pediatricians and surgeons the importance of adequate time for preparation and to gain their cooperation in admitting patients earlier.

After several revisions and trials, a manual of guidelines for teaching children of all ages was produced with specific instructions on approaches to working with various age groups, scheduling of teaching, content, the amount of information recommended for one session and actual explanations and terminology for each procedure.

As the program developed, we adopted a set of attractive body outlines and produced a number of tools that enhanced our efforts. Patient dolls (male and female, attired in johnny shirts) were made for us by the Volunteer Department and models of frequently used equipment were constructed (see Chapter 6).

During the first year, the greatest progress in reeducating the staff was made in several areas offering the least resistance. Initially the distribution of time and energy was unequal, and deliberately so. Those areas where personnel were uninterested or antagonistic were temporarily avoided. However, the passage of time and staff turnover (a mixed blessing) eventually opened up floors formerly not amenable to change.

Some of the staff complained that their patients had been neglected by the mental health team, an excellent sign of their readiness for the program. When this occurred, it was because the nurses were already motivated by the conviction that the new approach was important. Consequently, this attitude contributed greatly to their successful participation. A number of our nurses stated that they were encouraged through observing the success of colleagues in working with children. They were impressed by the actual demonstration of techniques and the discussion of principles involved. As students, they had heard repeatedly how important it was to support children and their families and to help them cope with the difficult experiences; however, they had not been taught how to do it, nor did they see it being done.

Others were convinced by the excellent results, which were common occurrences, consistently achieved. The children showed greater acceptance of staff members, ability to participate in treatments and ease in expressing their feelings. There was less preoccupation with procedures and illness, a greater capacity for socialization, and interest in play and tolerance for reasonable periods of separation from parents. The adjustment process for patients who were admitted repeatedly for chronic illnesses became easier because they had already mastered many of the fears hospitalization presented.

PHASE 3: INITIAL RESISTANCE

It would have been amazing had the program developed without opposition. Resistance occurred in many forms. At the outset, as long as the mental health consultant worked independently, there was little objection. Of course, there were a few who commented disparagingly on the need for a mental health service, but this was offset, for the most part, by those who were genuinely pleased to have assistance with patients. More overt resentment was demonstrated when tentative demands were made on the nursing staff for direct participation in the management of children with behavior problems. Resentment also occurred in response to the suggestion that much of the regressive behavior and disciplinary problems could be eliminated or modified by staff members themselves. The most common response to this was defensiveness—how could nurses be expected to carry out such functions when the pressures of work were already great?

Though they were never coerced into assuming roles they did not want, efforts were made to influence acceptance indirectly. However, a few of the nurses could not tolerate the discomfort they felt in witnessing the new approach, even though they were not actively engaged in it. Consequently, they resigned. This was balanced, fortunately, by those who were attracted by the program, which was reported in the professional literature, and joined the staff specifically to learn new skills in pediatric care.

Several children with whom the mental health consultant was working were the focus of early resistance. One instance concerned nine-year-old Mario, admitted for multiple operations to correct facial deformities. Prior to admission and during early hospitalization, he manifested severe emotional disturbance. He was referred for special attention because he was unmanageable and physically and socially repulsive to most people. During a five-month period, it was possible to win his trust and help him modify his behavior toward more acceptable standards. In comparison to previous behavior, he now developed remarkable control of violence and acquired the ability to verbalize his feelings and to postpone immediate pleasure. His change brought with it unfortunate repercussions. Whereas originally the plan for working with this child during the most trying periods won the full support of the medical and nursing staff, his improvement brought open resistance. Changes in his management were ordered without prior discussion. Those features and activities that were supportive in his care were suddenly eliminated. In addition, he was subjected to various provocative incidents that served to break down newly established controls.

The situation was analogous to that of resistance on the part of family members to a patient's progress in therapy—hospital personnel, in this instance, taking on the roles of family members. The staff was reluctant to accept the change evident in Mario. For some time he had been a useful scapegoat; and as is frequently the case in the treatment of a disturbed child, the family was unwilling to give up the gratification they derived from the child's negative behavior. One often sees parents attempting to devaluate the therapist or change agent by opposing his efforts. A similar attitude on the part of the staff was also evident toward the mental health consultant.

In Mario's case it was possible to work around the situation by enlisting the support of staff members who understood the dynamics and were willing to share in the responsibility for his care. In other cases, however, when support was not forthcoming it was necessary to abandon work with the children rather than to increase the resistance to the staff and stress to the child or to place the program in greater jeopardy. (See the story of Kate, Chapter 8.)

The most serious resistance developed with the medical staff. In the early phases, no organized effort was made to include them in the program except on an administrative level. It was hoped that enough support would develop among the nursing group to be influential in gaining their support and that a psychiatrist would eventually prepare them for participation in the program. This strategy produced the desired results. Whenever derogatory comments were made to the nurses about their "frivolous" work or about the mental health consultant's interference in medical care, the program and services were asserted to be integral to comprehensive care and not contrary to medical goals. By the time opposition grew, there were already small numbers of nurses, attending physicians and resident pediatricians who could defend the program. They were quick to grasp how the innovations could serve to support children and parents during periods of crisis. As a result, the program was sustained.

PHASE 4: THE MULTIDISCIPLINARY, ENVIRONMENTAL APPROACH IN ACTION

Within a year, the nurses were able to move from the passive stage of asking the mental health consultant to take over the complete management of burdensome patients to active participation in a program of preventive psychiatry—that is, they undertook complete responsibility for the psychological preparation of parents and children for diagnostic, medical and surgical procedures and became adept in the use of dramatic play techniques. This program became routine and was instrumental in reducing stress in most families.

Soon after the nursing staff was educated in this expanded role, both the psychiatry and the psychology departments grew in size and announced their willingness to provide a broad program of services to the pediatric department. The nurses and pediatricians greeted this event enthusiastically and saw in this the potential for a truly interdisciplinary approach to patient care. At this point, psychiatrists, psychologists, social workers and play staff were still working independently. However, discussion between the new liaison psychiatrist and the mental health consultant about this matter soon led to setting up regularly scheduled conferences for all these disciplines as a group in order to minimize the fragmentation of patient care and to expedite services.

At the onset, there was hope for the ideal in collaborative relationships in which a number of characteristics can be observed. One finds in such a group: (1) open-mindedness among personnel; contributions are judged by their relevance to the task or problem and not by the title and corresponding power of the contributor; (2) all groups affected by decisions are involved from the start in the decision-making process and, as a consequence, more relevant contributions emerge and the cooperation of the disciplines most affected is assured; and (3) support and encouragement are given to the discipline assigned to carry out the work.

With the beginning of multidisciplinary work, the program once again underwent a shift in focus from a preventive to an environmental approach. However, no one was prepared for what this would bring.

In the multidisciplinary patient-centered conferences, divergent points of view and basic difficulties in working relationships were exposed. All the traditional conflicts among disciplines were soon apparent. Initially, there was a clash between the child psychiatrist and the pediatricians. The pediatricians resisted some of the interpretations made by the psychiatrist, arguing that many of the theories were untestable and therefore unacceptable; that disturbed behavior could not be understood without considering the neurophysiological development of children, which they said psychiatrists were not doing.

The pediatricians were distressed by the psychiatrist's disinterest in details of physical management and often regarded him as less than professional. The psychiatrist obviously had a great deal to offer the pediatricians. He argued that they wanted magic, instant cures and pointed out that they were deficient in their knowledge of personality development since pediatric education had long neglected the nonhospitalized child. He believed that they were concerned about rare medical entities rather than the problems confronting them in daily practice. He explained that they needed more education in child development; but even so they would require specialists, since the needs of patients and families were too great for any one discipline. And furthermore, there was a substantial difference in the services each specialty had to offer.

The problem between psychology and psychiatry emerged early. The psychologist was new in the hospital structure and had just recently attained autonomy from psychiatry. He wanted recognition. He found himself in a power struggle with the psychiatrist, who showed no signs of deferring to him when their roles overlapped.

The social workers revealed that most of their discontent stemmed from lack of recognition for their role in family therapy. Everyone was willing to relegate to them the thankless jobs of finding placement for children, solving transportation problems, and counseling families with financial difficulties. They also found fault with the nurses who stepped into "their territory" when dealing with parents in the clinical area, even when the parents had not been referred to social work. Teachers, play staff and nursing assistants found that their observations and suggestions in problem solving were not given the same consideration as those of "professional" team members; this was not to their surprise, however.

The nurses had conflicts with almost every group. Once they accepted responsibility for the previously ignored aspects of psychosocial care, they were accused of abandoning their "proper" role. Nevertheless, over a period of months, contrary to traditional role expectations, they emerged as confident, knowledgeable and vocal participants. They lost their usual reticence in offering ideas and were proud to claim results and credit for their work. This view was shared by the parents, who gave the nurses enthusiastic praise when discussing their children with the medical staff.

The neglected area of pediatrics had begun to look appealing to others once techniques that obviously worked were developed. The program was receiving notice in the press and on television and was appreciated by parents, who communicated their gratitude in writing to hospital administrators and recommended the pediatric department to other parents who were interested in a child-centered approach.

The nurses realized what they had accomplished, and they weren't willing to pretend otherwise. They were unwilling to say that they were working under the auspices of other mental health groups. They saw themselves as the key force in change and in the modification of ward environment, although they were seldom credited with this. Their cooperation or lack of it in attempting a new approach with patients or modifying existing practice affected every discipline in the department. Even so, they did not have the status and prestige afforded others working in the area of mental health— psychiatrist, psychologist and social worker. There was a contradiction between status and importance, and the nurses refused to accept this. They wanted recognition for their achievements.

In actuality, there was just a veneer of teamwork, since all team members were not peers. Relationships were in the nature of a hierarchy—nurses subordinate to physicians; social worker, to psychiatrist and psychologist; recreation therapists, teachers and aides, to everyone; and the psychiatrist and psychologist vying for leadership.

Over months of working in this manner, there was a great deal of interpersonal tension and undermining of work, since each discipline was jockeying for leadership or a better position. The rivalry and extreme possessiveness in dealing with patients was most destructive. The needs of children and their families were secondary to staff's needs. The behavior exhibited was analogous to the territorial behavior of animals described by such leading animal behaviorists as Lorenz, Hall and Ardrey—that is, "behavior by which an organism characteristically lays claim to an area and defends it against members of its own species."[3] They assert that territoriality is a basic behavior of all living organisms, including man. Further, place and space are also functions of dominance and high status; the more powerful the animal, the larger and more choice his territory.[4]

In reality, the nurses' change in their traditional role was the basis for much of the disharmony in the department. The pediatricians were most offended by this change, as they were closest in their daily working relationships. (See Bates.) Few people accept changes readily, since change means a number of things to different people. It is associated with problems; it disturbs the equilibrium and necessitates readjustment, which most likely will be resisted. Change can imply that other disciplines are not doing a good job; that one discipline or individual is displaced; or that there is a loss of power or control for a person or a group. All of this applied in this particular situation.

During the years of interdisciplinary meetings, the mental health nurse consultant continued close contact with the nurses during orientation classes and during the six patient-care conferences held weekly. These contacts were used to teach the nurses how to fight constructively. During the crisis periods, the role of the mental health nurse was to help the nurses deal with each discipline so that they could survive in their expanded role.

This is how it was done. Before interdisciplinary meetings the nursing staff met with the mental health nurse to discuss grievances as a way of keeping them in perspective. One objective was to help them handle conflicts as they came up—that is, how to verbalize anger instead of suppressing it. This included not raking up former grievances even when it was tempting. As a result, explosions were kept at a minimum. They rehearsed how to interpret the nature of their work to those who felt threatened, communicating that actually they were offering services previously unavailable, that no one was displaced, and that their work was not contrary to medical goals. These preliminary sessions mobilized peer support, improved the group's ability to articulate their ideas and gave the nurses strength to withstand disapproval from many sides.

In addition, they looked for acceptance of their mental health activities by communicating with individual physicians, psychologists, social workers, play staff and teachers with whom they had good relationships. They talked about the necessity of withdrawing in the face of enormous odds. In some cases when support was not forthcoming, they reluctantly abandoned work with children rather than increasing resistance. (See stories of Calton and Michael, Chapter 8.)

Despite the bombardment the nurses were receiving, because of support they were able to continue their work. They were well on their way to acceptance when an unexpected development occurred: the arrival of a small but militant group of pediatric residents who refused to acknowledge the nurses' new role.

Tension grew. The residents accused the nurses of "taking over"—of resisting the physicians' leadership. Those nurses who also resisted change encouraged them in this point of view. Together, they were instrumental in convincing a number of pediatricians who had formerly accepted the program to withdraw their support. This period of resistance was most damaging, as it affected the treatment of several patients who were currently the subjects of controversy, polarized groups and weakened the influence of the nascent mental health team consisting of the mental health nurse and the liaison psychiatrist.

These physicians saw the contributions of others to patient management as a loss of control over medical care; and they saw the increasing application of psychosocial factors as a devaluation of their work in physical treatment. They then sought to discredit the mental health leadership and thereby to minimize the importance of the area in which they felt threatened.

They demonstrated their power by ordering the nurses to abandon their work; in fact, they actually wrote orders in the patients' charts to that effect, for example, "Discontinue Voodoo." To their amazement and everyone else's, their commands were absolutely disregarded. Instead, the nurses banded together to reaffirm their belief in the program and to insist on its continuation.

There was an impasse. In the power struggle that followed, no one was innocent; everyone took sides. The results were so crippling that top administrative intervention was required. Since the group could not respect and accept each other's roles and unique contributions, an external force was charged with mapping out areas of accountability. This was the Patient Care Committee, initially comprising medical and nursing administrators and attending physicians only. Over a period of months, they took testimony from each discipline involved in dispute, while work continued as usual.

There was a danger that the discord in relationships, as a result of the nurses' professional growth, would bring about the dissolution of the program; nevertheless, forces were working for it. Both nursing and medical administration gave support, and a number of pediatricians convinced their reluctant colleagues of the integral contributions of all members of the health team to comprehensive care.

Once the Patient Care Committee reviewed roles and relationships, the new rules for collaboration were made known in writing to everyone in the department. To ensure cooperation, a supportive pediatrician was named coordinator of mental health services.

Everyone gained from the open discussion that ensued, especially the nursing staff who won acknowledgment for their work. Had they known they had the psychological advantage, they would have been more confident of the outcome. According to Ardrey, possession of a territory offers some mysterious advantage to the defender: the defender is imbued with sufficient energy to fight to guarantee victory.[5]

BEYOND TERRITORIALITY

Once the furor subsided, good things began to happen. There was a tacit acceptance of each other's expertise and professional identity. Conflicts diminished, and the various disciplines moved from competition to cooperation.

The staff learned from these involvements. They found that working in small groups proved advantageous because they were able to trust one another quickly and consequently were more open in expressing their feelings and conflicts. This was possible because consistency of positions and the definition of areas of accountability for each specialty led to predictability of behavior and certain expectations regarding work with families.

As group members became less guarded and less protective of their "rights," they began asking one another for help in difficult situations. Not surprisingly, they found that some individuals were more effective in working with a particular problem or child or that one discipline had more time or better resources for problem solving in other areas. With increased security came increased tolerance for ambiguity, role blurring and an unanticipated by-product of the internal strife—the democratization of the Patient Care Committee to include membership from every group intimately involved in patient care.

The mental health team realized that they were working in an institution, similar to many, in which innovators are seen as people trying to gain power at the expense of others. They saw, too, that some of the disharmony and power struggles as the result of the nurses' professional growth might have been averted had they been able to foresee the extent to which change in the behavior of one discipline would affect its relationship to any closely allied group— just as treatment of one family member brings about counteraction in the total family. In retrospect, a more constructive approach would have been first to prepare each discipline for working with others as collaborators; then to offer similar educational opportunities for all, especially the medical staff. Aside from their basic foundation in the social sciences, the physicians' continuing education in the psychosocial aspects of patient care was limited to participation in multidisciplinary conferences. The nurses had the advantage. Because of additional education in emotional development as applied to the hospitalized child, close clinical supervision and continuous support of their work, they performed beyond expectation—the expectation of themselves and the expectations of others.

Long-term experiences showed that the staff required more than consultation services. It became obvious that the most effective mental health personnel participated directly in the clinical management of psychological crises, serving as role models and demonstrating that their work promoted staff development and the efficient operation of the department; they demonstrated that their presence or absence made a difference.

And the most important lesson was that a long-established program could not be taken for granted. Although it operated successfully for close to a decade, in spite of periodic setbacks, in the end it succumbed to economic pressures and a change in administrative leadership to one that did not value emotional care.

No program exists without administrative backing. Administration defines philosophy, sets standards, allocates money, recruits personnel to implement departmental objectives and determines the priorities of patient care. Is it not logical, then, to influence the administrative leadership to ensure that the emotional care of children is given equal status with physical health? This would consequently entail the selection of pediatric administrators based on their understanding of comprehensive care. What is needed is the clout to declare that emotional care is valued and that environmental change—to becoming emotionally therapeutic—is a priority. Unless such a trend emerges, and until professionals are prepared in their basic education to think about total child care, supportive research literature will remain on the shelves where it has been for several decades and the environmental approach will have to fight continually for survival.

REFERENCES

1. Schowalter, J. E.: Working together—is a children's hospital for children or staff? JACCH 3:3, July 1974.
2. Freud, A.: The role of bodily illness in the mental life of children. *In* Eissler, R., *et al.* (eds.): The Psychoanalytic Study of the Child, vol. 7, pp. 74–75. New York, International Universities Press, 1952.
3. Hall, E. T.: Hidden Dimensions, p. 7. Garden City, Doubleday, 1966.
4. *Ibid.,* p. 20.
5. Ardrey, R.: The Territorial Imperative, p. 48. New York, Dell (Laurel Edition), 1971.

BIBLIOGRAPHY

Ack, M.: Considerations governing the organization of a children's hospital. JACCH 4:27, 1975.

Bates, B.: Doctor and nurse: changing roles and relations. New Eng. J. Med. 283:129, 1970.

Bennis, W. G., Benne, K. D., and Chin, R.: The Planning of Change. New York, Holt, Rinehart & Winston, 1969.

Finch, S. M., and McDermott, J. F., Jr.: Psychiatry for the Pediatrician. New York, W. W. Norton, 1970.

Georgopoulos, B. S., and Christman, L.: The clinical nurse specialist: a role model. Amer. J. Nurs., 70:1030, 1970.

Glaser, H. H.: The hospital as an environment for children and families. Pediatric Annals 1(3):10, 1972.

Gordon, M.: The clinical specialist as a change agent. Nurs. Outlook 17:37, 1969.

Harragan, B. L.: Games Mother Never Taught You: Corporate Gamesmanship for Women. New York, Rawson Associates, 1977.

Haslett, N.: Environmental contributions to the care of hospitalized children. JACCH 5(2):14, 1976.

Lindheim, R., Glaser, H. H., and Coffin, C.: Changing Hospital Environment for Children. Cambridge, Mass., Harvard University Press, 1972.

Petrillo, M. (ed.): Hospitalization for Children. Pediatric Annals, 1(3), 1972.

Petrillo, M.: Preventing hospital trauma in pediatric patients. Amer. J. Nurs. 68:1468, 1968.

Prugh, D. G., *et al.:* A study of the emotional reactions of children and families to hospitalization and illness. Amer. J. Orthopsychiat. 23:70, 1953.

Vernon, D. T., *et al.:* The Psychological Responses of Children to Hospitalization and Illness: A Review of the Literature. Springfield, Ill., Charles C Thomas, 1965.

2

A Working Knowledge of Childhood

INTRODUCTION

The challenge of caring for children is to combine knowledge of the individual child with an awareness of the relevant facts and theories of the past 80 years in order to achieve a synthesis that could be called an adaptive developmental assessment.

One cannot know everything about a child. Observation, history and interview supply a portion of the picture; this is the raw data. A more comprehensive and complete "profile" of an individual exists when data are interpreted in the context of professional experience and theoretical knowledge.

General knowledge works in two ways: it tells us what to look for, and it helps us to make sense of what we find. The various theories of this chapter added to clinical experiences gathered over time will lead to a structured general knowledge needed by professionals. Unorganized experience, however fascinating, can lead to chaos. But knowledge of theories alone is dull and empty. However, when clinical experience is integrated with a theoretical foundation and the two are combined, the possibility for creative and constructive evaluation of children exists. On this evaluation rests the innovative, environmental planning of subsequent chapters.

Before proceeding to an outline of the major theories of growth and development, practitioners wishing to gain a background in emotional care need to consider the factors that follow.

Psychological Factors Can Become Preeminent

There are numerous occasions when the attitudes and behavior of children and their families have precedence over medical necessities.[1,2] One has only to think of hemophiliacs who purposely hurt themselves or take undue physical risks, thereby requiring multiple admissions, transfusions and rehabilitation of hemarthritic joints. There are diabetics who, through purposeful neglect, anger or bravado, will enter extreme states of hypo- and hyperglycemia to the point of coma and death. Asthmatics, colitics, children with eczema and nutritional peculiarities can often precipitate recurrences of manifest disease. Congenital heart disease sufferers may become accident prone or so cautious that fractures or lack of athletic development causes greater concern than the underlying primary illness. Donation of a kidney or a skin graft from one member of a family to another can engender such psychological rivalry, closeness or guilt that the family structure itself is destroyed even though the patient survives.

Scientific-Technical Developments Have Pros and Cons

Progress has mixed benefits: The need for so many blood tests to determine the nature of hepatitis is increasingly difficult to explain to the nonprofessional. With more precision in diagnosing bacterial infections, patients become less tolerant when their fever remains ''of unknown origin.'' Because of antibiotics, bed rest and isolation procedures are abbreviated, and it then becomes harder to tell a child why he must remain in the hospital at all. Since more premature neonates are now being kept alive, subtle forms of neurological brain damage may evidence themselves months later. The effects on body image and emotion because of organ transplants are often unrecognized.

Professionals need to keep up with science. Progress in preventive medicine has made professionals more aware of: insult to the fetus from tobacco, alcohol and drugs; the subtle need in newborns for quiet contact with the mother, early bonding, cerebellar stimulation, and childhood atherosclerosis, to list a few.

Adults Have Some Natural Difficulties when Working with Children

It has been called the conflict between the generations, adolescent rebellion, oedipal rivalry; nonetheless, it needs to be said that, for their part, adults are often threatened by the young, who want grownup privileges without responsibilities. Children express feelings that embarrass adults by their accuracy. Adults who think themselves to be "good with children," and who invest many years of training to become expert in some aspect of the young, may find that they are not as talented as they thought. Others who hold confident opinions of themselves as good parents may be surprised when their children disagree. A complicated pattern often follows in which the adults become both disappointed in themselves and angry at the child. Since most adults value shielding "innocent" children from their anger, they feel guilt instead and hide their anger by either withdrawing from or becoming overly solicitous of the child. Situations of chronic illness, genetic damage or preventable accidents have the potential to heighten this end result of withdrawal or oversolicitude.

Briefly summarized in this chapter is a theoretical and development overview of childhood. There is much additional knowledge that a professional caring for children must have. For example, many of the children seen in inner-city hospitals come from economically disadvantaged families. Though each person is unique, belonging to a disadvantaged minority affects individual and group reactions in a predictable way when relating to an authority figure who represents the advantaged majority. To familiarize oneself with the black or Hispanic experience is helpful.[3, 4, 5, 6]

It is common knowledge that the TV set exerts a strong influence on children. Violence on the screen is often followed by increased aggressivity. Passivity and shallowness are some other effects. In the hospital there is a dramatic increase in television viewing. The tendency to deny the reality of illness is helped while the necessary adjustment to the facts of life on a pediatric floor may be blunted severely by the influence of so many electronic events offered by television.[7, 8, 9]

Family organization and vulnerability to detachment are affected by illness in children. A fragile marital adjustment may progress to open conflict. Sickness gives opportunity for blame, for sudden desperate emotional flare-ups. At times, separated or disunited families will come together at the bedside, fulfilling the child's secret wishes that his parents stop arguing and/or reunite.[10, 11, 12]

The growing literature in child abuse reflects a national concern concomitantly with an increasing incidence. Summary articles[13, 14, 15, 16] can yield a basic framework for an understanding of some of the usual etiologies and necessary interventions.

Finally, every professional concerned with the care of hospitalized children ought to know the new and burgeoning literature on neonatal development. The field is so new that the fragments of knowledge have not been completely integrated. The newborn can see, hear, sense and remember events and has many behaviors that influence the caregiver. A "dance" occurs between infant and mother wherein each adjusts to the other, resulting in a reciprocity that leads to competence for the infant, gratification and attachment for both. Hospital procedures and practices can drastically warp this harmony. Too much light, noise; changes of caring nursery personnel, too soon or too delayed responsivity to the infant's needs; different styles of touching, vocalizing and smiling are a few examples.[17, 18, 19, 20, 21, 22]

In the following pages, many of the important theories of growth and development are outlined. Presented are the beginnings for a basic, organized approach to children at different ages. The Bibliography contains the most recent reviews and writings of these theorists. However, no summary can do justice to the rich clinical and theoretical material that will reward the reader who goes beyond this chapter.

CONCERNS OF THE HOSPITALIZED CHILD

Hospitalization can be seen as a series of tasks that a child must experience and deal with:
1. His body is now imperfect and in need of diagnosis and remedy.

2. Parents are concerned enough to call a doctor, who in turn is concerned enough to arrange for hospitalization.
3. The threat and actuality of separation from family and home, often for the first time, are real.
4. Except for rooming-in arrangements, he is to spend time with completely unfamiliar people.
5. To maintain contact with siblings and friends will be difficult.
6. Being at the mercy of nurses and lab technicians who carry out instructions for procedures that may be painful is stressful.
7. Contact with unfamiliar routines, equipment and confinement is frightening.
8. There is disappointment and anger at self and parents if the hospitalization was caused by human failings. The majority of children under six think that the illness resulted from something they or their family did.
9. In spite of missing and/or being angry at parents, the child may discover that parents need to be supported themselves. For the first time in the child's experience, they look helpless compared to the professionals to whom they have turned.
10. He must fit in with the patient role, yet be ready when discharged to become once more as independent as before.
11. He has to relate to doctors and nurses whose stereotypes may fill him with fear rather than confidence.

There is also the consideration that some hospitalized children may be drawn from a less emotionally healthy population and so professionals are not relating to a representative group of normal children, but rather something closer to children seen as psychiatric outpatients, or at least an atypical group. Still, if a child is working through some of his deeper anxieties and problems during a hospitalization, preparations prior to, during, and after hospitalization are all the more necessary.

("An Overview of Growth and Development" begins on the following page. References for this chapter begin on page 51.)

AN OVERVIEW OF GROWTH AND DEVELOPMENT

Developed by Sirgay Sanger

THE FIRST YEAR

Developmental Landmarks Central Nervous System Maturation (Gesell)

1 day to 1 month: Responds to bell; makes crawling movements

1 month: Follows an object to midline; coos, gurgles, makes a fist; shows tonic neck reflex

2 months: Social smile; 180° visual pursuit; transitory reflexes—Moro, suck, grasp

4 months: Reaches for objects

5 months: Rolls over

6–8 months: Raking grasp; sitting, crawling

9 months: Crude purposeful release of objects grasped

10 months: Pincer grasp

10–14 months: Walks; knows 3 to 4 words

Interactional, Field and Systems Theories (Spitz, Escalona, Sander, Lewis)

When baby sends a cue to mother (cry of distress), how appropriate is her response? This is also called the degree of fit between mother and child.

Development of mutual regulatory and reciprocal interchanges between mother and child; e.g., synchrony of sleeping, eating, elimination—between mother and baby.

In the first few months, the baby gradually takes more of the initiative in signaling his needs.

With time there is an increased intensity in the baby's expression of needs.

Stages of Intellectual Development (Piaget)

Sensorimotor stage from birth to 2 years:

"Neonatal reflex" substage: complete self-world undifferentiation

"Primary circular" substage: simple acts are repeated

"Secondary circular" substage: there is repetition of acts that affect an object

"Secondary circular" substage: actions become committed to memory

Psychosocial Tasks or Crises (Erikson)

Basic Trust or Mistrust: The first year encompasses the time when confidence in having needs met and in feeling physically safe takes place. When needs are consistently met, anticipation of satisfaction occurs. The result is optimism. When a child anticipates frustration, pessimism about the world develops.

Individual Differences

Shortly after birth it is possible to note differences in vision and audition, activity and temperament that remain as preferences for months to come. Some activity temperament types are: (chess)

Active/passive
Regular/irregular rhythmicity
Intensity of movement (high/low)
Approach/withdraw
Adaptation/nonadaptation
High/low response to stimulus
Positive/negative mood
High/low selectivity, attention span, persistence
High/low distractibility

Certain combinations are less successful, such as passive, high intensity or withdrawal and nonadaptation. Other combinations are adaptive; for example, mood is positive, adaptation high, and strong approach.

Psychosexual Stages (Sigmund Freud)

Infant wants the mother and fears her loss lest body needs go unsatisfied and create increased tension. Mother gives satisfaction and relieves tension. From birth to 18 months is the ORAL stage. This includes respiratory, sensory and kinesthetic responses. The mode of relationship is incorporative. With a good mother, baby's energies gradually decrease in concentration on the self and increasingly are directed toward the mother. The threat of losing the mother produces increased tension in the infant who is left without the object (mother) on whom he has placed all his energies. This is primary anxiety. Defenses that the infant and toddler use to cope with anxiety are imitation, avoidance and denial.

(Continued)

THE FIRST YEAR (Continued)

Brazelton[23] describes an inflexible infant severely affecting the mother. Mother's anxiety early affects infant's temperament. Infants with a low sensory threshold had many more sleep disturbances (Carey). Subtle maturational differences may have an effect—for example, visual attention to size and pattern is different at birth.[24, 25, 26]

Ego Psychology (Anna Freud et al.)

0–3 months: Normal autism: Complete self-absorbing without awareness of the world

4–18 months: Symbiotic phase (Mahler); mother seen as an extension of child's body and needs (and vice versa)

6–10 months: Stranger anxiety begins; shows that infant can distinguish between the symbiotic object (mother) and all others

Ego/Instinct Accommodation-Developmental Lines (Anna Freud)

A. From dependency to emotional self-reliance and adult relationships:

In the first year, there is a biologic unit with mother. This symbiosis then evolves toward separation and individuation.

B. From body dependency toward body independence:

1. May have difficulties in feeding and in achieving synchrony with the mother—for example, oral deprivation may be consequent to abrupt weaning, with rejection of new tastes in foods. By the end of the first year, child begins to feed himself.

2. Has complete freedom from bladder and bowel control.

3. Has no responsibility in body management—the mother does everything.

Positive feeling toward his own body protects the infant from self-damage.

4. Infant is totally egocentric (selfish or narcissistic). Other persons are a disturbance of the relationship to mother and are treated as lifeless objects.

5. Infant's own body is the source of orientation and play; e.g., interest in mouth and skin sensation of self and mother. Transitional object begins at this time.

8–24 months: Separation anxiety: Reluctant to lose sight of mother; beginnings of transitional objects (Winnicott)—partly the representing mother, partly the self, partly the self, (e.g., an animal or security blanket)

ONE YEAR TO THREE-AND-A-HALF YEARS

Developmental Landmarks Central Nervous System Maturation (Gesell)

1½ years: two-cube tower; scribbles with crayon; knows ten words; capable of bowel training

2 years: 6-cube tower

2½ years: Three-word sentences; names six body parts; pronouns

3 years: Tricycle; copies O; matches four colors

3½ years: Talks to self and others; takes turns; walks on a line

Interactional Field and Systems Theories (Bowlby, Lorenz)

From birth to age two, the mother is the central integrator of attachment behavior. Social releasers from baby such as sucking, crying, following, clinging, smiling—all lead to behavior responses in the mother. Stranger anxiety between approximately 6 to 7 and 24 months coincides with the height of this adaptation to the mother. Aggression is the opposite to attachment and needs discouragement, not punishment. Aggression is heightened by mother's teaching this to the child, or by forced weaning.

Stages of Intellectual Development (Piaget)

2 years: By this time the child performs mental combinations by trial and error. There is relatively coherent organization of sensorimotor action. The child learns that certain actions have a specific effect on the environment. There is beginning symbolic activity. There is recognition of constancy of external objects. The world is represented primitively. Symbols and figures stand for objects. Egocentric thinking predominates (The child refers every event to himself; for instance, if mother leaves, it is because of his action.)

(Continued)

ONE YEAR TO THREE-AND-A-HALF YEARS (Continued)

Psychosocial Tasks or Crises (Erikson)

Autonomy vs. Shame and Doubt: By the age of 3½, there is established on the basis of previous adaption a general attitude of initiative illustrated by—"I am what I imagine I can be." Each effort is preceded by fantasy play. Failure at this stage is shown by guilty reluctance to explore, by doubt, by sense of uselessness.

Psychosexual Stages (Sigmund Freud)

One-and-a-half to 3½ years is the anal and urethral stage when elimination and retention are the modes. Muscles are used to express control and inhibition. Feelings are displaced onto objects or symbols and projected onto others—for example, "If I feel this way, others must also."

Ego Psychology (Anna Freud et al.)

From 12 to 28 months the infant and toddler are in the separation-individuation phase (Mahler). This is seen in self-feeding from 17 to 30 months. This is the height of the oppositional syndrome (assertiveness to begin differentiation of the child from the mother [Levy]).

From two to three, there is messiness, exploration, parallel play, pleasure in looking and being looked at. At approximately 3, a self-concept begins. Early conscience occurs—by way of identification with parents. Orderliness, disgust, masturbation and curiosity are expressions of instinct development. There is also cooperative play, fantasy play and imaginary playmates based on magical-thinking (that things happen when they are wished.)

Ego/Instinct Accommodation-Developmental Lines (Anna Freud)

A. In second to fourth year, the mother is a part-object, or an instrument, who captures the child's interest because of his needs. By the third year, the child has a constant mental representation of the mother regardless of her absence or lack of gratification. The child acts as if he remembers, misses her, and, doubts that she will return. Toward the end of the third year, the ambivalent (anal-preoedipal) stage is exemplified by love alternating with hate, clinging with defiance.

B. In developing toward body independence:

1. Though there is self-feeding, food is the battleground in differentiation from mother—("battle for the spoon"—Levy). There is a craving for sweets, food fads and food refusal that is always aimed at mother.

2. Body products become invested with sexual and aggressive energy. There are swings between love and hate, curiosity and neglect, emptying and hoarding. The instinctual drives in going from the oral to the anal zone lead to increasing oppositional behavior (stubbornness).

3. With increasing ego functioning and awareness of cause and effect, the body is protected and dangerous wishes are controlled under the reality principle; for instance, fire, heights, water are facts that must be respected.

4. From 1 to 3½, the toddler sees other persons as helpers in carrying out his wishes. By 4 years they become partners and objects in their own right—to be feared and admired. At the same time, earliest friendships begin.

5. In progressing from interest solely in his own body and in play, the toddler changes from one specific transitional object to other inanimate objects that are treated with love, hate and invested with sexual and aggressive energy. By the middle of the third year, cuddly toys fade out except at night. Play helps direct drive energies to socially useful pursuits.

(Continued)

THREE-AND-A-HALF TO SIX-AND-A-HALF YEARS (PRESCHOOL)

Developmental Landmarks (Gesell)

4 years: Copies X; throws overhand; develops early right/left orientation

4½ years: Copies □

5 years: Copies △; ties knots in string

6 years: Prints name; ties shoes; makes single-function similarities; rides two-wheeler; copies ◇

Psychosocial Tasks or Crises (Erikson)

Initiative vs. Guilt: Attempts to seek who he really is by attempting to be like his parents. Environment is increasingly explored and behavior is initiated. New mastery of physical and of social environment. Locomotor skills increase. Verbal

Stages of Intellectual Development (Piaget)

Between 3 and 7 is the stage called "pre-operational" or "preconceptual." Thought is intuitive, prelogical (magical). There begins the first relatively unorganized and fumbling attempts to grasp the new and strange world of symbols. Thinking is still egocentric—conclusions are based on feelings or on what the child would like to believe.

Psychosexual Stage (Sigmund Freud)

Four years old—the phallic stage (loco-motor). Intrusive and inclusive modes—there is much interest in competence, prowess and dominance. Oedipal is the last phase. The child in this phase likes the parent of the opposite sex and tends to turn away from the parent of the same sex. There is a fear of castration by the parent of the same sex. This leads to repression of original oedipal wishes. Ambivalence occurs toward both parents. The resolution is the renunciation of the heterosexual incestuous object, and later a search to find someone like the parent of the opposite sex. (Normally occurs after age 6.)

skills flourish with language sufficiently developed to initiate considerable questions. Occasional discomforts when task obstructed leads to guilt and disappointment. Family the primary group but increasingly explorative of outside groups such as neighborhood play group and nursery school peers.

Ego Psychology (Anna Freud)

4 years: Mastery is most important as shown by task completion; magical-thinking decreases; rivalry with parent of same sex continues

5 years: Follows rules; prelatency type play gives way to latency play in which skills count

6 years: Shows problem-solving achievements, voluntary hygiene, competition, hobbies and ritualistic play

Ego/Instinct Accommodation-Development Lines (Anna Freud)

A. The phallic period (4 to 5 years):

Closer to true mutual relationships, though still wishes for exclusive rights with each parent. Castration anxiety at its height, also exhibitionism.

B. In developing toward body independence:

1. 4½ to 6½—food representing mother fades out, though food retains a magical quality—that is, overeating leads to getting fat and having a baby. Eating can become sexualized (anorexia). It may become involved in reaction formation—that is, food refusal is a way of denying wish to devour the mother.

2. By 5, attitudes toward bowel and bladder control come to resemble mother's through identification and ego-superego maturation. Ego develops inner defenses against urethral and anal wishes (total freedom to mess), which now get channeled into such patterns as punctuality, neatness and miserliness.

[Continued]

SIX-AND-A-HALF TO ELEVEN YEARS (SCHOOL AGE)

Developmental Landmarks (Gesell)

7 years: Makes simple opposite analogies; knows days of the week

8 years: Counts 5 digits forward; defines brave and nonsense

9 years: Knows seasons, rhymes

10 years: Counts 4 digits reversed; expresses and defines pity, grief and surprise

Psychosocial Tasks or Crises (Erikson)

Industry vs. Inferiority: Between 6 and 11, the child's skills and values expand to include those of the neighborhood and school. Successful adaptations here lead to industry (I am what I learn); unsuccessful to inferiority.

Stages of Intellectual Development (Piaget)

Seven to 12 years is the stage of "Concrete Operational Thought." Conceptual organization takes on stability and coherence. There are rational, well-organized adaptations. Conceptual framework is brought to bear on objects in world. Physical qualities are seen as constant despite change in size, shape, weight and volume.

Psychosexual Stages (Sigmund Freud)

Latency occurs between 7 and 11 years. The sexual drive is controlled and repressed. There is use of the unconscious mechanisms of isolation (separation of an idea from its accompanying feeling), pseudocompulsion (repeated rituals and mannerisms as foot tapping, hair pulling, avoiding stepping on cracks), turning to the opposite (a child will deny her hatred of the new sibling by saying she loves him), and sublimation of instinctual wishes (channeling of drives into socially acceptable outlets; e.g., oral needs may evolve into gourmet interests). Emphasis during latency is also on development of skills and talents.

Ego Psychology (Anna Freud)

The 9-year-old is: Rational about food; companionable; invested in nonfamily relationships

Autonomous ego functions develop—automatically behaves in areas that formerly created conflict—for example, uses words instead of violence, comfortably obeys most rules, can postpone immediate gratification

Ego-Instinct Accommodation-Developmental Lines (Anna Freud)

A. In relationships:

The 6- to 11-year-old transfers interest to others outside the family. This and the normal disillusionment with parents lead to the feeling of having been adopted (the "family romance" where an idealized set of parents is envisioned).

B. In developing toward body independence:

1. There is the final phasing out of the sexualization of eating with a rational attitude.

2. In bowel and bladder control, cleanliness becomes disconnected from object ties and becomes an autonomous ego-superego concern.

3. Body management completely taken over by child.

(Continued)

ELEVEN TO EIGHTEEN YEARS (ADOLESCENCE)

Developmental Landmarks (Gesell)

11 years on: Knows where sun sets, about microscopes and nitrogen, why oil floats. Divides 74 by 4, makes abstract similarities, understands COD. Repeats six digits forward; five reverse.

Stages of Intellectual Development (Piaget)

Twelve years—formal operational thought: Deals effectively with reality and also with abstract propositional statements and the world of possibility. Cognition is adult type. Deductive reasoning developed. Can evaluate logic and quality of own thinking. Increase in abstract powers leads to capacity to deal with laws and principles. Still egocentric at times. Important ideals and attitudes develop in late adolescence and early adulthood.

Summary of Piaget

Overall: Adaptation and coping change and reorganize the mind. Complex stimulation in a favorable environment causes accommodation of mental structures to the nuances of reality.

All mental function derives from motor actions on objects. Growth of intelligence is based on the transformation of these motor patterns into thought. Incorporation of the novel is assimilation; reorganization of past thoughts and memories to more closely approximate the assimilated novelty is accommodation. Development is the interplay between assimilation and accommodation. When accommodation stops with respect to an assimilation, behavior is adapted or a balance then exists between assimilation and accommodation. It is a human tendency to assimilate all possible novelty. It is novelty that motivates repetition of circular reactions in order to give more contact and exposure to the unfamiliar.

Psychosocial Tasks or Crises (Erikson)

Identity vs. Role Diffusion: Between 12 and 17, the youth seeks to "know what I am." The predominant values are those of adolescent peer group and leadership. Identity is the outcome. If the individual is unsuccessful, there is "identity diffusion."

After 17, ability to love is paramount with success being shown by intimacy. Lack of success leads to isolation and alienation. Values at this time: fidelity, friendship, and cooperation. Sexual behavior and competition approach the adult type.

Psychosexual Stages (Sigmund Freud)

Eleven to 13 years (Puberty): Importance of peer group, recapitulation of oedipal struggle consequent to resurgence of sexual drives. Contact with the opposite sex is once more seen as potentially dangerous as it leads to competition with others of the same sex and possible defeat. In addition, seeking a new idealized self to replace the parents, who are now discredited, often causes attraction to another of the same sex who has admirable qualities ("normal" homosexual phase).

Thirteen to 18 years: Adolescent-adult modes of leadership. Coping mechanisms are intellectualization, rationalization, asceticism.

Genitality achieved with the primacy of heterosexual orgasm. Ability to love and work are the culmination of these stages.

Ego Psychology (Anna Freud)

Adolescent revolt loosens ties to family. Cliques develop with friends. Responsibility and independent work habits solidify.

Late adolescence: Heterosexual interests lead to marriage and parental readiness. Recreational and intellectual activities prepare the young adult for vocational choice and later commitment.

(Continued)

ELEVEN TO EIGHTEEN YEARS (ADOLESCENCE) (Continued)

Ego/Instinct Balance–Developmental Lines (Anna Freud)

A. In relationships and self-reliance:

Eleven- to 13-year-old preadolescents have a return of ambivalence and weakening of phallic and latency accomplishments.

Thirteen- to 15-year-old adolescents loosen ties to parents.

Fifteen years on: Genital supremacy. There is an active, healthy struggle to finally control the impulses of the first six years. Relationships acquire give and take qualities—mutual self-help.

B. All developmental lines toward body independence continue to solidify. During adolescence there is a final voluntary endorsement of the rules of hygiene and medical necessities. The ability to work is the culmination of the developmental line that began with play, task completion, and the use of inanimate objects. Control of destructive impulses, frustration tolerance, and living by the reality principle (future gratifications may involve short-term renunciations) are also necessary for adult work.

Comment on Anna Freud's Developmental Lines

Each area described represents an intra-psychic balance between ego-superego and the id. No one of these developmental lines is to be used exclusively in assessing a child. It is more of a clustering or profile of different intrapsychic dynamics that gives the true picture. Thus a 14-year-old boy could have several close friends, be over-eating, be sloppy, brush his teeth, practice body building, have several hobbies, and be doing mediocre work in school. He would have attained different stages in his separate developmental lines. From this data, the conclusion is drawn that he just approaches emotional adolescence.

REFERENCES

1. Stocking, M., Rothney, W., Grosser, G. and Goodwin, R.: Psychopathology in the pediatric hospital; implications for the pediatrician. Psychiatry in Medicine 1:329–38, 1970.

2. Jessner, L., Blom, G. E., and Waldfogel, S.: Emotional implications of tonsillectomy and adenoidectomy on children. The Psychoanalytic Study of the Child 7:126–69, 1952.

3. Bolling, J. L.: The changing self concept of black children: the black identity test. J. Nat'l Medical Assn., Jan. 1974.

4. Ward, S., and Braun, J.: Self-esteem and racial preference in black children. Amer. J. Orthopsychiat. 42:644, 1972.

5. Comer, J. P., and Poussant, A. F.: *Black Child Care*. New York, Simon & Schuster, 1975.

6. Taylor, R. L.: Psychosocial development among black children and youth. Amer. J. Orthopsychiat. 46(1), Jan. 1976.

7. Singer, D. G., and Singer, J. L.: Family television viewing habits and the spontaneous play of preschool children. Amer. J. Orthopsychiat. 46(3), July 1976.

8. Winn, M.: The plug-in drug: Television, Children, and the Family. New York, Viking, 1977.

9. Sheikh, A. A., and Prasad, V. K.: Children's TV commercials, a review of research. In Chess, J., and Thomas, A., Annual Progress in Child Psychiatry and Child Development. New York, Brunner/Mazel, 1975.

10. Anthony, E. J.: Children at risk from divorce: a review. In Anthony, E. J., and Koupernik, C. (eds.), The Child in His Family, vol. 3. New York, Wiley-Interscience, 1974.

11. Wallerstein, J. S., and Kelly, J. B.: The effects of parental divorce: the adolescent experience. In Anthony, E. J., and Koupernik, C. (eds.), The Child in His Family, vol 3. New York, Wiley-Interscience, 1974.

12. Magrab, P. R., and Alter, E. B.: Divorce. In Magrab, P. R. (ed.): Psychological Management of Pediatric Problems, vol. II. Baltimore, University Park Press, 1978.

13. Gelles, R. J.: Violence toward children in the United States. Amer. J. Orthopsychiat. 48(4), Oct. 1978.

14. Newberger, E. H., and Bowine, R.: The medicalization and legalization of child abuse. Amer. J. Orthopsychiat. 48(4), Oct. 1978.

15. Pelton, L. H.: Child abuse and neglect, the myth of classlessness. Amer. J. Orthopsychiat. 48(4), Oct. 1978.

16. Williams, G. J.: Child abuse. In Magrab, P. R. (ed.): Psychological Management of Pediatric Problems, vol. II. Baltimore, University Park Press, 1978.

17. Walters, C. E.: Mother–infant interaction. New York, Human Sciences Press, 1976.

18. Rexford, E. N., Sander, L. W., and Shapiro, T. (eds.): Infant Psychiatry. New Haven, Yale University Press, 1976.

19. White, B. L.: The First Three Years of Life. Englewood Cliffs, N.J., Prentice-Hall, 1975.

20. Stone, L. J., Smith, H. T., and Murphy, L. B. (eds.): The Competent Infant. New York, Basic Books, 1973.

21. Lewis, M., and Rosenblum, L. A. (eds.): The Effect of the Infant on Its Caregiver. New York, Wiley-Interscience, 1974.

22. Ringler, N., Trause, M. A., Klaus, M., and Kennell, J.: The effects of extra postpartum contact and maternal speech patterns on children's I.Q.'s, speech, and language comprehension at five. Child Dev. 49:862–65, 1978.

23. Brazelton, T.: Observations of the neonate. J. Amer. Acad. Child Psychiat. 2962 1:38–58.

24. Carey, W. B.: Night waking and temperament in infancy. J. Pediat. 84(5):756–58, 1974.

25. Carey, W. B., Lipton, W. L., and Myers, R. A.: Temperament in adopted and foster babies. *In* Chess, S., and Thomas, A. (eds.), Annual Progress in Child Psychiatry. New York, Brunner/Mazel, 1975.

26. Fantz, R. L., and Fagan, J. F. III: Visual attention to size and number of pattern details by term and pre-term infants during the first six months. Child Dev. 46:3–18, 1975.

BIBLIOGRAPHY

Blos, P.: The Young Adolescent, Clinical Studies. New York, Free Press, 1970.

Erikson, E. H.: Childhood and Society, 2nd ed. New York, W. W. Norton, 1963.

———: Identity: Youth and Crisis. New York, W. W. Norton, 1968.

Freud, A.: The Ego and the Mechanisms of Defense, rev. ed. New York, International Universities Press, 1966.

———: Normality and Pathology in Childhood: Assessments of Development. New York, International Universities Press, 1965.

Gesell, A.: The First Five Years of Life. New York, Harper & Row, 1940.

———: The Child from Five to Ten. New York, Harper & Row, 1946.

Gesell, A., *et al.*: Youth: The Years from Ten to Sixteen. New York, Harper & Row, 1956.

Hollitscher, W.: Sigmund Freud, An Introduction. Freeport, New York, Books for Libraries Press, 1970.

Josselyn, I. M.: The Happy Child: A Psychoanalytic Guide to Emotional and Social Growth. New York, Random House, 1955.

Levy, D. M.: Oppositional syndromes and oppositional behavior. *In* Hoch, P., and Zubin, J. (eds.): Psychopathology of Childhood, vol. X. New York, Grune & Stratton, 1955.

Lewis, M., and Rosenblum, L. A.: The Effect of the Infant on its Caregiver. New York, Wiley & Sons, 1974.

Lidz, T.: The Person: His and Her Development Throughout the Life Cycle, rev. ed. New York, Basic Books, 1976.

Mahler, M. S., Pine, F., and Bergman, A.: The Psychological Birth of the Human Infant. New York, Basic Books, 1975.

Mussea, P. H., Conger, J. J., and Kagan, J.: Child Development and Personality. New York, Harper & Row, 1974.

Neuhauser, C., Amsterdam, B., Hines, P., and Steward, M.: Children's concepts of healing. Amer. J. Orthopsychiat. 48(2), April 1978.

Piaget, J., and Inhelder, B.: The Psychology of the Child. New York, Basic Books, 1969.

Prugh, D., and Eckhardt, L. O.: Children's Reactions to Illness, Hospitalization and Surgery. *In* Freedman, A. M., and Kaplan, H. I. (eds.): Comprehensive Textbook of Psychiatry II. Baltimore, Williams & Wilkins, 1975.

Report of the Joint Commission on

Mental Health: Crisis in Child Mental Health: Challenge for the 1970's. Chap. 8. Social-psychological aspects of normal growth and development: adolescents and youth. New York, Harper & Row, 1969.

Rheingold, H. L.: General issues in the study of fear. In Lewis, M., and Rosenblum, L. (eds.): The Origins of Fear. New York, Wiley & Sons, 1974.

Sander, L. W.: The regulation of exchange in the infant-caretaker system. In Lewis, M., and Rosenbloom, L.: Interaction Conversation and the Development of Language. New York, Wiley & Sons, 1977.

Solnit, A. J., and Provence, S. A.: Modern Perspectives in Child Development. New York, International Universities Press, 1963.

Spitz, R. A.: The First Year of Life. New York, International Universities Press, 1965.

Sugarman, M.: Paranatal influences on maternal infant attachment. Amer. J. Orthopsychiat. 47(3), July 1977.

Summit, R., and Kryso, J.: Sexual abuse of children. Amer. J. Orthopsychiat. 48(2), April 1978.

Thomas, A., et al.: The origin of personality. Sci. Amer. 223:102, 1970.

Tyossem, T. D. (ed.): Intervention Strategies for High Risk Infants and Young Children. Baltimore, Johns Hopkins University Press, 1976.

White, B. L.: The First Three Years of Life. Englewood Cliffs, N.J., Prentice-Hall, 1975.

Winnicott, D. W.: Collected Papers, Through Pediatrics to Psychoanalysis, pp. 229–42. London, Tavistock, 1958.

Wolff, P. H.: The role of biological rhythms in early psychological development. Bull. Menninger Clin. 31:197, 1967.

Child, Parent, Staff Interactions

ENCOUNTERS WITH PARENTS—TEACHING HOW TO PREPARE CHILDREN FOR HOSPITALIZATION

In most instances, preparation for admission to a pediatric hospital is a well-organized event involving the collaboration of physician, parents and child. This expectation is the result of a growing acceptance among pediatric staff of expanded roles that include the assessment of the family's ability to deal with crises and the implementation of new approaches to minimize hospital trauma. Such an orientation is reflected in a willingness to assume responsibility for guiding parents by explaining illness and hospitalization and by an attitude which presumes that parents need or deserve help during this vulnerable period.

BEFORE HOSPITALIZATION

It is important to determine in early conferences with parents what has been said to the child and how realistic a picture he has received. Such questions as "How much does your child know?" and "What do you plan to tell him?" require in-depth responses that help expose behavior patterns for coping with anxiety-producing events. Usually there is a need for correction or clarification according to the child's developmental level. When mothers and fathers have been unable to tell their children that hospitalization is required, or have gained their child's cooperation by deceit, the task is more difficult. (See also Chapter 4 on family assessment.) These shortcomings may be caused by a variety of reasons—often the parents' own nervousness.

In the instance of planned deception, effort should be made to convert parents to honest, open communication. One must be aware, however, that long-established behavior patterns are rarely changed by lecturing or moralizing. A more productive method is through investigation of how underlying parental anxieties cause destructive behavior. One way of accomplishing this is to ask what the parents believe may have caused the child's illness. Replies such as "I had bad thoughts during pregnancy" or "It happened because I weaned her on her third birthday" reveal the guilt many parents experience, which may be assuaged by their overindulging the child or protecting him from the knowledge of coming events.

The nature of parental reactions and the degree of distress observed are not necessarily related to the seriousness of the illness: A minor problem can precipitate as much anguish as a severe cardiac anomaly. Accordingly, it is important to find out what lies behind an unexpected response. Once fantasies are exposed, the type of intervention required becomes clearer.

It is also profitable to explore the parents' anticipation of the child's reaction to truthful preparation. A common belief is that the child will be overwhelmed by anxiety (an indication of the parents' own feelings), which in turn may trigger anger against the parents or provoke unmanageable behavior.

When parents are encouraged to take the initial steps of preparing their child and are given the tools with which to do so, it is rare to find that they resist following through; however, the incidence of unprepared patients is still too high. In addition to specific information regarding illness and treatment, therefore, anxious and deceptive parents need to be told how detrimental their reactions are to the child's sense of security: lack of preparation subjects the child to perplexing experiences, deprives him of sufficient time for coming to terms with painful events and forces him to bear the burden without support. Eventually he will know the truth, and the deception will be all the more shocking, leading him to distrust his parents and everyone involved in his care. If they cannot change, arrangements should be made for the parents to talk with a mental health specialist before forming further plans for the child.

Some parents believe that young children do not have the capacity to understand or to cope with the knowledge once it is given; others do not know what to say and abdicate responsibility altogether.

When parents withhold explanations because of insufficient knowledge, the staff needs to play an active role to help them perform more adequately before and after admission. This aspect of parental inadequacy may be remedied with the help of personnel of the clinics or by private pediatricians. Guidance and information can be dispensed verbally or in printed form. Two examples of the latter are *Preparing Your Child for Hospitalization and Eye Surgery (page 59) and Preparing Your Child for Hospitalization and Tonsillectomy (below).*

PREPARING YOUR CHILD FOR HOSPITALIZATION AND TONSILLECTOMY

Developed by Madeline Petrillo

Usually a first hospitalization is an unpleasant and frightening experience. The following steps can be taken to help you and your child understand the procedure and hospital routine, thereby making your child as comfortable as possible.

Some guidelines are proposed below which can help you answer your child's questions before he or she arrives at the hospital. We will carefully explain the admission procedure and preoperative routine to you and you will receive printed instructions as well.

Before admission, it is important that the child be told why he or she is going to the hospital and what is likely to happen while he is there. Once he is a patient, the medical and nursing staffs make every effort to explain procedures to both you and your child.

Children need to know that the tonsils are two little lumps in the back of the throat; that because the tonsils sometimes cause trouble (for instance: sore throats, ear aches or whatever symptoms common for your child) and are no longer needed, they are going to be removed. For this reason, he will be coming to the hospital to have an operation. Also tell him that no other part of the body will be operated upon.

Tell your child that he or she will be receiving a sweet-smelling medicine through a "space mask" which will keep him from feeling the operation. Afterward, however, he will have a sore throat; he needs to know this. Tell him, too, that doctors and nurses know how to make his throat feel better and that in a few days he will be completely well.

For children between 4 and 7 years, it is a good idea to inform them of the admission date 4 to 7 days in advance. This will give your child the opportunity to think about it and to ask questions. For very young children, between 2 and 3 years, telling them 2 to 3 days before and on the morning of admission is ample time. For children over 7, frank discussion a few weeks ahead and actual participation in the planning is advisable.

In order to help children discuss the coming operation, it is helpful for parents to ask simple questions to determine how much information the child has retained. For example:"Why do you have to have your tonsils out?" "Where are they?"

The younger the child, the more important it is for his mother to remain with him. Mothers are encouraged to stay with young children the day and night of surgery. When this is not possible, do not promise. When a parent is unable to stay with the child, we encourage her to be present before the child goes to the operating room and when he returns to the floor. Visiting hours are liberal. Your child should know when you are leaving and when you may be expected to return. Good-byes may be difficult and tearful, but evasive answers only increase the child's anxiety and make him mistrust everyone. The emphasis should be on the certainty of your return.

To help your child understand hospitalization better, try reading some books to him concerning a hospital experience such as *A Hospital Story* by S. B. Stein or *Curious George Goes to the Hospital* by Margaret and H. A. Rey. Also, allowing him to play with a doctor's kit may be helpful. Telling your child about your own experiences with hospitals, if they were fortuitous, is also anxiety relieving.

PREPARING YOUR CHILD FOR HOSPITALIZATION AND EYE SURGERY

Developed by Madeline Petrillo

Hospitalization is a new and often bewildering experience for a child, but careful preparation helps him to understand and accept necessary procedures. Because we know that parents frequently have questions regarding this preparation, we are proposing some guidelines for making this task easier for you.

Before admission, it is important that the child be told why he is going to the hospital and what is likely to happen when he gets there. Once he is a patient, the medical and nursing staffs will make every effort to explain procedures to him and his parents.

Your child needs to know that he is coming to the hospital because he has an eye condition which the doctor knows how to correct. Tell him he was born this way (if true); that you don't know why but no one is to blame. Often children think that their condition or hospitalization is a punishment. Make it clear to him that this is not so.

Try to explain his eye condition in terms of what he can visualize. For instance, if his eyes turn in or out too much, tell him that the doctor knows how to do an operation to make his eyes look straight so that he will look better. Tell him, too, that he will be receiving some sweet-smelling medicine through a "space mask" which will keep him from feeling the operation or any hurt, and afterward, he will have a bandage on his eye (eyes) because the doctor will want his eye to rest for a while. After a day or so, he may go home. Also tell him that no other part of the body will be operated upon.

You have probably given your child some explanation of his eye condition in the past—for visits to the eye doctor, when his tests were given or when eye patches or glasses were used to treat his condition. At this time, it is helpful to remind your child of past explanations or treatments and to relate this information to surgery.

It's a good idea to begin 4 to 7 days before admission if your child is 4 years or older, so that he will have time to think about it and ask questions. For very young children, between 2 and 3 years, telling them 2 to 3 days before and on the morning of admission is ample time. For children over 7, a frank discussion a few weeks ahead and actual participation in the planning is advisable.

In order to help your child discuss the coming operation, it is helpful for parents to ask simple questions to determine how much information the child has absorbed. For example: "Why do you have to have an eye operation?" or "What will you have on your eye afterward?" For the very young group, explanations can be given more easily by doll play—that is, pretending the doll is going to the hospital to have his eyes fixed and having your child put bandages or eye patches on the doll. We are constantly amazed at how much the child learns from this little drama.

The younger the child, the more important it is for the mother to remain with him. It is advisable for one parent to room-in or to visit as much as possible. Visiting hours are liberal. Your child should know when you are leaving and when you may be expected to return. Good-byes may be difficult and tearful, but evasive answers only increase the child's anxiety and make him mistrust everyone.

In planning for hospitalization, bring some familiar sounds from home—a musical toy or records and any toys or security objects to give him comfort. A doctor's kit is helpful both before and after a trip to the hospital. Try reading a book to him concerning a hospital experience such as *Curious George Goes to the Hospital* by M. and H. A. Rey.

Prospective patients ideally should have a booklet that is specific for that particular institution, designed to acquaint the child with various and realistic aspects of hospital life in a nonthreatening fashion—taking into consideration physical structure, various personnel and their functions, equipment commonly used in caring for children and the daily routines. As substitutes, publications that accurately portray hospital activities in general would be acceptable. The reader is directed to such helpful examples as: Collier, J.: Danny Goes to the Hospital, New York, W. W. Norton, 1970; Rey, M. and H. A.: Curious George Goes to the Hospital, Boston, Houghton Mifflin Co., 1966; Shay, A.: What Happens When You Go to the Hospital, New York, Reilly and Lee (Division of Henry Regnery Co.), 1969; Stein, S. B.: A Hospital Story, New York, Walker and Co., 1974; Weber, A.: Elizabeth Gets Well, New York,

Thomas Y. Crowell, 1970; Wolff, A.: Mom, I Broke My Arm, New York, Lion Press, 1969; and Going to the Hospital, Having an Operation, Wearing a Cast. Let's Talk About It, Pittsburgh, Family Communications, Inc., 1977.

Another helpful preparation tool is parent–child play. Since children under seven could well distort what they are told, parents can either play out stories about dangerous situations, body damage, or even play doctor/hospital games with makeshift instruments in the home. Parents need to know that the impact of hospital procedures on children is far from innocent. Perhaps adults can better understand children's reactions of fear if they are told that the effect on the child is strongly similar to that which an adult experiences when he is told he has had a "mild heart attack," a "mild stroke," or a "small tumor." Even after a child has focused on and played out significant stressful themes in the home, certain recurrent anxieties will continue to be expressed if the home atmosphere allows it. In particular, mutilating operations will need as much advanced work as possible to minimize the shock of disfigurement.

The child with repeated hospitalizations will need just as much preparation. Perhaps more time, play and talk to review past memories will be needed. This child may often be neglected, as it is common for a family to think he knows all about what will happen from prior times. The referring physician can support the child indirectly when he takes the time to describe to the parents simply what is to be expected in the hospital and how playing it out with the child beforehand makes it clearly more understandable and provides the opportunity for ventilation and mastery of fears.

Repeated hospitalizations for the under four-year-old can lead to progressive maladaptation. But if such a child has an elective admission, a brief hospitalization, good preparation, a steady familiar person as the primary caregiver and parental support, much of the trauma can be averted.

Preadmission Visits

Effective preparation for elective hospitalization frequently includes the prehospital visit. Introductory programs scheduled close to the day of admission are designed to reduce fears of the unfamiliar by providing prospective patients, siblings and parents with an accurate preview of relevant experience. A typical tour, conducted jointly by professional and volunteer staff, would include a briefing on pediatric facilities—patient rooms, dining area, bathroom (and bedpans), treatment room, x-ray department, laboratory and anesthesia bedholding area—during which children try out wheelchairs and stretchers, and manipulate the equipment used in physical examinations. Follow-up discussions on the meaning and content of hospitalization and associated feelings help clarify misconceptions and alert the staff to children and families who may need continuous mental health services. A variation in program might include a slide show featuring children participating in all aspects of hospital life or the performance of puppets who voice the concerns of parents and children, reinforce concepts of preparation and serve as positive role models for the entire family.[1]

In the initial meeting, opportunity for supervised hospital play in which children take an active part is important for helping master

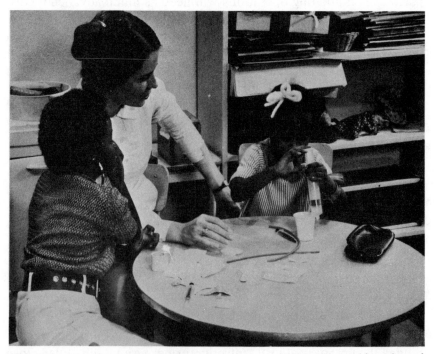

Fig. 3–1.   The therapeutic environment supports children's working through and achieving mastery of developmental tasks as they cope with the hospitalization experience. (From Play School Association: "Play in the Hospital, Campus Films")

fears related to procedures and equipment. (See Chapter 5 on Play.) Parents, too, require additional instruction and discussion with professional staff in preparation for their supportive role. A child's successful adaptation will be greatly influenced by his parents' perception of this experience. The mother's feeling state especially, is readily communicated to a young child. When parents are anxious, their ability to supply emotional care and sustenance is significantly reduced. By providing guidelines and knowledge for hospital preparation, focusing on special problems and encouraging verbalization of their own fears, their anxiety will be reduced, thereby allaying indirectly their child's anxiety as well. Thus, the ''extra'' time spent in the development of parental competence for the hospital setting is well justified.

A variety of methods is valuable in introducing the subject of hospitalization as long as there is always opportunity for discussion. These methods are geared to increase a child's understanding and to present hospitalization as helping the child to get well. All these factors serve to minimize distorted ideas that lead to anxiety.

THE ADMISSION INTERVIEW

The ability to conduct a competent interview is a basic skill useful in any area of professional life. The objective is to derive relevant and reliable information in a manner both efficient and considerate. To do this, one needs a planned approach along with a sensitive ear in order to survey the broad areas of the patient's life, without missing the subtleties. Obviously, an effective grasp of patients' life situations can directly affect the quality of their management. Feeling tones, incidental remarks and body language can give clues to the most meaningful attitudes and experiences. The following diagnostic procedure should not be confused with the more typical medical history taking that all too often approximates an interrogation for purposes of filling in a checklist. Such a traditionally modeled inventory dehumanizes the process.

The first step for an interviewer to keep in mind when seeing a child and his family is that this may not be the family's initial experience with a caretaker or professional. It is essential for the interviewer to discover the family's past relationships with health care personnel and the impressions they have made—particularly on the child. Knowing the child's previous encounters does justify the extra effort needed to obtain this information because the present reaction—whether favorable or unfavorable—is strongly colored by those earlier contacts.

Richard, an obese teenager hitherto known by the staff as "the slob," had a previous colectomy during which his appendix was removed as a part of the standard operating procedure; however, it was removed without his knowledge. Now he was resisting further surgery, which included revision of the colectomy and an ileostomy. He was also ready to sign out of the hospital. His submissive parents were powerless to influence him. He was either belligerent or stubbornly silent with the pediatrician; however, he gave clues to several staff members that indicated his deep sense of having been betrayed and his subsequent mistrust of surgery (for what might be done to him without his permission). Fortunately, one of the members of the original surgical group responsible for the removal of his appendix was invited to attend an emergency meeting of the mental health team. This doctor then reviewed with Richard the previous surgery and tendered an apology for the oversight of not informing him of the appendectomy. They also discussed in detail the impending surgery. Richard was proud of his assertiveness and pleased with his importance; as a consequence, the outcome of this newly established rapport and belated apology was his acceptance of surgery.

Ms. D, mother of Tommy, had had multiple hospitalizations and openly complained to the nurses about past mistakes the doctors had made in her care. Yet she was bewildered by her son's excessive fears about hospitalization and his aversion to doctors and nurses "because he had never been in a hospital." Discovery of his mother's negative reaction and influence regarding medical "mistreatment" allowed the staff to intervene successfully. First Tommy was encouraged to describe his knowledge of hospitals and then to describe what he imagined would happen there. Finally, his actual illness was described to him, and it was emphasized that he had a different diagnosis from that of his mother. Tommy also learned that his treatment and recovery would not be the same as hers.

The interviewer should avoid making promises that cannot be fulfilled or making predictions that cannot be anticipated with certainty. Experiences over the years have shown a need for caution in giving the child ideas that may lead to magical expectation of improvement or cure. Parents, out of guilt, and doctors, out of anxiety, despite the best of intentions, can (particularly with preschoolers) have the child imagining strange consequences—to become muscular and stronger than a sibling, to be more acceptable to parents, to be taller. Unreal hopes are also likely to occur in the child who is confused on arrival at the hospital because of inadequate preparation.

Nonetheless, even with the parent's observance of this caution, a child often develops his own notions of what will happen to him during hospitalization. These need to become known to the staff. Children will have fantasies particular to their age. (See Preoperative fantasies, pages 69 to 73.)

Deaths in the family that were preceded by a previous hospitalization can be associated in the child's mind in such a way as to cause panic at the prospect of a severe illness. Children, especially those under six years, may associate going to the hospital with other morbid outcomes, particularly mutilation.

The above possibilities need to be considered before a formal interview takes place. In this first phase, the all-important rapport with the child and family needs to be solidified before any further information is solicited. The roles of the various professional and paraprofessional workers with whom the child will be in contact should be explained.

The next step for the interviewer is to decide on the general areas to be covered by the interview. These differ with various syndromes; for example, in the immediate posttrauma period for a burned child, interest in the safety of the home, the guilt of parents, and the circumstances of the accident would be more pertinent to elucidate than whether the child has a history of the common childhood illnesses, or whether he is usually battling with a certain sibling. With the readmission of an asthmatic, the interviewer should be alert for triggering events such as arguments, new people in the home, separations and recent lapses in the home treatment of minor respiratory ailments.

The interviewer should ask the parents such open-ended questions as: "How have things been with your family these last few weeks? What has gone on? How did this happen? When did you first notice a change in the child's health and what happened after that? What should we know that would help us make your child more comfortable in the hospital? Who and what will he miss by being away from home? What are his likable qualities?"

People prefer to say things in their own way: these open-ended questions make that possible. As long as the answers they give appear to have relevance to the management of the child, parents welcome the opportunity to be candid about their lives.

The third step for the interviewer is to take the usual, careful medical interview, which contains details on present illness, history, review of systems, physical examination, and diagnosis.

The fourth step should be taken by that interviewer who has the beginnings of a solid relationship with the family. For this step he follows up leads from the preceding steps and begins to inquire about issues that may be threatening. Such things pursued are overt and covert complaints, topics glossed over, omissions, and any oddities. For example, the following responses may be significant: if the only thing Johnny is missing is the vacuum cleaner, if the father is never mentioned, if it is passingly stated that things have been awful for months, or if the obvious hardships of a chronic illness are denied.

Fifth, it is highly desirable to interview others in the same family by using this same general approach. The assessments described in Chapter Four are brought in at this time. (See The Family Diagnostic Interview, page 151.)

Sixth, and finally, the interviewer should explore those specific issues generally known to challenge and upset most individuals and families because these issues often form the foci of further difficulties. Examples of nonthreatening inquiries that elicit information and uncover problem areas are: "Who is supportive in the environment? To whom do you turn when you need help? Who helps with the children? How do the different individuals in the family respond to the illness? Does the family as a group find stressful events pulling them together or apart? Are there typical difficulties? Is this child different from siblings or cousins? What has been his most difficult area of growing up? How do you think this illness started? Does this illness bring relatives into the family who are not usually seen? Do you like this? How are the remaining children being cared for? What do they know of the patient's illness and about hospitals? Is this illness interfering with plans the family has made (economically, geographically and socially)?''

Also much valuable information for the effective management of the child can be learned by the following interview questions: "Is the marriage harmonious? What is the prevailing form of punishment? Do the parents have a life of their own? What is the overall emotional atmosphere? How secure is the family financially? What are their pastimes? Was the patient born at a convenient time in the family history?''

The above questions elicit information that leads to the formation of a judgment about the family adaptation in the past and in the present. Furthermore, with some degree of confidence, the family's capacity to take in new information and follow through on instructions can be predicted. Prior to discharge, plans could thus be made regarding the type of help specific to carrying out a therapeutic regimen—visiting nurse, homemaker, social worker and outpatient care. These steps given the initial guidelines and direction to the mental health team and to everyone in the pediatric unit who interacts with this patient and his family during their first days in the hospital. This interview procedure should be applied with each readmission, as new family experiences may have caused significant changes in the child's needs.

PARENT PARTICIPATION IN THE HOSPITAL TEACHING PROGRAM

Most parents have given their child an initial explanation for hospitalization prior to admission. It is helpful for them to receive advance briefing so that they may employ the same principles and techniques used by medical personnel. (See Chapter 6.)

Once the child has been admitted to a pediatric unit, responsibility for additional emotional preparation rests with the staff. Ideally, parents should participate in the stories, games and explanations that help the child anticipate and understand diagnostic, medical and surgical procedures.

Whether or not parents actively participate in the preprocedural teaching, they must be cognizant of what the child has been told in

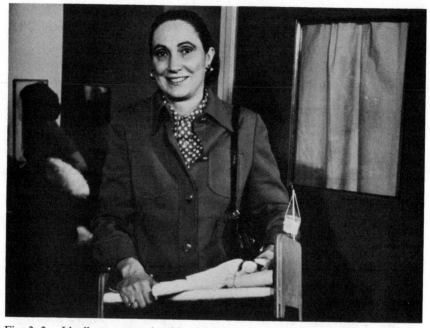

Fig. 3–2.   Ideally, parents should participate in stories, games and explanations that help the child anticipate and understand procedures. To do so, they require advance briefing so that they may employ with confidence the same principles and techniques used by the staff. (From Staff Development Filmstrip Series: "Preparing a Child for Herniorrhaphy," Campus Films)

order to be able to reinforce it. Clinical judgment must be made on when and how the parents are to be included. When parents demonstrate cooperative attitudes and are in control of their emotions, their presence during a teaching session can be beneficial for them and supportive for the child. However, when parents are obviously anxious or uncooperative, it is wise to exclude them from the instruction. In this case the child is likely to perceive the parents' anxiety or staff–parent conflict and associate this with the efforts to help him cope. A better method under these circumstances is to plan separate sessions for parents and child.

Occasionally parents are openly opposed to the psychological preparation of their children. One of the most frequent objections is to telling the children "so much." This might be a valid point if explanations were not geared to the needs of the individual child—that is, if the manner of "telling" were not related to age, family situation, illness, intellectual and emotional development. Parents need to know that whenever reasonable explanations concerning the nature of illness and treatment are absent or unclear, it is characteristic of the child to formulate his own conclusions about what is taking place as his way of coping with threats to his body. This often results in fantasies reflected in the child's current preoccupations. Distorted ideas, if unclarified, may be more frightful than realistic presentations and can become obstacles to healthy emotional development. Clarification was possible in the following cases once the fantasies were disclosed.

> Soon after two-year-old Amy acquired a sibling, she was admitted to the hospital for repair of an umbilical hernia. She explained to her nurse that she was brought to the hospital because her mother did not want her any more.

> When the nurse started an IV on two-year-old Danny in preparation for chemotherapy, he screamed over and over again, "I'm sorry; I said I'm sorry." As a way of explaining that the procedure was not a form of punishment, he was introduced to needle play in which the puppet who had a similar view of treatment was reassured by the nurse. (See needle play, p. 198.)

> Ms. K refused to allow preoperative teaching for Douglas, age three, who was hospitalized for repair of hypospadias. She thought that too much attention had been given to the congenital anomaly already, and she wanted to play down his problem. No amount of discussion deterred her from this position. On the day before surgery, Ms. K became enraged on hearing from Douglas that his nurse had told him he was going to have his "pee pee" cut off. This statement was interpreted to the mother as her son's preoccupation and fear. The nurse again offered to explain events so that Douglas could be helped to understand, but Ms. K remained opposed. Hours later an evening nurse heard a similar tale—that a janitor told Douglas his penis would be cut off. The nurse was skeptical, explaining that it was the child's fantasy, but she promised to investigate. On the

following morning when Douglas reported that the dietitian told him that his penis would be taken off that day, it finally occurred to Ms. K that the child was asking for reassurance. She apologized to the staff and asked for help in preparing him for the operation.

Ricky, three and a half, was admitted for a tonsillectomy. After a briefing in preparation for surgery, he was asked to show on a body outline where the tonsils were located. He anxiously pointed directly to the genital area. This annoyed his father, who said that his son knew better, but the nurse said it was not unusual for children to wonder about other parts of the body. After repeating the explanation, she questioned Ricky again. Once more he revealed his preoccupation, pointing to the genitals. Realizing his concern, the nurse became more specific, pointing out that the tonsils were in the throat, not on his head, nose, ears, arms, chest, belly or penis, nor on his thighs, legs or back. He was finally reassured.

Christina, age four, was hospitalized for evaluation of adrenogenital syndrome. Her clitoris was quite prominent. Although this child spoke no English, her fantasy was clear enough. She frequently attempted to urinate in a standing position and was found in the boys' bathroom on numerous occasions. The older boys found her annoying and sought to keep her out.

Jenny developed precocious puberty and an insatiable appetite at age four because of a brain tumor. She attributed these symptoms to a little man in her stomach who ate her food and caused her trouble.

Four-year-old Sandy said he had a cyst. When asked what it meant, he was quite clear about it. "I got a cyst from my sister. She hit me in the eye." Hearing this, his nurse said it sounded as though his sister gave him trouble. She encouraged him to talk about the sibling rivalry and sympathized with his plight, acknowledging that it was hard to get along with brothers and sisters all the time and that it was okay to get angry with people we love. She stressed that even though he was angry with his sister for what she did, the cyst wasn't her fault, nor was anyone else to blame for his condition.

Ms. P complained that it was completely frustrating to care for Craig. He whined continuously, and it was impossible to understand what distressed him, since he would not answer her questions. The mental health nurse facilitated communication with this five-year-old by using a body outline. She said to Craig, "I'm telling a story about a young boy who worries a great deal about what is happening to him. He wants to ask a question, but it scares him to think about what he wants to know. So he doesn't ask it. Instead of using words, he sounds like this (imitates his sounds). But no one can understand what he means, even though his mother and nurses try hard to help him. They say, 'What could be the question; what is it that worries this boy?'"

In response, Craig took the pencil from the nurse's hand and drew a urinary stream from the boy into a urinal below. The mental health nurse observed aloud, "It seems that everything is working fine, just the way it should. I bet the boy wonders, then, why he needs to be in the hospital." Craig nodded yes. He was then told about neuroblastoma in terms of "bumps" he could see on the body that were causing him trouble (symptoms). The whining stopped. And immediately afterward, in reply to an invitation to join the hospital play groups, he said, "My turn first."

At age five, Audrey required a nephrectomy for treatment of Wilms's tumor. After a five-year remission, she was readmitted with metastatic disease. Her nurse asked the reason for the large surgical scar on her abdomen. She explained, "Parts of my body get rotten."

After admitting Leo, age five, for a cardiac catherization, Ms. L asked if there was anything she could do to make hospitalization less traumatic for her son. The nurse suggested that she reinforce the teaching repeatedly since children in Leo's age group were frequently fearful that other parts of the body might be involved in whatever procedure was described. "Oh," she said. "Now I know what that was all about. This morning as we were getting ready to come here, I saw Leo holding his penis in front of the mirror and saying to himself, 'I wonder what could be wrong with it.'"

Ruby, age six, required periodic transfusions because of a rare congenital blood dyscrasia. After a particularly severe nasal hemorrhage, she told her nurse a story of a mother and father who placed candles around a coffin in their living room for a little girl who finally ran out of blood.

Will, age seven, developed visual disturbances and was hospitalized for diagnostic studies. His parents were so overwhelmed with the realistic possibility of brain tumor that they could not discuss the illness with him. Will told his nurse he had figured out by himself that he was admitted to have his eyes removed.

Just before surgery for a bone replacement in the lower arm, seven-year-old Danny chatted with his social worker, who casually asked him what was new. He told her about the tumor that was worrying him. Ms. A wondered how such a problem could happen, and Danny told her how. "Well, you know when you do something bad and your mother doesn't punish you? Then God has to do it."

Beth's mother reported that her nine-year-old daughter, who was admitted to the hospital after a large cabinet fell on her, was adjusting exceedingly well after her ordeal, although she required diagnostic studies to rule out the possibility of a bladder injury and was on complete bed rest. Ms. L jokingly said that Beth liked the attention, as did her younger sister who had a tonsillectomy two days before. However, she was startled when Beth confided that she believed she might have caused the accident in order to be treated as well as her sister.

When his nurse asked Keith, age ten, what he knew about undescended testicles and how they might have developed, he was quick to tell her the family myth. "I was dropped by my older sister when I was two months old. That's when the testicles happened." It was suggested to him that the problem, which existed at birth, was discovered after his sister dropped him. His response was, "She never liked me." The story was discussed with his mother, who supported Keith's beliefs. She agreed that the incident was the basis of much of the anger Keith harbored against his adolescent sister. Unwittingly, the family had reinforced sibling hostilities and guilt in their children. They were surprised when they realized that the blame could not be put on anyone.

When parental cooperation is lacking, the staff will most likely make progress in obtaining consent for teaching if they focus first on the needs of parents. If the staff ignores the parent's wishes, there is a greater possibility of open hostilities, resistance to preventive programs and greater stress on the child.

Charles, age seven, was scheduled for cardiac surgery. His cardiologist unwillingly agreed to the parents' conditions for treatment—that the child remain unaware of what was happening to him. Otherwise they threatened to leave the hospital. Mr. and Ms. Y were determined to protect their son from the knowledge of coming events. They believed that they alone understood what was necessary to keep the boy alive. Charles was told that he was undergoing a yearly checkup as were the other patients. The father invented ludicrous stories to answer his son's questions regarding equipment and procedures he saw on the unit. Although the staff assured the parents that their wishes would be respected (while making it clear that they were not in agreement with the parents' management), the parents were still uncomfortable and guarded Charles day and night for fear that someone might divulge the secret.

The staff was reluctant to allow the child to undergo such a harrowing experience without first attempting to influence the parents' views. The approach decided on was to support the parents' decisions but to inform them that they themselves required preoperative teaching in order to avoid the shock of Charles's postoperative appearance.

They were briefed in the same manner used for children—with drawings, dolls and miniature equipment. As the sessions proceeded, the parents became less antagonistic, asked intelligent questions and confessed that they had no idea of the complexity of the situation. The nurse interjected that Charles would also be surprised and that it might be wise to prepare explanations in advance. Before long, the staff noticed that Charles had acquired a doll with a chest tube attached. Mr. Y claimed that it was the only concession he would make.

Luckily for the boy, his operation had to be rescheduled in order to accommodate another patient who required emergency cardiac surgery. In the interim, the parents met a mother whose child had just been prepared for a similar procedure. She was lavish in her praise of the staff—complimenting them on their sensitivity to the needs of children and on the techniques they used to introduce traumatic events in advance as a way of enhancing a child's coping abilities. This chance meeting raised serious doubts in their minds concerning their approach. They were completely shaken soon after when Charles told his father that something terrible was about to happen to him. The futility of pretense was obvious. Subsequently, Mr. Y undertook the teaching assignment himself.

Surgeons, operating room personnel and hospital policy may at times deny parents closeness to their child on the important day of surgery with the excuse that parental anxiety will transmit itself to the child and make the child uncomfortable. Instead of hiding the parents at that time, it is better to have someone from the mental health team who is known to the family stand by and show both the parents and child how they can make use of their common feelings of fear. Such a professional can at this time teach the family that, though uncomfortable, at least they are together facing a common stress as a family unit.

Parents receiving staff support are capable of being part of the mental health team that makes a positive experience of the hospitalization. The idea for the professionals who work with the emotional health of children to keep clearly in mind is that the child returns home and continues to live for many years in a family group. A little more time in helping that group cohere and help itself may go a long way in assisting them with future, as yet unseen, stresses. Hospitalization ought not to be considered a unique experience, but one of a series of life stresses when the family has the opportunity to interact meaningfully and constructively. There is no question that preparation for hospitalization and surgery reduces the stress and aftereffects of fear, confusion and depression. But adequate care of children now *demands* pre-, during, and posthospital play and talk. This represents an investment of time for families and staff.

CHILDREN'S COPING STYLES

In struggling to adapt to and master the overwhelming life experiences presented by illness and treatment, children demonstrate various coping patterns. The attempts at mastery that follow include identification with powerful figures (the aggressors), regression in the service of the ego, intellectualization, recapitulation, reversal or turning to the opposite, denial and humor.

Seven-year-old Freddie was treated for severe asthmatic attacks. When he was physically improved, he made no effort to participate in school or recreational activities, and he refused to care for himself or to wear daytime clothing as was the custom for children on his unit. On making rounds one morning, the head nurse impulsively gave Freddie a toy mouse she had found. He accepted the gift without comment, carelessly putting it aside. The mouse appeared on the following day, popping out from under the blanket as the nurse made his bed. She was startled by it and ran from the room screaming. Freddie picked up the mouse, examined it carefully and said, "But it's only a mouse." In a matter of minutes, he mischievously placed the mouse in another nurse's uniform pocket. When she found it, she convincingly pretended to be startled and frightened.

Two similar reactions made a deep impression on Freddie. He observed that these powerful women were made vulnerable by a small, defenseless creature like himself. Magically, he identified with the mouse that tamed people who hurt children, and thus felt stronger himself. As a result, he underwent a dramatic change in behavior, becoming interested in other patients and activities and dressing in his best clothes. From then on, he worked actively to master the environment, instead of passively sitting by.

Since Israel was so undisciplined, he had a difficult time adjusting to hospital rules and routines. It was typical for him to provoke fights, steal and disrupt school and social activities. Naturally, he was uncooperative with treatment.

Dr. G thought the nurses were too soft on him; that their plan of setting clear limits, expelling him from activities when he was disruptive and providing a role model (volunteer as father figure) was futile for a nine-year-old boy who had no parental guidance and different social values.

When Dr. G found Izzie bullying a smaller patient, he demonstrated what he considered appropriate management: Dr. G paddled him firmly and told Izzie that he would be accountable to him directly for any misconduct from then on. This discipline impressed many of the staff because of Izzie's reaction to it. He complied immediately in every way and, what's more, began policing other children as well. He allowed no swearing, stealing or uncooperative behavior. Out of fear, he had identified with the aggressor and maintained self-control at least for the duration of this hospital stay.

Since he was 14 and quite mature in appearance, Mike was thoroughly prepared for cardiac surgery in a sophisticated manner. During convalescence, he noticed that several of the younger boys were playing with models of cardiac monitors, suction machines and other equipment. After observing this, he made an appointment to see the mental health nurse on a confidential matter: to report his nurse. He explained that although she was kind to him, she did not know how to teach, nor had she given him the things he needed, as the others had. He complained that he would not be able to demonstrate to his friends all that had happened because of her neglect.

It was comical to hear the tall adolescent demanding toys. However, the mental health nurse agreed that it was most important to give a full and accurate account of events and feelings. She suggested that he and his nurse prepare a dummy with all the appliances he recognized and gave him a great deal of equipment he was allowed to keep as his own—dummy, electrodes and leads, chest and Foley catheters and miniature IV sets. But he was annoyed to learn that the more intricate teaching tools, not easily replaceable, were not included. So he sulked and said he would make his own. And so he did, with the help of the recreation staff during the last two days of hospitalization. He pulled himself together and left with several shopping bags full of well-made equipment. Mike knew what he needed to help him integrate the experience. And a temporary regression (regression in the service of the ego) allowed him that opportunity (to play with "toys") though he had also regressed to a stormy tantrumlike state concomitantly.

George moved into the hospital armed with textbooks, graphs, body diagrams and diaries in preparation for cardiac surgery. From the first day, he kept meticulous records of intake and output, vital signs and physical sensations in response to treatment. He said with considerable pride to one nurse, "I suppose you wonder how someone my age (17) could have such extensive knowledge." Indeed, his questions and observations indicated that he made an in-depth study of his cardiac problem and was well prepared intellectually. On the other hand, the staff wondered how he would fare emotionally since he was so elusive in any discussion of feelings.

A psychiatric consultation revealed that intellectualization was very much a part of George's basic defense pattern, which he needed to maintain his adjustment during hospitalization. Therefore, understanding that it strengthened his capacity to cope, the staff relaxed their concern about this matter. George responded well to this "hands-off" approach.

Eight-year-old Arthur received no preparation for ileoconduit surgery. Because he was so emotionally disturbed preoperatively, his parents sought to protect him from further knowledge of the procedure.

Postoperatively, as their anxiety lessened, they were convinced of the folly of their behavior and consented to giving Arthur appropriate explanations. Since it was obvious that he had regressed, preparation equipment ordinarily reserved for younger children was employed. His nurse made numerous attempts to engage him in conversation and to determine his understanding. However, he made no sign of acknowledgment, so she continued in a monologue.

The nurse wondered if the toys were too young for him. She made it possible for him to save face by saying, "I brought these models, even though some of them are too young for you, because I know that your four-year-old brother, Russell, has been asking about your operation. The equipment and dummy will make it easier for you to explain." Although this brought no response, his later behavior showed that a great deal had happened.

When his nurse was not present, he secretly manipulated the toys and talked about what Russell needed to know. After discharge from the hospital, his mother reported that he had established a twice-daily routine for Russell's education, dealing primarily with where the urine comes out of the dummy. Through this constant replay, Arthur was incorporating a new body image. After a six-month period, however, Russell had had enough education. He said to Arthur, "Now let me show you how I make pee pee." Russell, who initially had avoided talking of Arthur's operation, had now adjusted. This story illustrates the need for sibling education. (For other examples of mastery through play, see Chapter 5.)

The staff and his family marveled at how well twelve-year-old Ross adjusted to amputation of his leg. Before and after surgery his nurses tried to focus on feelings about body mutilation and its significance in his future development. But he denied any difficulties and said, "If it has to be, it has to be. My doctor said it was necessary and that's it." By the use of denial, he was able to defer coming to terms with this devastating event until a later time. He appeared to make a remarkable recovery: he refused to acknowledge that he was different by learning to ski and keeping up with his swimming.

Harry, the ward jester, had quite a following among his nine-year-old peers. Because of his skill in telling jokes and relating gossip about the staff, he held their attention and became the leader of the group. His humor had a sharp edge to it, however, and the troubled children on the unit felt the sting; he would taunt them in areas where they were most vulnerable—for example, laughingly teasing youngsters who were afraid of needles.

Harry demonstrated soon enough that he used humor as a way of avoiding discussion of problems or situations that increased his own anxiety. In preparing him for kidney biopsy, it was not possible to hold his attention for more than a few seconds. Mention of the procedure brought gales of laughter. And the persistence of his nurse led to his falling to the floor and rolling out of the room into the hallway, still laughing all the way.

Since a direct approach was too threatening and confronting him on the meaning of the behavior would have increased his defensiveness, a roundabout way was used to deal with his problem. In a regularly held group meeting with the children, the nurse leader directed the discussion to the reactions and fears of another child who had had the same procedure. Harry was uncharacteristically mute. His behavior later indicated that he had benefited: the laughing subsided and he was able to tolerate the diagnostic procedure without excessive anxiety.

ENCOUNTERS OF STAFF WITH PARENTS WHO "ROOM-IN" AND PARTICIPATE IN CHILD CARE

One of the great concerns of parents on a child's admission to the hospital—visiting and rooming-in privileges—will have been previously and arbitrarily settled by the institution's policies. Despite research findings that indicate conclusively the damaging effects on young children of separation from their mothers,[2, 3, 4, 5] the application of this knowledge is lacking in some pediatric departments, and the merits of parent participation in the care of hospitalized children remains a controversial issue.

However, there is an increasing tendency in many communities to challenge the regulations that prevent close interaction of families during periods of stress. Existing knowledge favors more flexible approaches. Also, for a growing number of pediatric personnel the issue is no longer whether it is wise to permit extensive interaction of families during hospitalization, but rather how this interaction can be accomplished when facilities are inadequate.

Hindrances to this trend are noteworthy. Even today, few institutions are sufficiently spacious to accommodate comfortably the presence of family members and their personal effects. The staff frequently complains that it takes time and effort to answer questions, to teach child hospital care and to deal with challenging statements from parents.

Fortunately, the disadvantages of time, space and staff–family conflict are balanced by the obvious positive aspects. Evidence of these positive aspects is given by the absence of separation anxiety as described by Robertson and Yarrow (see Phases of Separation Anxiety, page 91); the greater sense of security that children feel when accompanied by their parents; the comfort mothers give to one another and the greater absorption of the teaching program by these families. Also, rooming-in affords the opportunity for evaluation of the mother–child, and other family, relationships.

Davey, nine months old, was admitted to the hospital because he was failing to thrive. During the admission interview, the pediatrician observed a loving, concerned mother who derived gratification from caring for her son. Her only complaint was the amount of time each meal required. Subsequent observations of the mother as she participated in his care during the following week altered the initial impression. The feeding process as described by the staff consisted of a one-and-a-half hour "shooting-in" process— that is, the mother took aim from a distance of a few inches and threw food at the infant's mouth. Very little food hit the target. Repeatedly the mother berated the nurses for the ease with which they fed the child successfully, although they made every effort to underplay their success (in order to minimize the mother's jealousy). Their suggestions only frustrated this mother and confirmed her inadequacy to herself and to others. On two occasions Ms. M revealed her deeper concerns—disappointment over the sex of the child and his resemblance to his father. These findings altered the approach in this case. Instead of proceeding with medical investigation of each physiologic system, as had been planned for Davey, the staff realized that the mother needed assistance to resolve her fear and dislike of males and to develop confidence in the maternal role. She was encouraged to see a social worker regularly.

Ten-month-old Gregory was admitted to the hospital for investigation of a seizure disorder. Although he had his parents' exclusive attention, it was obvious that he was a very unhappy baby, especially at mealtime. This observation came to the attention of the staff during a mental health conference. One nurse described Greg's behavior as:

screams after finishing his bottle, followed by a blank stare. A nursing aid suggested that the baby wasn't getting enough to eat; she had seen the mother eating his breakfast. The head nurse described a conflict with the father, who sent back Greg's lunch on the grounds that his wife was in the habit of overfeeding. He said it was up to him to eliminate meals regularly in the baby's interest. Although the nurse protested this, citing Greg's obvious hunger (he began howling at the appearance of food), it did not impress the father.

The situation required further observation to determine whether the child was actually having seizures or reacting to the deprivation of food. It was also necessary to evaluate the parent's adequacy in the light of new information elicited from the staff's observations.

Greg was assigned exclusively to two nurses, who put the following plan into action: They explained to the parents that it was a nursing responsibility to feed the child in order to make firsthand observations of the problem that was so evident after meals. Greg was allowed to indicate when he had enough to eat. At first, he panicked when the nipple was removed from his mouth. Therefore, his caretakers eliminated rest periods in between feedings and supplied as much food and sucking gratification as he demanded. And he needed a great deal. He devoured meat, vegetables, fruit and three bottles in record time. He behaved as though the food would not return (this had been his experience). To increase sucking time, very hard nipples with small holes were used. This slowed him down, and eventually he was able to relax. It took many days before he became more trusting and comfortable with this new technique. The so-called seizures disappeared.

The next step was to include the parents in the plan. But this was a bigger problem. They became confused on learning that diagnostic testing was negative and that they should revise their child care practices. Further investigation of the family disclosed a history of psychosis in the mother and maternal grandmother. The father's behavior was no less disturbed. With much difficulty, social work was able to make limited plans for follow-up of this family. Psychotherapy was reactivated for the mother, and the baby was enrolled in a nearby infant day-care center. The father was not amenable to treatment.

Whenever a parent program is to be established, care in planning can avoid professional resistance later on. A pilot effort in a small pediatric unit is one way to find out the impediments to this idea. Before hospitalization or during the admission interview, parents can be informed of any existing program for young children. The types of activities in which the staff would welcome family involvement with patients need to be made clear—for example, bathing, dressing, feeding, accompanying to diagnostic procedures, participating in recreation, preparing for bed, and assisting with procedures that will eventually require home follow-up.

Caution should be taken to avoid further arousal of guilt in a mother who already has conflicts about separating from her child because of responsibilities to her other siblings. Also to be avoided is the participation of parents whose prolonged presence in the hospital life stifles the patient's involvement with peers and interferes generally with his adjustment.

> Henrietta, age 14, balked at her parents' continuous presence during the day and her mother's sleeping in her room overnight. She was delighted when the staff intervened on her behalf by convincing her family of her good adjustment in the hospital. With this assurance they were able to leave this budding adolescent increasingly to her own resources.

> Harry, age seven, was bewildered by his mother's concentrated attention. Normally, he was cared for by servants and saw his parents at rigidly scheduled periods during the day. After his admission, his mother was convinced by other parents of the importance of her participation. With obvious discomfort, she complied. This unfortunately worked against Harry, who believed that he must be sicker than he thought to warrant such unfamiliar togetherness. Discussion with Ms. B regarding the advisability of a regular visiting pattern for children in Harry's age group brought immediate relief for this mother, who was released from an imposed maternal role; consequently, her absence allowed him to seek out friends and a mother substitute from the nursing staff.

Children under six should routinely have parents stay. When a child is critically ill, rooming-in should be related to the parents' and the patients' wishes.

While the majority of parents pose little difficulty for the staff, the few who become nuisances are long remembered and supply the ammunition for personnel who oppose increased parent participation. The potential for staff–family conflict is great, considering the pressures under which medical staffs work and the anxieties of parents with sick children. Not to be forgotten is the fact that many individuals are difficult even under ideal situations. In stress everyone demonstrates an intensified version of his everyday self; consequently, illness shows us people at their best or at their worst. Realistically, staff and parents need to be protected by enlightened policies and guidelines that are designed to curb interpersonal friction and that permit parent programs to exist alongside the usual routines of ward management.

Firsthand experience with parents who participate in child care or stay overnight demonstrates the importance of having policies clearly specified in writing, and particularly indicating the limits of family involvement. A brochure prepared for parents stating what to expect often prevents major collisions with staff. The pediatric department needs to emphasize the philosophy that overnight accommodations have been made available because the staff recognizes that hospitalization is less traumatic for young children when a family member is consistently present, and that this conviction has prompted the institution to initiate a parent program in the face of inadequate structural facilities. A realistic description of accommodations—sleeping, bathing, and dining arrangements—is essential. Pediatric departments can rarely offer the conveniences of home. An honest presentation will influence parents' expectations and curtail the number of complaints regarding the facilities. At the beginning of hospitalization, those individuals who require the kind of "deluxe" services that are beyond the staff's capacity could be smoothly discouraged from rooming-in.

Parents always need to know that regardless of their presence or absence, medical and nursing personnel observe their child and carry out procedures on a 24-hour basis; that whenever indicated, they will enter the child's room, possibly disturbing a parent sleeping in the same room. It must also be understood that the staff assumes responsibility for the child's welfare even though parents ask for and are delegated some procedures.

A guide for parents needs to include the regulations that make for harmonious living conditions among children, other parents and staff. These regulations—proper attire (nudity in public areas causes embarrassment for everyone), smoking and alcohol restrictions, and the number of family members or guests allowed for one patient—are often neglected until they become a problem. When limits are set early, applied equally and firmly, there is less likelihood for rules to be abused.

Rules on a pediatric unit are designed to facilitate the smooth functioning of a program, yet they must be flexibly applied; it may be just as appropriate to withdraw privileges as it may be to increase them in the interests of patient care.

> The evening nurse on a busy private unit found herself the scapegoat for a number of anxious mothers after a seemingly minor incident. This occurred when Ms. Z returned from dinner to find her infant's diapers soiled. She immediately sought out the nurse in charge and berated her for her negligence. The nurse replied, not too pleasantly, that mothers were permitted to room-in with the understanding that they participate in their child's care, that other more urgent matters required her attention, and that she expected Ms. Z to cooperate. However, cooperation was not this mother's game; retaliation was. The tale of the nurse's rudeness and "incompetence" spread rapidly to several mothers whose children were critically ill. They, along with Ms. Z, decided that they could not safely leave the unit unless one of them remained on guard. The task of the mother in charge was to supervise the nurse and to report her findings regularly to the others by telephone. Soon no medication or treatment could be delivered without a challenge. A matter of personality conflict between the mothers and this nurse had now become a situation where patient care was in jeopardy. The mothers' hysteria grew to the point where they were demanding replacement of the nurse.
>
> Fortunately, this nurse was particularly competent. It was clear that she had to be supported and that the floor personnel together needed to regain the goodwill and

cooperation of Ms. Z. After many fruitless efforts at trying to regain her cooperation by long talks and explanations, it was necessary for the head nurse and chief pediatric resident to place firm limits on Ms. Z by allowing her to choose between staying in her room or leaving the hospital altogether. This had a calming effect on Ms. Z. The other mothers required an intense group session with the staff before they were convinced that their children were well cared for. A few days later, Ms. Z appealed to her private pediatrician for support. However, as a result of being present at a mental health team conference, he concurred with the staff, thus reassuring Ms. Z that everyone agreed about her child's requirements and that the quality of care from all the nurses was excellent.

Atypical in this incident was the lack of conflict between the staff and the attending pediatrician in resolving the problem. A departmental policy, established in advance, and specifying how staff–staff and staff–family conflicts are to be handled is necessary to avoid seemingly unprofessional conduct. It seems reasonable that the authority should rest with those who bear the brunt of the problem—namely, the nursing and medical personnel who manage the unit. Decisions cannot be left to those who disregard the implications for total patient care or ignore the effect the decision has on the direct caretakers of the patient.

The negative aspects of a parent participation program should be presented to the staff to sensitize them to the areas that require advance thought and planning. Success does not depend on the parents' awareness of staff goodwill alone. Goodwill is quickly eroded when, for example, the staff regards parent assistance as a time-saver and a way of relieving them of these routine duties that are chores. Under the circumstances, they can expect mothers to complain of being exploited or to believe that their children will not be cared for during their absence. To avoid this possibility, staff must check frequently to determine the outcome of delegated functions and to ascertain whether a parent needs periodic relief from responsibilities. Good feelings are also quickly dissipated when a parent has the attitude that the cost of hospitalization entitles her to personal services beyond medical and nursing care for her child.

Any of these complaints demonstrates a need for discussion and possible reorientation of the staff and parents.

> A nurse who emerges quite irritated from the patient's room reports that it takes her longer to instruct a mother in the technique of applying leg bags to urinary drainage tubes than it does to just apply them herself.

> A physical therapist excuses herself for not looking in on a parent and child because she "knows" the mother will call if assistance is needed for the child's exercises. The therapist does not understand that her failure to look in is interpreted as neglect by families, whereas short, conveniently planned appearances would eventually save her from being interrupted by complaints at inopportune moments.

Dissatisfaction in parents usually indicates that they may be asking to be appreciated for their efforts or may be conveying the need for increased support in order to cope with illness and hospitalization. When viewed from this perspective, parent participation can seldom be considered a method of relieving staff shortages. Quite the opposite—parent participation may require more staff time, but be well worth it.

Initial staff enthusiasm sufficient to begin parent participation is not enough to sustain such a program. Mental health workers (psychiatrist, mental health nurse, social worker or psychologist) should be available in the treatment team to facilitate communication and mitigate the negative feelings of the staff. Overt and covert negative attitudes about children, child patients, and their families should be exposed and dealt with.

It is through multidisciplinary conferences that a sensitive communication system can be maintained. Often, nurses will acknowledge and seek help for their apprehension, angry feelings and sense of depletion in their relationships with patients. Physicians, who may spend considerably less time with the children, are correspondingly less involved, though their decisions can be far-reaching and influential. Through group discussion a more complete picture of staff–patient–family interaction can be elicited and a more unified approach to patient management can be developed. Physicians may therefore be motivated to gain more knowledge of the child's world.

The nurse assigned to Mr. S's ten-month-old daughter (who was admitted for treatment of respiratory distress) reported that she found it difficult to understand what was going on with the child's father. He called her to the infant's bedside four times within an hour, indicating quite innocently that the intravenous infusion had almost stopped. On the last occasion, it occurred to Ms. M that something was amiss when she found that the IV clamp was adjusted to obstruct the flow of solution altogether. She asked Mr. S if anyone else had been in to regulate the infusion. He denied this vehemently. However, another nurse had seen Mr. S tampering with the clamp and had stopped him.

At the team meeting, which included the pediatric resident, head nurse, child psychiatrist, attending pediatrician, as well as all the floor nurses, more evidence of Mr. S's interference in his child's treatment emerged. The previous day Mr. S was seen removing the restraints from the infant's wrists. When reproached for this action, he became quite defensive, stating that he would not allow his baby to be tortured in this manner. The nurse asked him if he really understood that the purpose was to keep the baby from pulling the needle out of the vein. He replied by telling her at length about the movie *Midnight Express,* which he had just viewed, and told her how he associated the movie's torture scenes with the methods of treatment being given to his daughter by the staff. Discussion temporarily helped Mr. S to gain perspective.

Nevertheless, the pediatric resident's experience with this family indicated that the difficulty was far from resolved. Shortly before a second conference, the baby developed an asthmatic attack. An injection of Adrenalin was ordered. When a nurse attempted to administer the medication, Mr. S flung himself across the crib and declared that he would not allow this kind of treatment. While the mother stood by wringing her hands, the father continued with his loud protests. The pediatric resident, having unsuccessfully tried to reason with this father, finally gave up. He told Mr. S that as a father he had to take the responsibility for whatever happened. Fortunately for the baby, the attack subsided. Unfortunately for the father, the incident reinforced his distrust of the staff, and as a result his anxiety and bellicosity markedly increased.

Information supplied by the head nurse gave the staff

some insight into this man's own daily adaptation. Being a successful business executive, Mr. S was accustomed to making decisions, issuing orders and demanding immediate action—in short, always exercising complete control over any situation. His wife remarked that few people ever challenged him. He assumed a similar role in the hospital environment; however, here it became a significant hazard to the child's health.

The staff was unanimous in supporting the following plan: that the head nurse and attending physician on separate occasions (a) acknowledge the father's executive talents and ability to get action in his work situation; (b) sympathize with his need to help his child and with his feelings of helplessness in the hospital; (c) determine the father's medical background (if any) and experiences with illness and physicians in the past; (d) elicit the father's opinions on the management of the child and inquire on what basis he makes the judgment; (e) make it clear that his intentions, however good, are interfering with the child's treatment, and that his behavior indicates he has lost perspective between his own sense of helplessness and that of his child; (f) explain that the medical staff is competent in areas in which he is not and that the staff will be in charge, taking complete responsibility for the child's medical care—otherwise, medical care could not continue.

Not surprisingly, once Mr. S understood the firm determination and unity of the staff and realized his own overprotective behavior, he acquiesced. Secure in the fact that responsible others were in charge, he no longer felt that he had to manage the case.

Another facet of parent participation in patient care that deserves attention concerns fundamental interdisciplinary problems, often aggravated by the presence of nonprofessionals. The manner in which nurses and physicians react to complaints made by parents illustrates these difficulties.

Traditionally, nurses tend to defend and protect the physician's actions in order to maintain his reputation in the eyes of the patient and his family. This characteristic behavior is the result of the indoctrination of basic nursing education, supposedly in the interest of the patient. The reverse is unfortunately not true. Doctors usually do not support the work of nurses and other paramedical personnel when it is criticized by parents. Both of these attitudes are detrimental in managing problems that involve parents, as is illustrated by the following incident.

Ms. B's distrust of the nursing staff became quite apparent when Judd was transferred from the Intensive Care Unit to a pediatric floor. She challenged the nurses about the child's diet, the frequency of treatments on the respirator and his position in bed. When the child's nurse explained that she was following the doctor's orders and that she had confidence in him, the mother blurted out that she thought the nurses did not know what they were doing, and that she could not leave her son unprotected. At first the staff believed that she was reacting to the gravity of the child's condition and to the fact that he no longer had the extraordinary attention given by the staff of the Intensive Care Unit.

The relationship between the mother and nurses deteriorated further after Judd reported to his mother that the night nurse had awakened him to give him a sleeping medication. Ms. B was so agitated that she proceeded to inform anyone who would listen of the nurse's "bizarre" behavior. The head nurse asked this mother to withhold her judgment and her statements to visitors until the night nurse could be consulted about this alleged incident. This request was interpreted by both mother and son as a cover-up. They summoned their pediatrician, who agreed with them that the nurse had acted irresponsibly. The pediatrician appeased her without considering either the facts or the impact such a statement would have on interdisciplinary and staff–family relationships.

Therafter, tension grew between Ms. B and the nurses, as did the nurses' anger with the medical staff. They requested intervention of the nursing mental health consultant. As the facts came to light, it was learned that the nurse did in fact awaken the child to take vital signs and to give him a treatment. She gave Judd sleeping medication when he complained that he was unable to fall asleep again. These facts only incensed Ms. B further. She pointed out, quite correctly, as was discovered, that her pediatrician had informed her that he had discontinued all treatments. Investigation disclosed that the pediatrician was giving verbal instructions to Ms. B at the same time the surgeon was writing orders that did not coincide. This mother was justifiably alarmed about inconsistencies and the lack of coordination of services.

This incident had a positive side: it led to administrative examination of the policies governing requests for consultation, more service coordination, and to new methods for writing orders.

The participation of a mother in her child's care only brought to the surface what had been a basic problem in communication and interdisciplinary relationships. The staff can avoid this kind of conflict when they realize that both automatic blame or support of one discipline by another constitutes mismanagement of a problem. Every complaint, however minor, needs serious consideration, that is, acknowledgement, acceptance of the feelings expressed and understanding of the basic issues. This does not imply automatic agreement with the parental opinions stated. If these precepts are followed when staff conflict does occur, it will create positive opportunities for role redefinition, mutual understanding and cooperation.

Unfortunately, in too many institutions where the staff has not developed a cohesive therapeutic atmosphere, programs of parent participation have been abruptly terminated. Preparation for parent participation takes time and the support and assistance of mental health professionals to deal with the interpersonal and professional conflicts that always arise. Whenever there is conflict over a program, one can predict an immediate return to the traditional method of dealing with families: eliminating them from the hospital environment.

VISITING AND SEPARATING

Where parent participation and rooming-in are not permitted, or families are unable to take advantage of facilities that are offered, the best alternative in managing separation anxiety in young children is by instituting lengthy and flexible visiting privileges.

It was not too long ago that medical personnel saw parent visiting as detrimental. That their apparently serene patients became difficult (screaming and unable to accept the departure of parents) gave evidence to support this view. Frequent management problems following visiting hours led to the practice of severely curtailing or prohibiting visitation in order to hasten the ''settling'' process.

Separation Anxiety

Actually, separation from parents initiates in young children a process described by Robertson that progresses from protest to despair to denial of longing for the parent.[6] Characteristically, in Phase 1 the child is restless, cries a great deal, looks eagerly toward sights and sounds that may indicate the presence of his parent; he may reject comforting by the staff. In Phase 2, the child makes fewer attempts to alter the environment; crying diminishes and apathy sets in. It is a mourning state that is frequently misinterpreted as a positive sign. With the onset of Phase 3, the child demonstrates interest in his surroundings and acceptance of new persons, seeming to have forgotten the parent altogether. Cheerful, he may show ''homesickness'' only at night.

Research of the past two decades has taught professionals that ''settling'' was a false adjustment, easily reversed by the arrival of parents, and that visiting did not cause the child's discontent, but rather exposed the distress that lay behind the calm exterior.[7] Furthermore, the young child who eventually ceased to react negatively to infrequent visiting was showing an impaired relationship to his parents. Subsequently, evaluation of children suffering severe maternal deprivation demonstrated persistent, long-term manifestations of this deprivation: impaired trust leading to difficulties in establishing close relationships, distractibility, diminished intellectual functioning and self-centeredness.[8]

The Management of Separation Anxiety

From the newborn to three-month group there is little apparent separation anxiety, although it may be observed by using special instruments recording sleep/wake/fussing patterns. While a young baby can discriminate between mothers and others, he also readily accepts substitutes as long as his need for food, warmth and human closeness are met and dependable routines for care are established. However, once the infant develops a strong attachment to his mother, substitute mothering cannot adequately compensate for her absence. This occurs at approximately six to seven months.

The infant indicates displeasure whenever his mother is out of sight and rejects the attention of strangers. His reactions may range from minor episodes of crying to periods of terror. He cannot understand, and will not learn for months to come, that objects continue to exist when they are out of sight. This fact poses a difficult problem when a parent is not available during hospitalization of the infant from 3 to 18 months.

Parents and staff need to work together to minimize the difficulties. Certainly, frequent and regular visiting must be emphasized so that family relationships are maintained and the parents' sense of adequacy in caring for their child is preserved. The lack of a stable parent figure imposes greater staff responsibilities. Parent visits, with their strain of separation and reunion, are worthwhile no matter how upsetting. The staff needs much support to tolerate the constant anger of children protesting separation from their parents. For babies, especially from birth to six months, there is a greater need for consistent assignment of personnel in order to develop trust (the anticipation that his needs will be met). The more time a nurse and infant spend together, the greater the likelihood that the infant's signals will be received, his individual needs met and his sense of confidence in the caretaker established. (See Guidelines for Working with Infants, page 212.)

A baby will be less fearful of strangers when he is given opportunities to regard medical personnel as safe people. He responds well to an indirect approach—for example, when the staff pays attention to others in his presence, works in his room away from his crib and avoids making facial contortions and loud noises. Ideally, the baby will make the first overture for attention, indicating that the staff member is being accepted.

Babies can be helped by parents and staff to cope with separation anxiety through repetitive games in which people and objects appear and disappear.[9] Peekaboo serves this purpose, as does hide-and-seek for toddlers. These games may also be initiated by the child. This "active mastery" of the separation brings presence and disappearance under the child's control and turns aspects of an unhappy, passive experience into happy, playful occasions.

For toddlers, as well as for other children under four years, sudden and prolonged separation can be overwhelming. Because these young children do not understand the concept of time, a few hours may seem like an eternity to them. These children can be reassured only by the actual presence of the parents. (See Guidelines for Working with Toddlers and Young Threes, page 218.) Beyond the age of four, there is some understanding and anticipation of the mother's return.

The amount of anxiety shown varies greatly with the individual child, depending on his developmental level, the extent of his social contacts outside of the immediate family and his former experiences with separation. Generally, the child with a strong and exclusive relationship with his mother will show a more severe reaction; those who do not have as strong one-to-one ties will have less to mourn and instead will form indiscriminate, hasty ties to the staff. (See the story of Philip, page 335.) Naturally, most children in this age range are somewhere between these extremes.

Parents may not fully understand that these reactions are normal, acceptable and the only way the child can tell of his sorrow. A regular visiting pattern can lessen a child's grief when it can be described to him in terms of the sequence of ward activities. Rather than setting the exact time that the parents will visit, one can say, "Mommy will be here after naptime tomorrow." Once a child finds parents predictably visiting, he will accept the reassurance that he will be going home again. These suggestions are most important for parents who stay away because they find the child's response too painful for them, or mistakenly believe that a subdued facade or rejection of them in favor of the staff indicates that they are not essential to the child. (See the story of Jack, page 339.) Most children will find some comfort in keeping nearby personal articles belonging to their parents and in showing family photos to the staff. Even a very young child is reassured by a photograph of his mother taped to his bedside table. Mother substitutes may be required for children whose parents visit irregularly, and it is particularly important that such children have the same nurse giving them care each day. Favorite toys, special objects from home and their own clothes reinforce some permanence for the child at this traumatic time.

As the child matures, his dependency needs decrease, and he is better able to tolerate parental absence. Even though the school-age child will still be lonely and homesick, he often finds some comfort in peers and new interests. Evidence of separation anxiety is usually shown by regressive tendencies, such as baby talk, petulance, irritability, bragging, or bed-wetting. Coping styles change: the older and more verbal the child, the less need he has to act out his feelings. The following examples indicate some of the foregoing age-specific reactions.

>Sean, age three, had a gigantic tantrum on his mother's departure. Rallying, he sought the company of his favorite nurse, whom he found in the nurses' station. She acknowledged his presence but indicated that she also was not free to be with him. Sean's rage was reactivated on being disappointed again. He proceeded to pull down his pants and "deposited" a large stool in the middle of the floor. His communication was direct and visible.

>Josh, age six, confidently told his mother that she could leave him during his nap-time. Once she was gone, he regretted his bravado. He buzzed the nurses' station and over the intercom told the staff in a quivering voice that his mother had just left and he needed someone to stay with him right away. Fortunately, his request was quickly fulfilled. When the incident was brought to the attention of his mother, and Josh was praised for his ability to communicate his needs, his mother said that she had advised her child that medical personnel were always on hand to help children and that he could rely on them. This child had promptly put the information to a test. The favorable response to his request greatly influenced Josh's development of positive feelings toward the staff throughout his hospitalization.

Before this discussion of separation anxiety concludes, one should be reminded of another aspect of the bonding-separation phenomenon: the psychology of the parent expecting a baby who faces the stress of separation when the baby has to remain in the hospital. Early separation studies show that the mother is at risk for not knowing how to calm her baby, for feeling herself inadequate, for becoming depressed, for early feeding disorders, and for later potential of abuse and neglect. Yet generally the infant remains in the hospital and the mother goes home.

To arrive home without a baby after nine months' waiting must be a very searing disappointment indeed. The natural joys of parenthood are gone, and in their place is the aching concern that years of difficulty may lie ahead. When the least blemish in any newborn causes upset, how much more distressed are parents who learn that their infant is underweight, is being observed for signs of neurological damage, or has cardiac, hematologic, GI or respiratory complications. More painful still to parents is to see a physical defect such as hemangioma, hydrocoele or jaundice. It is important for the mental health team to arrange for immediate work with these parents. It is only a beginning to give factual knowledge about genetic causes, probability of outcome, statistics of the disorder or the efficacy of rehabilitation methods.

What has to be addressed is the guilt, the sense of loss, the disappointment and anger, the depression and feelings of isolation and alienation. The parents' hopes of recreating themselves in an improved form, of sharing a happy growing child, of validating the meaning of their relationship to each other and to themselves have come crashing down. The grieving is assuaged by facts and assurances to a limited degree. Mostly, however, the mental health team has to be prepared for a long process of working through how this profound shock has affected a particular individual and family. Siblings of the neonate are also deeply affected by the continuing hospitalization as well as by the moods of their parents. Self-damaging fantasies in under-six siblings is frequently noted in the analyses of adults who reported that the loss of a sibling through death or placement, or the presence of a damaged sibling, had the profoundest effect on family life.

As with the dying child, dealing with parents of a hospitalized newborn infant requires the utmost cooperation and mutual support among the members of the mental health team and all other concerned hospital disciplines. Whoever from the staff begins to have a good rapport with the family should consult with the psychiatrist or mental health consultant about the specialized interviewing and interpretive techniques that are called for.

Ms. Leonard's first baby, a boy, was mongoloid. Her husband first learned this from their pediatrician, who had examined the infant its first day. Mr. Leonard became so depressed that he had to leave the hospital lest he cry in front of his wife. As he passed the window of the nursery, his signs of distress alerted a nurse who beckoned him to wait. He was met in the waiting area and there then began a supportive relationship that enabled him to tell his wife. The Leonards' decision to keep the infant in their home as long as they could was encouraged in the staff conference, as it was thought that Ms. Leonard could not tolerate the separation from her newborn. She began psychotherapy outside the hospital and was able to place the baby in an institution two years later when she was pregnant and amniocentesis showed no abnormality.

Ms. Clark and her husband had many visitors in the first days after delivery of a premature girl and there was almost a party atmosphere in her room. After Ms. Clark left, it was not a complete surprise when she failed to visit the nursery. A visiting nurse was sent to the home to find what might be the trouble. In a crowded, inner-city apartment, the three other Clark children were busily taking up their mother's time, and there was no sign of any preparation for the new baby. The nurse concluded from her interview—over the noisy TV—that the pregnancy was unplanned. The mother had continued to take sleeping pills and to smoke marijuana throughout and seemed slightly guilty about this. She would accept an appointment to come in to talk to the social worker only for the end of that week. Because the infant was a candidate for adoption, a nurse was appointed as a surrogate mother.

Ms. Clark was belligerent as she began her sessions with the social worker, having already been accused of being a bad mother by her mother-in-law. In her third session she began to speak of how much she had wanted a daughter after having had three sons. However, she wished a daughter to go further than she had in school and to become a professional instead of a housewife. That the infant was premature meant to Ms. Clark that it would be prevented from fulfilling her plans for herself that she had projected onto the infant. Two interviews later, without any prompting from the social worker to visit the infant, the mother said as she "had the time," she "might as well take a look." It was love at first sight, and Ms. Clark was inseparable from the baby girl from then on. The person who needed some working through after this was the nurse, who in two weeks' time had become so attached to the infant that she had named it and begun buying toys!

The concept of comprehensive pediatric care must include attention to preventive care as well. Not all parents and families respond pathologically when their newborn needs to stay longer in the hospital. It is helpful if every discipline pools its knowledge in a team conference about a family's way of handling the infant—or its separation from the newborn infant. Mothers should be enlisted to do as much caring for their infant as possible and to assist the doctors and nurses as well. Telling the mother as many positive things as possible about her baby not only builds a supportive relationshp with her but also builds her self-respect as a new mother. From this position it may then be possible for her to talk of her guilt about how the baby came to need to be hospitalized or her fears that all may never be quite right again. Mothers and fathers can so easily feel left out when they are on the pediatric floor or "just visitors" to the newborn Intensive Care Unit. They may also have concerns about family and work that they may be neglecting. Showing them how significant they are to their newborn infant has important consequences for their future interaction with him or her.

These particular references to articles and books where infants were not emotionally considered[10, 11, 12, 13] or articles and books that show the long-range effects of events and characteristics of infants[14, 15, 16, 17, 18] are significant additions to the developing literature.

THE THERAPEUTIC RELATIONSHIP

In providing comprehensive care, pediatric staff of all disciplines are called on frequently to work therapeutically with troubled children and parents, even though they lack the formal education and clinical skills of mental health experts. Because the emotional needs of families are great and the number of specialists too few to meet these needs, other professionals—pediatricians, nurses, play staff, teachers, clergy, occupational and physical therapists—of necessity assume counseling functions with varying degrees of self-confidence and ability to withstand the added stresses inherent in the helping role. The challenge, then, for developing professional staff who are sensitive to psychosocial needs and capable of assisting patients to cope more effectively with illness is two-fold: to teach the nature of the therapeutic process (a theoretical framework) and also the constructive management of strong feelings that are common to all who invest emotionally in the lives of others.

As a fundamental point, staff must be clear on the definition of a professional role—the demands and constraints on the individual as a counselor—as opposed to the expectations of the social role. Social bonds develop primarily for reasons of companionship, identification, respect, affection, dependency needs and mutual sharing of experience, without the expressed intent, but with the implicit benefit, of problem solving. The professional relationship, on the other hand, has a beginning and an end and exists solely for the purpose of one person's helping another toward a specific goal through explicit, planned interventions.

Discussion of role definition is bound to create some controversy among staff. The inexperienced especially, are often fiercely opposed to a professional model, believing that being professional imposes rules of conduct that stifle spontaneity and the development of warm feelings toward patients. Actually, this is not the intention. Spontaneity and caring are vital components of the therapeutic process. However, the professional relationship does require a self-discipline. It involves the maintenance of a perspective that enables the counselor to see simultaneously what happens to a patient and what happens to himself within the relationship as it progresses. This dual focus is essential to the understanding and management of reciprocal feelings that always exist in any helping interaction: the patient demonstrates the tendency to displace on the staff helper feelings (negative or positive attitudes) that were appropriate to significant persons of his past. Knowledge of this phenomenon of transference helps the counselor realize that they are not directed to him personally, but rather to the various others he represents. The counselor must be prepared, too, for the counter-transference phenomenon of strong negative or positive reactions toward the patient which may contain frightening or irrational elements that disrupt his equilibrium or comfort.

Objectivity is dependent on the ability to identify and face these feelings squarely, as distinct from those of the patient. By so doing, the counselor brings them under conscious control and thus avoids being directed by them without awareness. As a result, a distance is established that allows the counselor to perceive clearly what the patient is saying and doing.

Counseling within a social relationship creates a conflict in roles. Contaminating the interaction with a patient by intimacy renders it more difficult to know the patient. Exchange of confidences between friends obliterates the creative distance, makes the assessment of feelings difficult and increases the risk of identification with the patient. All this negates a therapeutic result.

Several pediatric nurses were immediately drawn to Wendy, an attractive, intelligent 17-year-old who developed osteosarcoma of the femur. Before long, they were socially involved and behaved very much like family members: they spent off-duty hours in her company and openly discussed personal and professional affairs. Over a period of months, it became obvious that the nurses' identification with the patient, close to their own age, was affecting her nursing management.

In addition to the femur replacement in the left leg, Wendy later required amputation of the right leg and additional chemotherapy for widespread metastatic disease. She became a recluse as a result, demanding to have the curtains drawn around her bed and the room darkened. She dropped school and recreational activities and, to the distress of everyone, refused dressing changes, regardless of the foul odor. She was allowed what she wanted without thought to what she needed.

The new nursing administrator questioned the appropriateness of this plan. Her primary caretakers did not recognize that their relationship to the patient had any bearing on their judgments. (The therapist's, or the helpers', inability to acknowledge the significance of this behavior is a clue to detecting countertransference.[19]) In a grim determination to continue the same course, they sought the support of colleagues, parents and visitors.

As time passed, the original caretakers withdrew from the patient. Wendy complained, "They don't have time for me any more." The staff had led the family to expectations they could no longer fulfill. Being emotionally drained, they guiltily abandoned Wendy to the care of new nurses in the process of orientation, who were in turn overwhelmed by what they found.

The danger of countertransference is not that it happens, but that it may go unrecognized. Even experienced mental health counselors are not immune to this possibility, although generally maturity, the understanding of psychodynamics, and of the professional's role are safeguards against its going unnoticed. Adolescents are particularly skillful in exploiting staff who fall into role playing.

A pediatric social worker was chided by the nurses and Wendy for not answering personal questions about herself in counseling sessions. This adolescent wanted specific details of Ms. A's love life. Instead of complying, the social worker turned the questions back to her to open discussion on the obvious preoccupation of a teenager in Wendy's situation: sexual attractiveness and the prospects for a love life for someone with a femur replacement in one leg and amputation of the other. Ms. A explained to the nurses that answering personal questions would involve her more personally in the patient's life and could compromise the professional relationship. Also, to have satisfied her curiosity by giving this information could have created envy and resentment, thus working against a therapeutic atmosphere.

Wendy accepted Ms. A's limits and responded to a refocusing of the discussion, although grudgingly at first. Because the relationship was quite positive, Wendy felt secure that she could express her negative feelings without fear of rejection. In future discussion when she expressed this curiosity, she would add in a good-humored way, "I know you won't tell me, but that's okay. Well, back to me..."

The demands for self-discipline in a professional relationship protect both the patient and the counselor. For example, addressing parents by surname (children's first names are always used) and referring to one's self as Dr., Ms. or Mr. makes a strong statement; it defines the interaction as professional. Clarification is important, particularly in the early phases when interest in the child or family may be misunderstood and lead to expectations for social involvement. Misunderstanding can be easily avoided and the direction of the relationship reaffirmed by this simple formality.

The staff may complain that this is an unnatural style in a permissive age and may often suggest that the approach should be one of personal preference on the part of the counselor or the patient. It may be workable for the *highly* experienced; but for novices, this can become a trap, especially in regard to manipulative patients who quickly usurp control. The most common countertransference problem of staff occurs when the patient sets up a situation for staff to rescue him from "bad" parents or from a "deprived" life. In maintaining a professional model, the helper must retain control. To this end, staff need all the help they can get. They need to understand that any aspect of a social model, in which the counselor maintains contact with the patient apart from the helping relationship, accepts gifts and divulges his personal life, works against the neutrality required for straight thinking and accurate perception. Therefore, to take a position in favor of personal involvement is counterproductive.

There are other safeguards for avoiding the blind spots that result from lack of perspective. In multidisciplinary conferences or individual supervision with a mental health specialist, attention to the interaction of counselor and patient leads to the recognition and correction of the countertransference feelings that impede progress and increase feelings of stress among staff. An atmosphere of trust and acceptance encourages reflection on feelings and behavior that would otherwise be difficult to face: depression, anxiety, aversion to or excessive interest in the patient, extraordinary measures taken on the patient's behalf and dominance over patients are some signs that alert the counselor and others to overinvolvement. Expanded vision is the requirement for understanding one's behavior and for continued close interaction with patients without getting "burned" or burned out. Assistance in gaining this understanding lessens the danger that sensitive and caring people will become overwhelmed by feelings and will withdraw from patients in self-protection.

Ms. D wondered if she could continue to work in pediatrics; she was emotionally torn by the problems she encountered. "Sooner or later," she said, "I see everyone of my patients as a brother, sister or cousin." This realization was a significant step toward the mastery of these painful reactions.

Dr. W made himself available to the parents of dying children. Because he had lost a young child himself, he said that he could tell families how to cope with grief and separation. He was surprised to hear from his colleagues that his way might not be appropriate for everyone and that telling others to grieve according to his own expectations is a way of controlling them, providing a vicarious experience for him. No one can possibly know the meaning of the death of a child in a family unless those parents are allowed the opportunity to express their feelings in their own way.

In mental health conference Ms. L said that her primary concern was to make ten-year-old Nina's last weeks of life happy ones. "I work hard at getting a smile from her. It's worth so much to me that I will bring her anything she wants to get it," she said. Examination of the child's circumstances revealed that because the nurse's expectations and needs dominated in the interaction, she was making it impossible for the child to talk about her own concerns: Nina was placed in a double bind with the nurse and her parents—that is, encouraged to pretend happiness although she received terrifying messages that undermined her security. The parents argued with the nurses who started the IVs, indicating that the technique was incorrect or brutally performed; they examined every medication and challenged laboratory reports they knew nothing about. And in moments of extreme duress, they talked inappropriately, in Nina's presence, of her impending death while, at the same time, denying the seriousness of neuroblastoma in response to this child's direct questions.

As a result of the staff's attention to this family, a plan was made whereby the child psychiatrist would help the parents cope more constructively with their anxiety, and would guide the nurse in discussing with Nina feelings related to her parents' perception of the staff and their response to her illness.

The staff's reactions to the displacement of anger of parents and children indicate how well they are able to maintain a measure of objectivity in the face of seemingly personal attacks.

Ms. H ordered hot cereal for her seven-month-old baby and angrily reported that it was missing from the breakfast tray. The dietitian promptly supplied the cereal, remarking casually, "I could swear that it was sent." Further difficulty was reported on the following day: the cereal was missing again. On this occasion a bewildered dietitian spoke directly to the distraught mother to assure her that the problem could be solved. She said she had personally prepared the tray, remembering the confusion of the previous day, and would continue to do so.

After several occasions of missing cereal over a three-week period, the nurses reported their impatience with Ms. H, citing the cereal caper as the basis for their disaffection. They had not been able to determine how the cereal disappeared, but it was now no longer the issue. They wanted an end to the personal attacks Ms. H was making on them.

The mental health nurse directed the group's thinking to the meaning of the mother's outbursts: could they be related to her anxiety about the baby's illness? Alan's prognosis was poor (promyelocytic leukemia), and his condition was deteriorating rapidly despite heroic efforts.

On the assumption that the anger Ms. H expressed so righteously made her feel powerful and more able to cope than did the anxiety for which it was substituted, a new plan was made to help the nurses deal more objectively with the problem. Opportunity to test it came immediately when the mother complained that the baby's lunch was cold, and as she made more disparaging remarks about the staff's competence. The nurse standing by, as planned and without defensiveness said, "It must be difficult to accept inefficiency when your baby is so sick. How is Alan today?" The mother crumpled, crying, "The bone marrow showed that nothing is working in spite of all the chemotherapy. I don't know what to do."

Thereafter, the nurse's availability and caring attitude helped Ms. H ventilate her feelings and face directly the anxiety she felt about Alan's approaching death. Thus, by using her energy to deal with the problem, instead of avoiding it through the displacement of anger, she moved along in the mourning process. Knowing this, the staff began seeking her out compassionately instead of avoiding contact, as they had done previously.

As demonstrated by these common difficulties encountered by professionals, the ability to remain warm, spontaneous and human in working closely with troubled children and families, without getting lost in the process, is dependent on maintaining perspective on the interaction. Successful outcomes and satisfaction are dependent on self-understanding, self-discipline, an understanding of the therapeutic process and the noncritical guidance of colleagues.

COUNSELING PARENTS

Rooming-in, extended visiting, and parent participation in child care increase the probability that medical personnel will be called on to discuss with families not only the illness of the child, but also various aspects of growth and development, along with adjustment problems of the patient and his siblings. Frequent topics include the preparation of children at home for the arrival of newborns, coping with congenital anomalies and the death of the hospitalized child. (See Chapter 7.) Parents also ask for advice in managing general behavior problems of their hospitalized children after their discharge and for help in reintegrating the child into family routines if the hospitalization has been lengthy.

Counseling sessions can be a help on a one-to-one basis at a planned time, in an ad hoc fashion on a contingency basis or in a group. The bonding together of a group of parents who are experiencing the same problems is supportive in and of itself.

Preparing a Sibling for the Arrival of Premature Twins

Ms. G was offered little hope for the live birth of twins. She had suffered numerous stillbirths and miscarriages as a result of erythroblastosis. Polly, age six, was her only child;

Howard had died of leukemia a few months previously at age eight. The pregnancy itself was difficult. Mr. G, who regarded the pregnancy as one more failure to be endured, did not give support to his wife and was openly hostile toward her.

Much to the amazement of the family and medical personnel, Ms. G delivered living twins prematurely. It was an event that held little prospect for celebration. The boys were frail and required heroic measures to sustain life. Within a month, however, it became evident that the infants would survive. Mr. G praised his wife's bravery and wisdom in the face of such odds. The parents bought clothes and toys and finally named the twins.

Eventually it occurred to the mother that because of the pessimism surrounding the birth and because she was immersed in the process of dealing with her own feelings, she had not discussed the existence of the twins with her six-year-old. Now she asked for help on how to proceed with the explanation. She could not believe that her daughter had any idea about what had occurred.

Before Polly's visit to the Premature Nursery, where sibling visiting was allowed behind a glass barrier, she was told about the babies and their need for hospitalization until they grew stronger and bigger.

When Polly arrived, the occasion was used to evaluate her reactions and understanding of the events. She told the nurse who was nearby that she was waiting to see her twins. The nurse said that she knew a set of twins named Tim and Tom. Polly became quite excited, saying "Them's the ones. They're mine." Thereafter, she was easily engaged in conversation regarding their appearance, size and attitudes prevailing at home. "They thought I didn't know, but I heard Mommy on the telephone; I sneaked out of bed to listen. Daddy was very mad at her." The description of what she expected to see was so accurate that the nurse wondered how she knew so much. Polly was eager to tell. "My friends at school didn't believe that we had babies because they aren't at home. So I took the pictures of wee babies to school [referring to a booklet given to Ms. G showing prematures in isolettes] and my teacher told us all about them. So everyone believed how little they were."

Ms. G was mistaken in assuming that her daughter was unaware of her pregnancy. When questioned about her knowledge of reproduction, Polly claimed that she had known babies were coming because her mother had gotten fat. She was also proud to reveal the difference between boys and girls, explaining that she had seen her friend Johnny's "thing-a-ling." She accepted the genital differences between boys and girls and rejected the idea that some children thought that girls had lost their "thing-a-lings." "Naw," she said, "girls are like their mommies."

Polly had learned from her mother that the infants required treatment for a blood disease. She was asked if she knew anyone else who had a blood problem; consequently, this question led into a discussion of her dead brother. "Well, Howie died; he bled a lot. He finally went [she gestured thumbs up]." When pressed for details, she explained that he went up with the angels when he died. Polly believed that the infants had the same illness that Howie had. When this was clarified, and she was assured that no one else in the family was affected, Polly seemed more relaxed.

To check whether Polly felt responsible for the babies' illness and Howard's death, since children of Polly's age and under, and sometimes older children, tend to be egocentric, thinking that the world revolves around them and that things happen because of their personal actions, aspects of sibling rivalry were touched on. She was told a story about Henry, a boy who sometimes liked his baby brother and sometimes really hated him. When the baby was cute and wanted to play, he was fun; when the baby cried and took so much of their mother's time, Henry did not want him to be part of the family. When Henry could not have his mother to himself, he was jealous and had some pretty bad thoughts—he wanted to get rid of that baby. This boy was just like everybody else—sometimes he loved a person, and sometimes he did not. When the baby became sick, Henry got the idea that the baby was sick because he had wished it. This boy did not know that you cannot harm people by thoughts. Polly's response indicated that she understood quite well and experienced some guilt at her own wish to be rid of rivals. Soon after she allayed her guilt by saying, "Aw, wishes never come true."

Happily, it was possible to report to Ms. G that Polly was coping exceptionally well and that it was a tribute to her parents that this was true. Although their current crisis had temporarily overtaxed Mr. and Ms. G's capacity to deal with their daughter's needs, it was obvious that Polly's straight thinking, extensive verbal abilities, and skill in obtaining the help she wanted indicated a solid child–parent relationship and good family adjustment.

The parents were advised to convey to Polly the fact that all subjects were open to discussion, especially sibling rivalry; to encourage her to express her thoughts about the twins and her dead brother; to assure her that nothing she could imagine or think would eliminate her special place in the family.

Explaining Congenital Anomaly

A question frequently raised is the advisability of telling the siblings of a hospitalized child about the illness or obvious congenital anomalies, and what to say. A significant point to consider is that children always come to some conclusions on their own whenever information is withheld. These conclusions are usually erroneous and painful to endure. With diplomatic assistance, most parents can be helped to present the facts with words appropriate to the child's emotional and intellectual level while offering reassurance at the same time.

Ms. R did a creditable job in preparing her three-and-a-half-year-old daughter for the arrival of a sister. However, the homecoming was delayed when the newborn developed a bowel obstruction that required a colostomy. Although the parents wanted to present a factual picture to their older child, they hesitated in discussing the subject, thinking it was too complex for her to understand. They were relieved to hear that a simple explanation was possible and suitable. The parents told Annie that after her sister was born, she had trouble making "do do" from her "coolie" (parent's jargon), and that the doctors had helped her by making a small opening on her belly for the "do do" to come out. They also told her that eventually the doctors could fix it so that she could make "do do" from below. She was told that no one knew why the baby was born that way, but that no one was to blame (to counteract egocentric thinking). Because the mother was admitted snortly afterwards to a neighboring hospital for a hysterectomy, the father was asked to tell Annie that she was not going to be the next one to have an opening made in the tummy, nor was he. Putting a "reasonable doubt" into the mind of a child about their egocentric way of thinking can frequently offer some instant relief.

Suggestions Particular to Parents of Children with Congenital Anomalies and Exceptional Children

Parents of children with congenital anomalies need long-term support and counseling from the member of the health team whom they know best—whether this person be the physician, nurse or social worker. Too often, the parents are so preoccupied with the child's adjustment to adulthood—the world of adults and its demands—that they exclude giving attention to his contemporary adaptation. A change from their focusing on the long-range goals (which may be revised in the light of new knowledge) to appropriate age developmental tasks, such as trust, autonomy, initiative, etc., is required. Handicapped children still have the emotional and developmental concerns of other children alongside their special needs. This change in approach frequently depends on the parents' resolution of anxiety related to the birth of such a child. Anxiety causes these parents to deny the immediate emotional impact by concentrating on the future, but the price is too high. Neglect of normal developmental aspects of coping and behavior eventually costs in the form of immature behavior as adults.

Parental use of egocentric thinking can cause them increased guilt. They place blame on themselves or project this blame onto a spouse. Even worse, they may project it onto the child himself.

Ms. W explained her toddler's congenital heart defect in relation to "bad thoughts" during her pregnancy. Her husband agreed with her.

Ms. F regularly claimed her family to be free of blood diseases, so that her child's blood disease had to come from her husband's side of the family.

Although these parents need the utmost of compassion, the mental health team should encourage all staff members to avoid the pitfall of oversolicitous reinforcement of parental self-pity. The parental marriage will be strained by the birth of an abnormal child. And such families have a disproportionately high record of marital breakup. Only through the total assessment of the family can staff members know when to intervene between parents who have started to drift apart. There is a discrepancy between what the parents expected and reality; the reality contrasts unfavorably with the ideal image, leading to denial, shock, disappointment and anger. This wish to be rid of the strange child before them leads to tremendous parental guilt. This dynamic universal and normal reaction must be accepted, explored and explained as very human before the parents can deal with the knowledge of science's ways of helping the child overcome his inborn deficiencies. They need to be helped to mourn the loss of the perfect child "that might have been."

Developing Parental Competence

Although she was not the primary caretaker for her ten-year-old severely retarded daughter, Ms. B was determined to nurse Pansy when she developed leukemia. The mother insisted on taking responsibility for the mouth care Pansy required to treat oral ulcerations as the result of chemotherapy. However, the nurses soon discovered that the care was seldom done and that Pansy's mouth was in poor condition. They decided to relieve the mother of the task altogether, but she became angry, saying, "I want to do the job because I can't feel guilty after she dies. But Pansy won't cooperate with me."

Indeed, the more the mother tried, the more resistant Pansy became. She clenched her mouth and gritted her teeth so that it was not safe to try mouth sprays under these conditions. In an attempt to reduce Pansy's fear of the procedure and to coach Ms. B into establishing a more satisfying method of communication with her child, the nurses planned puppet play appropriate for a two- to three-year-old.

A large rubber hippopotamus was selected as the most suitable puppet, since it had a large mouth and was sturdy enough to survive hard wear.

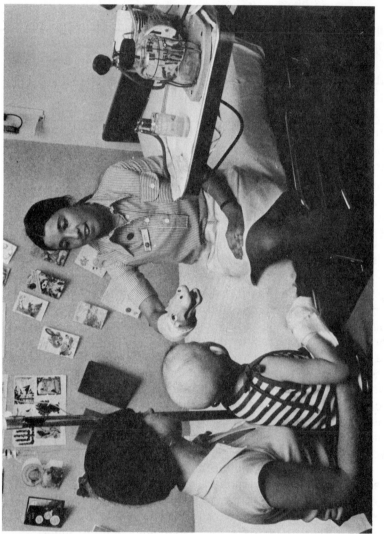

Fig. 3–3.   To reduce a young child's fear of the procedure and to coach the mother in more effective communication with her child, a pediatric nurse introduces mouth care on a large-mouthed rubber hippo. (Photo by George Uibel)

Scene: Pansy and Ms. B are watching as a young hippopotamus is discussing Pansy's problem with their primary
nurse.

Hippo: "Pansy looks very unhappy. She won't open her
mouth for you, Nurse."
Nurse: "Yes, that's right. But her mouth is so sore that she
needs medicine. She won't let me show her how it's done. I
want to help the hurt go away."
Hippo: "I think she's afraid of the machine. It's very noisy
and scary when you turn it on. It's not easy, Nurse. Once I
was afraid, too. I used to make funny noises with my teeth."
Nurse: "I really do know how scary it is for little girls and
hippos. Really, I do."
Hippo: "You do?"
Nurse: "I certainly do understand, little hippo."
Hippo: "Nurse, my name is Dandelion. You may call me
Dandy, the way my friends do."
Nurse: "Thank you, Dandy. Now I have something to ask
you. Will you let me show Pansy how to do mouth care on
you?"
Hippo: "I'll let you if you spray my paw first. I love the way it
tickles."
Nurse: "Of course, Dandy." [Turns on machine.]
Hippo: [Giggles as paw is sprayed.]
Nurse: "Now I'm ready with the mouth spray. Open wide.
First a little mouthwash. Then a little water. Now swish a little
of this yellow medicine around your mouth. You're doing a
fine job, Dandy."
Hippo: "Swish, swish [makes exaggerated noises]. Okay,
Pansy, it's your turn now. First a little spray on the hand."
Pansy: [Giggles as her hand is sprayed.]
Nurse: "Now, open wide. I'm ready with the mouth spray."
Hippo: "You're doing a fine job, Pansy."

Pansy did cooperate quickly and was seen later cleaning the sores painted in the hippo's mouth with foam sponge
toothettes left at the bedside. Before long, Ms. B was participating more frequently in her role as nurse and deriving a
bit of satisfaction in caring for a child toward whom she had
so many ambivalent feelings.

Two days after discharge from the hospital, two-year-old Joey was readmitted because he was unwilling to take oral chemotherapy. His mother was impressed with the seriousness of the problem and demanded compliance by threatening to leave or bribing him. Joey steadfastly refused medication and often referred to himself as a bad boy, as did his parents. The nursing staff were equally frustrated in their attempt to medicate the child and were eager to accept direction.

As the result of a nursing mental health consultation, a puppet dramatization was developed in which Joey's concerns, feelings and questions were articulated: Puppets Billy Mouse and Ally-gator were used to express what the child could not, while Nurse and Mama puppets instructed Joey's mother in more effective interaction.

Scene: Billy Mouse is readmitted to the hospital and introduced to his roommate Ally-gator.

Ally: "I'm happy to have a roommate. It's been lonely here. Why are you in the hospital?"

B. Mouse: "I'm a bad boy."

Ally: "Listen to that mouse! Don't kid me. Nobody comes because he's a bad boy. What's the real reason?"

Mama: "He didn't take his medicine so the doctor says he needs to be in the hospital."

Nurse: "But there are other reasons, too. What did the doctor say?"

Mamma: "He has black-and-blue spots."

Nurse: "Yes, that's why he needs medicines—to get well. Here are your medicines, Billy Mouse. Mama can help you take them."

B. Mouse: [Fights Mama Doll] "No, no, go away. I don't want any. Why are you hurting me, Mama?"

Mama: "Billy, the medicine is for helping, not for hurting."

Ally: "You know, nurse, that's what I used to do. When I first came here, I thought everyone wanted to hurt me. I was so scared I wouldn't open my mouth for medicines or mouth sprays."

Mama: "Hurry up, Billy Mouse, or I'm going to leave. You're a bad little mouse."

B. Mouse: "No, no, don't go. I'm sorry. Don't go, Mama. I'm scared to be alone."

Nurse: "Billy, hear that? Mama's just teasing. She hopes you will take your medicine by pretending to leave. She wants you to take the medicines you need to get better. Sometimes she doesn't know how to help."

As a variation of the above was repeated, the medication nurse appeared, anticipating the usual protest. The actors signaled her to leave, since Joey was enjoying the drama (clapping his hands when Nurse puppet reassured Billy Mouse that Mother would stay). The medication nurse misunderstood the message and nonchalantly offered Joey medicine and juice. He took it. No one uttered a word until seconds later when Ally said, "Pretty good job. I couldn't do better myself." Nurse and Mama puppets agreed, "Very good job" (instead of good/bad boy).

Periodic reinforcement was required to help Joey remember the reason for medicines and to maintain an accepting attitude. As necessary, the puppets intervened with the mother's direct participation.

Preparing Parents for Discharge of the Child

Generally, a prediction of a child's posthospital adjustment can be made on the following criteria: the kind of preparation received before and during hospitalization, the extent of family involvement and support, the degree of emotional health prior to illness and the adaptation made in the pediatric unit. The length of the hospital stay may be a factor, but not necessarily so: long-term illness can be a maturing experience for the patient whose management has been ideal, while, on the other hand, short-term illness may be devastating for the child whose developmental needs have not been considered. Gross behavioral disturbance, present before admission or emerging under the stress of illness and treatment, can hardly be missed and will most likely require evaluation on an inpatient basis and professional follow-up. (See stories of Robinson, Whitney, Jill and Angela, Chapter 8.) As a rule the more subtle reactions do not command such specific attention. Nevertheless, parents still need help in coping with them.

Conferences with families regarding physical care and convalescence on returning home present excellent opportunities for the staff to interject comments and suggestions that further the emotional well-being of children. Personnel who have had the greatest contact with the family, and who have worked directly in helping the child with his feelings during hospitalization, are in the best position to counsel parents in preparation for the kinds of behavior seen so frequently at home. They need to know that phobias, nightmares, regression, negativism and disturbances in eating and learning are common aftermaths of hospitalization and indicate unresolved difficulties.

At the onset of the discharge conference, it is important to give parents support by acknowledging their distress and courageous behavior during the child's illness and then by expressing confidence in their ability to cope with problem situations when they arise. This praise can be elaborated on when hospitalization has been lengthy and parents have responded well to the crisis. In instances where the parents have not responded well, first an expression of understanding the parents' circumstances must be given; then these parents need to be given a list of behavioral danger signals that require a return to professionals for further help and guidance.

When problem behavior in the child, such as eating or disciplinary problems, is demonstrated even before discharge, the staff can indicate to the parents what measures they have taken and how parents can participate in the plan. Any practice they have with influencing behavioral change in their child is reassuring, especially since many are skeptical of this program. Parents are helped to realize that difficulties developing after discharge are the residual effects of hospitalization. While this knowledge may make them more tolerant of clinging, loss of recently acquired skills (bowel and bladder control), revengeful attitudes or fears of strangers, this does not imply that these manifestations should be passively tolerated. Confidence is buttressed when these parents are supplied with guidelines for the management of regression.

The following guidelines are helpful for all parents.

1. Return the child to integrated family life as soon as possible. This means giving the child responsibilities equal to his abilities.

2. Acknowledge the child's bravery but refrain from making him the center of attention because of sickness. There is danger in his using symptoms for attention (secondary gains). Lots of hugs and kisses can be lavished when the

hospital "veteran" does something that is cute or constructive, but is unrelated to his illness. Include pleasurable
activities in his routines.

3. Be kind, firm and consistent, especially in the management
of disciplinary problems.

4. Be truthful in order to preserve a child's trust.

5. Provide play materials such as clay, paints, doctor and
nurse kits and equipment given to him in the hospital. Allow
the child to play on his own.

6. Permit the verbal child to express his feelings regarding
illness and hospitalization. Clarify distortions in his understanding. This expression of feelings helps the child integrate experiences into his life rather than to deny them.

7. Avoid leaving the child for long periods or overnight until he
is well adjusted and trusting of his safety at home.

8. Allow the child to visit the staff in between admissions when
in the hospital vicinity or after clinic appointments.

ROUNDS

Careful observation of medical and nursing rounds will reveal in
most instances that they are oriented to the sickness or
pathophysiology of children rather than to children who are sick.
This happens in any hospital where there is the tradition of combining two major functions simultaneously: education and assessment
of patient progress. Understanding the effects of this practice on
children may lead to more constructive ways of implementing each
of these equally important functions. Any change from the traditional way rounds are conducted necessitates advance agreement on
the purpose of rounds, the implementation of these rounds and the
role of advocacy of the mental health team.

The first practical outcome of change is for all discussion to take
place in a location that respects both the child's right to be free of the
unnecessary distress of overhearing his "case discussed" over his
head and the professional right to confer in quiet, orderly dignity.
Much of the distorted information patients and parents obtain comes
by way of careless remarks and overheard semi-information during
rounds.

At 15, Carol, a sophisticated and knowledgeable adolescent who was admitted for the treatment of subacute bacterial endocarditis, quickly lost her cool facade when she heard the pediatricians discussing the mortality rates for her disease.

Eric, age four, overheard his doctors discussing arrangements for a bone marrow aspiration. After overhearing this, he asked his mother if he was to have a bow and arrow.

Jane's examining physician casually mentioned that she could not feel the child's ovaries. Not until much later did the staff learn from her father that this 13-year-old had interpreted the statement to mean that she had no ovaries.

Nancy, age ten, was quite depressed as a result of several setbacks following cardiac surgery. Her feelings of hopelessness were reinforced when, during rounds, her pediatrician said in an effort to be reassuring, "Well, there is nothing more we can do for you." Her anxious expression was picked up by the head nurse, who explained that what the doctor meant to say was that all the diagnostic tests he had ordered were already carried out.

The anxious parents of 14-year-old Carrie were present in the Intensive Care Unit when a surgeon checking the child's condition said to the nurse as he was making adjustments, "There is too much negative pressure in the chest tube." The parents became convinced that an error was made and that their child was incompetently managed.

A child who is hospitalized for the first time needs a special briefing on the meaning of rounds. Having a group of people surround his bed can be a frightening experience until he learns that it is routine procedure for doctors and nurses to see how each child is progressing. He needs to know that he will be examined by several people in addition to his own doctor, and that often there will be strangers who join the staff on their rounds. Naturally, the child would expect to be introduced. Parents, if included in this briefing, can repeat this explanation to their child so his understanding is clearer.

Although effective rounds should have a give-and-take quality between the patient and rounder, this is unlikely to occur unless the child feels safe enough to speak up. It helps to make personalized statements such as: "It's not easy for you to be here"; "I guess we interrupted your TV program"; "It's nice to see you again, though I wish it were outside the hospital"; "We'll try not to take too long." In other words, child patients should be included in the rounds as participants rather than being made to feel like specimens that are observed "under glass."

A common error of many professionals who have had limited contact with children is to be ebullient, overly familiar and coy. Sometimes the child is encouraged to call staff members by their first names. Although this first-name style of addressing the doctor and nurse might be appropriate for older children in certain cases, it is safer to assume that first names confuse the child: he believes that he can control the adult professionals, when in fact he has very little authority. What purpose first-name addressing serves the professional can only be guessed at. Young health-care professionals may think that the adulation of a child confirms their clinical skills. The child ultimately suffers because the allure of a close tie to an older, powerful figure on the ward causes him to have expectations that cannot be gratified. The professional's time exigencies and lack of a personal attachment to this child can result in disappointment for the child. This buddy approach encourages the child to test the limits of the new and unfamiliar relationship, often to the surprise of the professional who cannot handle the child's brashness. To trifle with a child in this manner complicates his adaptation to the hospital.

A medical student introduced himself to eight-year-old Billy, "I'm Jack," and continued, "I'm going to be examining and talking to you over the next few days." They told jokes together; Billy went through Jack's pockets. Within a few hours, Jack was being trailed by Billy, who was shooting him with his favorite water-filled syringe, and shouting, "Hey, Jack, come play!" The student asked his preceptor why he was having so much difficulty in enlisting the child's cooperation for any procedure. He complained of Billy's obstreperous and annoying antics. The preceptor, who knew Billy vaguely, advised the student to be very firm and to take the syringe from Billy. When this was done, Billy became quieter, but at the same time he muttered about his brother's strength to all who would listen.

Having considered the danger of overfamiliarity, and the need for orientation and circumspection in talk at the bedside, other common issues can be considered, such as the avoidance of giving the child the impression that he has a choice during the physical examination when there is in fact no choice. It is insincere to say "May I listen to your chest?" when the child has been kept waiting for rounds, and four staff members have their stethoscopes ready. It is better to say "We are going to listen to your chest." Also, allowing the child to stall a part of the examination, as with the partial obstruction of any procedure, only makes the child more anxious. It is best to proceed firmly with the examination and get it over with. Talking to the child while the examination is going on helps to humanize the process, so that the child is not treated as an inanimate object. He needs to know, in a simple way, what the doctors are looking for and what they have found. A child who is fearful of instruments might be allowed to play with one before it is used on him.

When the child is too young to understand what the nurses and doctors are discovering on the rounds, he can be told, "You may not understand what is happening here; we will tell your mother, who will explain to you what we're planning to do." An older child can be told, "You can tell your parents that we're going to be doing_____," and "We'll be talking to them ourselves."

Children constantly think about what the rounds evaluation means in terms of the possibility of their going home. It is better to keep this in mind and give them a rough idea of how long they will have to stay, rather than allowing them to think that the least improvement implies that they will be leaving the hospital; or contrariwise, that a new finding or procedure means their stay is to be prolonged.

Any grouping of beds in a unit should always be considered a dynamic environment—that is, when the staff tarries at the bedside of one child, the other children will wonder why he is getting special attention. The staff should explain that time spent by them at rounds has no relation to whether or not that child being considered has been bad or good, is liked more, or is getting better or worse. Rather, the children should know that the time spent with a child is related to whether he has just arrived, whether he needs extra attention to get to know him, or whether he has to have a new series of treatments. They should also know that those children who are completely passed by are not forgotten and neglected but are unchanged or progressing uneventfully, not needing medical work. These "passed by" children need to be encouraged to say if they are disappointed when someone on rounds does not say hello.

Then there is the child who is seen a second time by a few professionals after rounds are over because he has an interesting physical sign they wish to study. For this child, the rounds begin again, creating all the foregoing concerns in others who are in that unit. It also calls too much attention to the child's body, almost implying that now that he is sick, he has something of value. Unless absolutely necessary, this "doubling back" should be limited and carefully presented to the child in order to minimize these effects.

Children often regard the rounds as an unnecessary intrusion on their activities, especially when they have had to interrupt a wonderful play activity. In their beds quiet children may give no hint of their deeper feeling about a group of adults who invade the privacy of their bodies with hands and instruments. Also these grown-ups utter large words, snatches of which are easily distorted. Floor staff must remain alert to the extra stress rounds can cause. While it is routine for them, it is still unique for that individual child.

Periodically, there are larger, more formal rounds on the floor; then the atmosphere is usually more austere and the expectations even greater for the children to behave. These special rounds usually interfere with daily routines. Older children should be returned to their regular routine as soon as possible to respect their privacy and to free them for play activities. Very young children can tolerate waiting in their beds only when the bed is a regular place for them to be anyway. Efforts should be made to ensure that even these rounds are for the eventual benefit of the child and not merely to use him only as a curiosity or a learning tool.

Rounds create an occasion for possible staff dissension. Specialty doctors who are disease-oriented and short of time may be self-absorbed and unaware of the commotion they cause as they enter the scene. Parents, when present, solicit and welcome all the attention and reassurance they can get during rounds, and this could easily cause their demands to annoy the floor staff.

Another possible source of conflict within the staff is that orders for the care of children that are written by physicians affect other professionals, such as play therapists, teachers and social workers. In the mildly hectic atmosphere of rounds, these staff members rarely have the opportunity to contribute their experience. Other staff members who are not present at rounds will be instructed to treat the child in certain ways without participating in the decision-making process. This built-in conflict is so obvious that it must be one of the earliest areas of mental health team intervention in order to assure smooth functioning and interacting of the various professional groups, which must function as a team in the best interests of the child.

One way to ameliorate this problem is to have the nonphysician professionals on the staff regularly write notes in the medical chart. This is commonly done in areas where the Problem-Oriented Medical Record serves as a model. This information then could be included as part of the complete daily picture of each child. The mental health team teaches and encourages all professionals to speak up whenever their documented work is ignored.

If these aforementioned considerations are observed, it is likely that emotional disorders will be picked up for consultation at the earliest phases of hospitalization. Furthermore, certain medical and surgical procedures could be easily modified in the light of individual needs, thus combining the pathophysiological case with the emotional needs of the hospitalized child.

Once conflict is diminished on rounds, it might be possible to see this modification reflected in the furthering of each child's development. Rounds would then need to chronicle daily the atmosphere of each grouping of children, and of the floor as a whole. When this is achieved, the mental health team can recede in its activities. Because isolated needs of children are taken care of in separate ways, the maximum promotion of health in children requires the coordination of the total environment.

THE ROLE OF THE LIAISON PSYCHIATRIST

The psychiatrist who works with children in a pediatric setting can function in a variety of ways. One of the most effective ways is to integrate the traditional (liaison) consultation with primary and secondary prevention techniques. (Primary prevention is "intervention in order to lower the risk of the child's becoming ill"; secondary prevention, "prevention of the disability or a disorder through early and adequate treatment.") These are applied to the population of staff, patients and families.

In the traditional approach, psychiatrists often assumed that a healthy child did not need any individual attention for coping with the crisis of illness or for utilizing the hospital experience for furthering his maturation. Often the psychiatrist alarmed the staff with jargon and ominous pronouncements portending severe psychopathology. Psychiatric workers were seldom aware that their words had the power to create anxiety among the staff and families. Their use of complex terminology confused, upset, and very often intimidated the staff and the families.

In the customary approach, the usual service rendered was a psychiatric diagnosis based on data obtained from staff, parents and child. This diagnosis was a description given in a pathology-oriented context. Based on this description, a plan would be made that was individualized and limited to the disturbed child.

In a progressive program a psychiatrist and other mental health professionals can provide the opportunity for staff development— teaching them interview technique, play diagnosis and methods for establishing rapport with difficult parents and children. They can foster a team approach to observations, can teach how to discard the irrelevant and can recall similar problems and cases so that the staff can make connections with other examples of the same type. In this way generalizations are built up from clinical experiences. Such a psychiatrist or mental health professional shows how to make comprehensive assessments of family units and their interactions with the hospital environment.

Weekly rounds, with representatives from each discipline, can be an invaluable asset to maintaining the unified group approach. These discussions provide opportunities for teaching about children's reactions to illness. Establishing organized thinking about patient adjustment leads to practical programs of management and more rapid evaluation of the child's current emotional status.

The psychiatrist or mental health worker can give to a child and his family a sense of continued relationship with a medical person who does not cause him pain and who tries to focus on the child's point of view. Although the staff may emphasize the surface behavior (for example, that unless the child takes in x quantity of calories and fluid, he will physically deteriorate), the psychiatrist directs the staffs' thinking to underlying factors that influence the external behavior. In these ways the child and the staff are both directed toward treating the whole child.

When this program is fully instituted and with staff constancy, there is the opportunity to teach advanced concepts, such as operations of unconscious mechanisms, dynamic concepts of personality and techniques of crisis intervention.

In essence, the statement above is a job description for the mental health professional that should be expected by the pediatric staff and supplied by the department of psychiatry.

When the psychiatrist mistakenly assumes that he is the only one knowledgeable—the team leader and final authority—other members on the staff do not feel useful. He needs to show an openness to the contribution of all personnel—pediatric nursing, social service, aides, interns, residents, attendants, teachers, physical and occupational therapists, chaplain and recreation workers. The consultant psychiatrist's limited contact with patients and parents, compared with that of the regular pediatric staff, indicates that his most effective role is to rely on the latter's contributions rather than supplying and imposing his own ideas. For example:

> Mark, age nine, had a history of minor complaints as an attention-getting mechanism. The psychiatrist said to the resident pediatrician, "You handled that very well when you paid attention to the child's minor finger cut and put on the Band-Aid yourself, establishing a relationship with Mark that allowed him to sound off. This child obviously had ideas he wanted to express but required you to pass the test of handling the cut seriously."

The psychiatrist needs to make a conscious effort to avoid the shorthand formulations and abstractions of the field when working in another specialty such as pediatrics. To show the immense value and usefulness of psychiatric interventions and to encourage the staff to use their own talents for making children emotionally healthy necessitates avoidance of jargon and emphasis on real communication.

The psychiatrist functions better as part of a mental health team than as an individual. The follow-through and feedback from the floor personnel who are there continuously are absolutely necessary for successful psychiatric evaluation. For their part, the personnel need to have absorbed enough of the psychiatric approach to recognize its value and to utilize its expertise to the fullest extent possible. To have effective meetings without the consultant psychiatrist or mental health professional is a healthy sign that the value of mental health concepts are inculcated and being practiced by the staff.

The image of the psychiatrist may need to be clarified. He is often traditionally viewed as overpermissive, with the expectation that he will ask the staff to tolerate antisocial behavior—bad manners, sex play. The staff suppress their anger, thinking that the psychiatrist expects them to permit brashness. In fact, the psychiatrist is on the side of reasonable limit-setting to help pediatric workers do their jobs and also to reassure the children that adults are able to stop them if they lose control.

The psychiatrist contributes directly to professional staff development by teaching psychopathology and psychiatric treatment of special problems such as the antisocial, psychotic and withdrawn child. There is also a need to teach the attending pediatrician how to do a competent mental status examination, and how to recognize the indications for psychiatric consultation—for example, depression, threat of suicide, withdrawal, bizarre behavior, gender identity problems, hyperactivity, certain precocities, etc.

The integration of information from psychological testing is more conclusive when set in the context of staff assessment and total family evaluation. Furthermore, most children are in a stressful situation while in the hospital, and their performance on testing will reflect this stress by showing regression. A larger grasp of their adaptation to the environment is needed to arrive at an individualized treatment plan. The mental health professional can reinforce, teach and communicate integration of this testing data into the holistic care of the child.

The cognitive information gathered from psychological testing can be compared to expected norms for that age and family type. Certain test responses can give a precise account of the particular symbols that continually threaten a child. For instance:

•Abandonment and death themes in a child who ended animal stories with the dog being left alone, or the bird losing its way down a cold, dark passage.

•Deprivation themes in a child who visualized snow hiding the food.

•Castration themes in a child who visualized fallen trees and smokestacks, damaged motors and explosions.

The psychiatrist needs to avoid the psychopathological model that labels all strong reactions of sick children as disturbed. What needs to be demonstrated to pediatric personnel is the tremendous human variability and wealth of normal behavior patterns, which can be supported, modified or altered to promote greater resiliency, adaptability and ultimate strength. The art of medical management has always addressed itself to these ends, but with increasing specialization and scientific complexity, much of this art has been left by default to the psychiatrist.

Psychiatrists can humanize their own field by revealing the difficulties and removing the omnipotence and clairvoyance that other disciplines imagine. The purpose is not to convert pediatricians into psychiatrists, but to allow pediatric professionals to enrich their training with greater understanding of human nature. Much of the knowledge psychiatry has to offer can be taught once the self-consciousness common to people who are exposed to it for the first time is overcome.

Working with children who are under severe stress, or who are sick or dying, stirs up feelings that cause discomfort, thus impeding emotional availability. The psychiatrist can discern this. The problems of overinvolvement, or underinvolvement, or the "burn-out" signal a need for objective psychiatric support to the pediatric team. There is a need in these settings for people to meet, to support each other and to share experiences so they can return to the wards and maintain an optimal attitude toward their small charges. In their different reactions to discomfort, staff disagreements may also need the expertise of a psychiatric professional's intervention.

Problems in Liaison Work

Psychiatry tends to arouse extremes of feelings. On the positive side, there is the danger of oversell, wherein the staff becomes so expressive and emotional about their newly recognized and accepted feelings that floor conferences evolve into group therapy sessions where professionals "psych" each other. Every patient becomes a mental catastrophe, or the staff vies with each other to please and gain personalized attention from the psychiatrist.

On the negative side, pediatric personnel may come to reject psychiatric concepts completely. When a psychiatrist is critical, common words carry greater weight than intended because they are uttered by a mental expert. Hostile staff feelings rapidly degenerate without an intermediate person—a pediatrician interested in psychology, or a nursing mental health consultant, a head nurse with special growth and development training, or a social worker—to neutralize the criticism at its source or modulate the reaction.

> The psychiatrist wondered whether Nurse F had not been too harsh in removing Andy's syringe when he squirted it. She was hurt but did not defend herself. Only later did the head nurse, who missed the conference, take issue with the psychiatrist and explain that Andy had been kindly and repeatedly told not to use the syringe for that purpose. The next mental health conference raised the issue of staff reticence to defend themselves, and staff deference in asserting themselves to the psychiatrist. It emerged that they feared his criticism.

Negative reactions are also evoked when there is a lack of common courtesies such as late arrivals, lack of clear recommendations, exaggerations and lack of seriousness. The constructive approach for dealing with this is for the psychiatrist to have a continuous evaluation of his effectiveness. This can be done by soliciting the opinions of health team and administrative medical staff. The responsibility also rests with the pediatric department to spontaneously and regularly offer support and suggestions to the psychiatrist. Administrative acceptance is crucial to maintain a positive atmosphere about the value of liaison work. This is the only counterbalance at times of extreme resistance that can seriously impair the environmental program. (See Chapter 1.)

The entire staff needs to be treated as an entity. Those individuals who single themselves out by confidentially relaying information to the psychiatrist that illuminates a facet of the child's personality have to be skillfully shown how their observations and comments would benefit their colleagues.

Another delicate situation occurs when the staff utilize the psychiatrist for their own therapy. The staff member has to be given credence and assistance about the personal concern while being gently referred to the appropriate resource. At the same time, this person's work may be compromised by the personal issue expressed. The psychiatrist needs all possible diplomacy to support this professional's continued effectiveness.

People working in academic settings are often highly competitive and at times are under stresses not apparent to transient consultants. The latter can be drawn into internecine battles and unwittingly enlisted to give recognition or take sides in a power struggle. For example:

> Max's attending pediatrician sent him in for evaluation. Although he was reluctant to diagnose Max's grossly antisocial personality, he assumed that this difficult patient would be taken care of by the resource people. The pediatric resident found nothing medically treatable. Though Max's behavior was unremarkable for a ten-year-old, a radical change occurred when he was interviewed by the psychiatrist, who was trying to reveal the boy's basic personality and to expose the problem to the staff. The psychiatrist wanted to familiarize the staff with this kind of personality and to prepare them for managing the inevitable emergency situation that could develop without warning.
>
> Max refused to talk, rapidly became abusive and ran out of the room, returning to throw a hot teapot onto the conferees. Nurses claimed that they wanted protection from him, and the psychology intern insinuated that psychiatry was stirring up the patients. On investigation, nursing took advantage of the incident to request more staffing, pediatric residents criticized the outside doctor for an unnecessary admission and the psychology intern reasserted his plan to suppress the patient's emotions. Thus, each of the three groups used the patient's behavior to their own ends.

The care of any individual patient is, then, a coming together of many interests, and the challenge that it offers the psychiatrist may explain the fascination of this work.

The psychiatrist can promote the establishment of a team consisting of himself, the mental health consultant nurse, a psychiatric resident interested in liaison work, a pediatric resident, pediatric staff nurses, a clinical psychologist, a social worker, a recreation worker or play therapist, a chaplain and a teacher.

The success of such an enterprise might be demonstrated by the ability of the pediatric staff to characterize each child individually, as part of a family and a culture. The nurses would know the ability of the child and his environment to cope with the stresses of life, such as the effect of this illness. The administration would understand that certain problems in children would create conflicts between departments because of their complexity. People in medicine and surgery, nursing, pediatrics and psychology, who usually vie to a greater or lesser degree for the child's time, might now synchronize their skills.

The ultimate success is signified by each pediatric floor's operating as a therapeutic milieu in which the emotional growth of children, parents and staff occurs.

For the psychiatrist, there is the experience of being part of a mental health team. Collaboration with allied fields is rarely taught in medical school. The psychiatric role becomes clearer in working with a team. Contrary to the common misconception that close interdisciplinary work leads to a blurring of boundaries, the opposite is true: the identity of a discipline sharpens when it collaborates with another discipline.

REFERENCES

1. Johnson, B. H.: Before hospitalization: a preparation program for the child and his family. Child. Today 3:18, 1974.
2. Bowlby, J., *et al.*: Maternal Care and Mental Health: Deprivation of Maternal Care: A Reassessment of Its Effects, 2nd ed. New York, Schocken Books, 1966.
3. Bowlby, J.: Childhood mourning and its implications for psychiatry. Amer. J. Psychiat. 118:481, 1961.
4. Fagin, C. M.: The Effects of Maternal Attendance During Hospitalization on the Post-Hospital Behavior of Young Children: A Comparative Survey, pp. 61–65. Philadelphia, F. A. Davis, 1966.
5. Yarrow, L. J.: Attachment and dependency: A developmental perspective. *In* Gewirtz, J. L. (ed.): Attachment and Dependency. New York, Wiley & Sons, 1972.
6. Robertson, J.: Young Children in Hospitals, pp. 20–23. London, Tavistock, 1958.
7. Robertson, J.: Young Children in Hospitals, p. 14. London, Tavistock, 1958.
8. Bowlby, J., *et al.*: Maternal Care and Mental Health; Deprivation

of Maternal Care: A Reassessment of Its Effects, 2nd ed. New York, Schocken Books, 1966.
9. Fraiberg, S. H.: The Magic Years, pp. 76–83. New York, Scribner, 1959.
10. Gaylin, W.: Chapter on Separation. *In* Caring. New York, Knopf, 1976.
11. Spitz, R. A.: Hospitalism: an inquiry into the genesis of psychiatric conditions in early childhood. *In* The Psychoanalytic Study of the Child. New York, International Universities Press, 1945.
12. Rheingold, H. L.: The effect of environmental stimulation upon social and exploratory behavior in the human infant. *In* Foss, B. M. (ed.): Determinants of Infant Behavior 1:143–66. New York, Wiley & Sons, 1961.
13. Wachs, T. D., Uzgiris, I. C. and Hund, J. McV.: Cognitive development in infants of different age levels and from different environmental backgrounds: an exploratory investigation. Merrill-Palmer Quarterly 17:238–317, 1971.
14. Yarrow, L. J., Goodwin, M. S., Manheimer, H. and Milowe, I. D.: Infancy experiences and cognitive and personality development at ten years. Annual Meeting of the American Orthopsychiatric Association, Washington, D.C., March 1971.
15. Yarrow, L. J., and Pedersen, F. A.: The interplay between cognition and motivation in infancy. *In* Lewis, M. (ed.): Origins of Intelligence: Infancy and Early Childhood. New York, Plenum Press, 1976.
16. Walters, C. E.: Mother–Infant Interaction, pp. 30–55. New York, Human Sciences Press, 1976.
17. Leiderman, P. H.: Mothers at risk: a potential consequence of the hospital care of the premature infant. *In* Anthony, E. J., and Koupernik, C. (eds.): The Child in His Family, New York, Wiley & Sons, 1974.
18. Sigal, J. J.: Enduring disturbances in behavior following acute illness in early childhood: consistencies in four independent follow-up studies. *In* Anthony, E. J., and Koupernik, C. (eds.): The Child in His Family. New York, Wiley & Sons, 1974.
19. MacKinnon, R. A., and Michaels, R.: The Psychiatric Interview in Clinical Practice, p. 30. Philadelphia, W. B. Saunders, 1971.

BIBLIOGRAPHY

Abbott, N., Hanson, P., and Lewis, K.: Dress rehearsal for the hospital. Amer. J. Nurs. 70:2360, 1970.

Azarnoff, P., Bourque, L. B., Green, J. A., and Rakow, S.: The Preparation of Children for Hospitalization: A Final Report. Department of Pediatrics, UCLA, 1975.

Bailey, T.: Puppets teach young patients. Nurs. Outlook 15:36, 1967.

Becker, W. C., and Becker, J. W.: Successful Parenthood. Chicago, Follett, 1974.

Bergmann, T., and Freud, A.: Children in the Hospital. New York, International Universities Press, 1965.

Bernstein, D. M.: After transplantation—the child's emotional reactions. In Chess, S., and Thomas, A. (eds.): Annual Progress in Child Psychiatry and Child Development. New York, Brunner/Mazel, 1972.

Bernstein, N. R., Sanger, S., and Fras, I.: The functions of the child psychiatrist in the management of severely burned children. In Chess, S., and Thomas, A. (eds.): Annual Progress in Child Psychiatry and Child Development. New York, Brunner/Mazel, 1970.

Blake, F.: The Child, His Parents and the Nurse. Philadelphia, J. B. Lippincott, 1954.

Blom, G. E.: The reactions of hospitalized children to illness. Pediatrics 22:590, 1958.

Bowlby, J.: Child Care and the Growth of Love, 2nd ed. Baltimore, Penguin, 1965.

————: Attachment and Loss. Vol. 1, Attachment. New York, Basic Books, 1969.

Brenner, E.: A New Baby: A New Life! New York, McGraw-Hill, 1973.

Butani, P.: Reactions of mothers to the birth of an anomalous infant: a review of the literature. Maternal-Child Nurs. J. 3:59, 1974.

Callahan, S. C.: Parenting. New York, Doubleday, 1973.

Cherry, S. H.: Understanding Pregnancy and Childbirth. New York, Bobbs-Merrill, 1973.

Chodoff, P., Friedman, S., and Hamburg, D.: Stress defenses and coping behavior: observations in parents of children with malignant disease. Amer. J. Psychiat. 120 (8):744–45, 1963.

Coelho, G. V., Hamburg, D. A., and Adams, J. E. (eds.): Coping and Adaptation. New York, Basic Books, 1974.

Cofer, D. H., and Nir, Y.: Theme-focused group therapy on a pediatric ward. Int'l. J. Psychiatry in Medicine 6(4):541, 1975.

Erickson, F.: Nurse specialist for children. Nurs. Outlook 16:34, 1968.

Everson, S.: Sibling counseling. Amer. J. Nurs. 77:644, 1977.

Godfrey, A. E.: A study of nursing care designed to assist hospitalized children and their parents in their separation. Nurs. Res. 4:52, 1955.

Goldfarb, W.: Psychological privation in infancy and subsequent adjustment. Amer. J. Orthopsychiat. 15:247, 1945.

Gordon, B.: A psychoanalytic contribution to pediatrics. In Eissler, R., et al.: The Psychoanalytic Study of the Child, vol. 25. New York, International Universities Press, 1970.

Green, M.: Comprehensive pediatrics and the changing role of the pediatrician. In Solnit, A. J., and Provence, S. A. (eds.): Modern Perspectives in Child Development. New York, International Universities Press, 1963.

Gurwitt, A. R.: Aspects of prospective fatherhood: a case report. In The Psychoanalytic Study of the Child. 31:237–73. New Haven, Yale University Press, 1976.

Hamovitch, M. B.: The Parent and the Fatally Ill Child. Los Angeles, Delmar, 1964.

Hardgrove, C. B.: Working with parents on the pediatric unit. Pediatric Annals 1:44, 1972.

Hardgrove, C. B., and Dawson, R. B.: Parents and Children in the Hospital: The Family's Role in Pediatrics. Boston, Little, Brown, 1972.

Hardgrove, C. B., and Rutledge, A.: Parenting during hospitalization. Amer. J. Nurs. 75:836, 1975.

Hardgrove, C. B. Emotional inoculation: the 3 R's of preparation. JACCH 5:17, Spring 1977.

Hays, D. R.: Anger: a clinical problem. In Some Clinical Approaches to Psychiatric Nursing, p. 110. New York, Macmillan, 1963.

Hirschberg, J. C.: The basic functions of a child psychiatrist in any setting. J. Amer. Acad. Child Psychiat. 5:360, 1966.

Inei, E.: The identification of concerns experienced by fathers of hospitalized children. JACCH 4:43, 1975.

James, V., and Wheeler, W.: Care by parents unit. Pediatrics 43:488, 1969.

Jessner, L., *et al.*: Emotional implications of tonsillectomy and adenoidectomy on children. *In* Eissler, R., *et al.*: The Psychoanalytic Study of the Child, vol. 7. New York, International Universities Press, 1952.

Johnson, J. E., Kirchhoff, K. T., and Endress, M. P.: Altering children's distress behavior during orthopedic cast removal. Nurs. Res. 24(6):404, 1975.

Kennedy, E.: On Becoming a Counselor. New York, Seabury, 1977.

Kennell, J. H., and Bergen, M.: Early childhood separations. Pediatrics 37:291, 1966.

Kunzman, L.: Some factors influencing a young child's mastery of hospitalization. Nurs. Clinics of N. Amer. 18:625, 1971.

Levy, D. M.: Psychic traumas of operations in children. Amer. J. Dis. Child. 69:7, 1945.

Lickorish, J. R.: The psychometric assessment of the family. *In* Howells, J. G. (ed.): Theory and Practice of Family Psychiatry. New York, Brunner/Mazel, 1971.

Linn, S.: Puppets and hospitalized children: talking about feelings. JACCH 5:5, Spring 1977.

Lourie, R. S.: The teaching of child psychiatry in pediatrics. J. Amer. Acad. Child Psychiat. 1:477, 1962.

Mattson, A.: Long-term physical illness in childhood: a challenge to psychosocial adaptation. Pediatrics 6:176, 1965.

McDonald, M.: The psychiatric evaluation of children. J. Amer. Acad. Child Psychiat. 4:569, 1965.

Mellish, R. W. P.: Preparation of the child for hospitalization and surgery. Pediat. Clin. N. Amer. 16:543, 1969.

Menninger, K.: Transference and countertransference: the involuntary participation of the second party in the treatment process. *In* Theory of Psychoanalytic Technique, pp. 77–98. New York, Harper & Row, Harper Torchbooks, 1958.

Murphy, L. B.: Assessment of infants and young children. *In* Chandler, C., *et al.*: Early Child Care: The New Perspectives. New York, Atherton, 1968.

Murphy, L. B., and Moriarty, A. E.: Vulnerability, Coping and Growth from Infancy to Adolescence. New Haven, Yale University Press, 1976.

Nagera, H.: Children's reactions to death of important objects: a developmental approach. *In* Eissler, R., *et al.* (eds.): The Psychoanalytic Study of the Child, vol. 25. New York, International Universities Press, 1970.

Oremland, E. K. and J. D. (eds.): The Effects of Hospitalization on Children: Models for Their Care. Springfield, Ill., Charles C Thomas, 1973.

Petrillo, M.: Preparing children and parents for hospitalization and treatment. Pediatric Annals 1:24, 1972.

———: Staff Development Series: Preparing Children for Surgery or Teaching About Illness. Campus Films, 1975.

To Prepare a Child and A Hospital Visit with Clipper. Media Center, Children's Hospital Medical Center, Washington, D.C.

Provence, S. A., and Lipton, R.: Infants in Institutions. New York, International Universities Press, 1962.

Prugh, D. G., *et al.*: A study of the emotional responses of children and families to hospitalization and illness. Amer. J. Orthopsychiat. 23:70, 1953.

Ramos, S.: Teaching your Child to Cope with Crisis. New York, David McKay, 1975.

Schacter, S., and Singer, J. E.: Cognitive, social and physiological determinants of emotional state. Psychol. Rev. 69:379, 1962.

Schaeffer, A. J.: Advantages of mother living in with her hospitalized child. *In* Haller, A., *et al.*: The Hospitalized Child and His Family. Baltimore, Johns Hopkins University Press, 1967.

Schulman, J. L.: Management of Emotional Disorders in Pediatric Practice, pp. 109–239. Chicago, Year Book Medical Publishers, 1967.

Senn, M. J. E., and Solnit, A. J.: Problems in Child Behavior and Development. Chap. 8. Pediatric evaluation. Philadelphia, Lea & Febiger, 1968.

Shereshefsky, P. M., and Yarrow, L. J.: Psychological Aspects of a First Pregnancy and Early Postnatal Adaptation. New York, Raven Press, 1973.

Shirley, H. F.: Pediatric Psychiatry, pp. 642–45. Cambridge, Harvard University Press, 1963.

Shore, M. F. (ed.): Red Is the Color of Hurting: Planning for Children in the Hospital. Bethesda, Md., National Institute for Mental Health, 1967.

Silberstein, R. M., *et al.:* Autoerotic head banging; a reflection on the opportunism of infants. J. Amer. Acad. Child Psychiat., 5:235, 1966.

Skipper, J. K., Leonard, R. C., and Rhymes, J.: Child hospitalization and social interaction: an experimental study of mothers' feelings of stress, adaptation and satisfaction. Medical Care 6:496, 1968.

Skipper, J. K., and Leonard, R. C.: Children, stress and hospitalization: a field experiment. J. Health and Social Behavior 9:275, 1968.

Solnit, A. J., and Stark, M. H.: Mourning and the birth of a defective child. *In* Eissler, R., *et al.* (eds.): Psychoanalytic Study of the Child, vol. 16, p. 523. New York, International Universities Press, 1961.

Sperling, M.: Asthma in children. An evaluation of concepts and theories. J. Amer. Acad. Child Psychiat. 7:44, 1968.

Streepy, S.: Today He Can't. Tomorrow He Can! Your Child from Birth to Two Years. New York, The Learning Child, 1971.

Tabler, M.: Doing it better: a preview of coming attractions. Nursing '73 3:40, 1973.

Vernon, D. T. A., and Schulman, J. L.: Hospitalization as a source of psychological benefit to children. Pediatrics 34:694, 1964.

Visintainer, M. A., and Wolfer, J. A.: Psychological preparation for surgical pediatric patients: the effect on children's and parents' stress responses and adjustment. Pediatrics 56:187, 1975.

White, R. W.: Strategies of adaptation: an attempt at systematic description. *In* Coelho, G. V., Hamburg, D., and Adams, J. E. (eds.): Coping and Adaptation. New York, Basic Books, 1974.

Whitson, B. J.: The puppet treatment in pediatrics. Amer. J. Nurs. 72:1612, 1972.

Wolf, A. W. M.: Helping Your Child Understand Death. New York, Child Study Association of American Publications, 1958.

Wolf, R. E.: The hospital and the child. *In* Solnit, A. J., and Provence, S. A. (eds.): Modern Perspectives in Child Development. New York, International Universities Press, 1963.

4

Family Assessment and Management

Discerning the pattern of relationships in a family can be formidable. Interactions are complex; yet, unless the generally expected patterns are compared with the data from a particular family, a preliminary assessment cannot be made. This rough estimate of the current mode of adaptation helps to predict behavior under stress. Such anticipations are valid, since any group will retain its basic characteristics even in crisis.

In order to assess how any one family is functioning, one has to take into account the cultural factors operating on that family, where that family is socioeconomically, what stage of development they are in as a family unit and what their composition is.

CULTURAL FACTORS

One of the ways to deepen understanding of individuals and families is to have a knowledge of their cultural background. Many families will react to the stress of illness in character with their heritage. These reactions affect the child and also the hospital staff. For instance, Spiegel contrasts the time orientation of the foreign-born Italian working class with that of middle-class Americans.[1] He shows in basic ways how deep the differences can be—the Italians emphasize present, past and future in that order; Americans, the future, present and past. With this knowledge, professionals would be better able to understand the difference between the Italian grandparents, who would be concerned with the origins of an illness, and the American parents, who would consider how the illness affects the child's schoolwork and future. Thus the professional could anticipate an already existing conflict between parents and grandparents or between foreign-born parents and staff.

Because of the general American mixture of cultures,[2] there are no cultural patternings that exist in a pure form in America today. Since the differences within cultures are as great as those between them, it is best to rely on socioeconomic style and family development in addition to cultural type in order to make family assessments.

SOCIOECONOMIC FACTORS

The atmosphere in low socioeconomic homes is not only conducive to increasing incidence and prevalence of illness, but also to early pervasive impediments to the attainment of school success and sociability. Because of the large numbers of culture-of-poverty people in hospitals and clinics, a thorough knowledge is important. The Report of the Joint Commission on Mental Health of Children[3] outlines much of this information. (See chart, page 146.) The U.S. Government booklet *Growing Up Poor* shows how all races at the poverty level are affected by the stability or instability of both emotional and economic climate.

Hollingshead and Redlich describe five classes of people who are easily defined by residential address, occupation and years of schooling completed by the household head. Each class, furthermore, has cultural traits that cluster about it and sharpen its definition. These authors further demonstrate the type and prevalence of mental illness that occurs in correlation with class—for example, character neuroses are found most frequently in the highest classes (1 and 2) while antisocial and immature reactions are found in the lowest class (5).[4]

These distinctions are also true in the physical realm, in which the lowest class is found to have the poorest health—for instance, malnutrition, dental caries, obesity and accidental ingestions (in childhood).

Hospital personnel need to be attuned to their reactions to particular classes. Hollingshead and Redlich demonstrate that a bias does exist against certain classes in spite of "professional objectivity,'' which supposedly makes no distinctions. Because professionals come predominantly from classes 2 and 3, they have a natural unfamiliarity with classes 1, 4, and 5 and tend to have overcritical or oversolicitous attitudes toward them.

For example, bias on the part of professionals who wanted to demonstrate that child abuse existed uniformly in the population led them to say that in upper classes it was concealed by cover-up and underreporting, whereas the minorities and disadvantaged would be labeled as deviant by mental health professionals.[5, 6] Reports and studies, however, are increasingly pointing to the causal relationships between socioeconomic class and child maltreatment.[7] One strongly argued report goes further. It assigns professionals' and politicians' self-serving needs as the basis for ignorance as to the effects of poverty on the frequency and severity of child abuse.[8]

The National Academy of Sciences updates Hollingshead and Redlich in exploring the influence of socioeconomics and demography on the quality of life for families and on the identification of ''at risk'' children.

Turning the usual approach around by saying that child maltreatment indicates at risk neighborhoods, several researchers show the ecologic complexity of these issues. Maltreatment, they reveal, occurs in neighborhoods with few material and social resources.[9, 10]

FAMILY DEVELOPMENT

Families differ according to their development as a unit. A young family of under three years' duration, still settling marital roles, is insecure as to what tasks are masculine and feminine and often tries to ignore outside influences in developing its identity. The couple may turn to professionals as healthier influences than their relatives, who continue to treat them as they did before marriage. Money handling and financial planning are realistic issues. There is always the adjustment between what they expected from marriage and what they are getting. Inexperience with children may lead them to anxious overconcern with development and child care practices. They are often reluctant to rely on spontaneous feeling.

A family established for four to 10 years is less susceptible to outside influence and has routinized patterns of husband–wife roles and parent–child relationships. There is more stability in economic matters and with respect to relatives. The autonomy and independence of the children, and the relationships between the children and the school, are new issues. This more established family is not as prone to sudden mood fluctuation as the younger family is. In reaction to their earlier overconcern with growth and development, this couple may become so casual as to ignore important factors in the development of their children.

An older established family of 10 to 20 years has set patterns to the direction of their lives. However, they need to learn how to adjust to the difficulties of normal separation and emancipation of their children. These adjustments can be complicated by illness. For example, an adolescent who has been predominantly out of the home and involved with peer group activities can be quite a problem if he needs once again to be dependent on his parents because of illness.

FAMILY COMPOSITION

The size of the family and the child's position in it can alert the professional to certain probabilities. However, generalizations are misleading—for example, an only child can have regular, intimate companions, and a child from a large family can be isolated and lonely. Although a middle child may have neither the advantage of the oldest nor the immunity of the baby, he may avoid the high expectations imposed on a first child and escape the indulgence of the youngest. The youngest child may have to scramble and fight for love and attention, or he may become the spoiled family mascot. A large family may be able to give "each according to his needs" and provide a sense of unity and closeness; yet, on the other hand, it may lead to keen competitiveness, pugnacity, loneliness and confusion of generations.

With older siblings acting in parental roles, the younger child may form close attachments that are irregularly disrupted by the many changes in the lives of the "auxiliary parents." The elder children in a large family may be mature in the way of taking responsibility and doing chores, but may have missed developing such inner resources as imagination, generosity and spontaneity.

A small family may instill in the child a strict conscience and rigid patterns of relating to authority because of the absence of the moderating influence of other siblings. There is also the danger of narrow family alliances—for example, father–daughter, mother–son, which limit a broader identification with both parents' gender roles and those of siblings.

Special family experiences need to be included in any assessment. When a child has died, a parent is chronically ill, the family has moved frequently, or the children intermittently live with certain relatives, these events differentiate these families from the family unit that has never experienced loss or separation. Obviously, the effect of hospitalization on individual families will also differ.

If the professional keeps in mind the average characteristics for a particular patient with respect to culture, economic condition and family unit characteristics, he will look for confirmation or differentiation from this expectation. For example, a baby who had failed to thrive required multiple admissions and diagnostic procedures before the staff became aware that his eating and sleeping arrangements in a culture-of-poverty were affecting his growth. When these were altered, the child prospered.

It is important to avoid stereotyping a family because of its cultural or economic background, or other factors. This can be successfully overcome by the nurse and physician if more is learned about the family.

An example of professional bias is the result of the influence of the literature on the black family. Their low self-esteem was allegedly based on society's low esteem.[11] Familiarity with newer reviews of the subject can give a more balanced view that the black family is not simply reacting to the oppressive atmosphere but reflecting developmental and personal interactive forces.[12, 13]

Studies of Polish and Italian families show a difference in reaching out to professionals for children's behavioral problems from first, second and third generations of U.S. born. The first generation relies heavily on kinship supports for guidance even when the family clearly has exhausted their traditional resources.[14, 15]

Each family is unique, and generalizations about low income, large size, or culturally deprived families serve merely as a starting point in understanding the problems families face and in predicting how they will behave under stress.

PATTERNS OF FAMILY DYNAMICS

Family dynamics are complex and they do fluctuate, yet a classification scheme has recently been suggested for family pathology.[16] Divided into three sources of information, classification causes less mystery. The first source is the developmental history of the family: seeing the family as a small group experiencing its own historical stages and involving the pathological interactions and settings where problems have developed. The second contributor to family diagnosis is to take a mental status assessment of the family process. The family as a group can be asked to look at a series of ambiguous pictures, such as CAT cards, and tell a story together. The family is also observed building a model with blocks to see the quality of the family process in the present. Finally the family is studied, as is the child, when they are separated from each other. For example, do they tiptoe off, linger painfully or give elaborate guilt-relieving instructions when they depart from each other? With this classification system it is possible to group families into several categories.

In caring for the emotional health of children in hospitals where the majority of children have not been referred for psychiatric reasons and where mental retardation has not been diagnosed, it is not uncommon to find families whose *interactions are basically in reaction to the child's problems*. In the instances where this is so, the child usually is not changed during separation while the family is much improved; the family behaves pathologically only when the child is with them.

Walter is a seven-year-old who complains continually of having nothing to do. When the family visit, he makes them feel guilty that their toys and games are boring and quickly mastered. The least effort on his parents' part to show him how he might keep himself busy in the hospital is met with silence or a snap remark. By the time his parents emerge from his room, his mother is in tears and his father is morose. They appeared to be happy as a couple before they started their visit. They reported that at home Walter developed his self-centered personality after being with his grandmother for six months while the parents were working and trying to find a place to live. After his return from his grandmother he demonstrated these qualities, which seemed to remain.

Another category of family would be the one in which the *illness in one parent dominates the interaction, and the child patient may have been chosen to be the responder.* The history in this family is that of illness in the parent and a long, unsatisfactory relationship with the child patient. The other parent is often uninvolved and passive. During separation the child patient may attempt to recreate the disturbed relationship with the parent but usually stabilizes and improves dramatically. On the other hand, the family continues to be impaired in its atmosphere, and the pathological parent may choose another child for conflicted involvement.

Donna had the reputation even in the emergency room of taking things. Though only five, she covered her antisocial behavior by always requesting another item for her mother. She was apparently fond of pens attached to pads and would be seen trying to slip one into her basket in the waiting room. Her mother smiled and seemed to enjoy Donna's skill and apparently liked to acquire these pens and pads herself. However, for public consumption the mother would gently slap Donna's hand and ask her to give the items back. On the floor, Donna's room was the first place the nurses would look if anything was missing from the nurses' station, for her drawer was full of an assortment of pens and pencils, paper clips and pads. Donna gradually, over the course of her treatment for a fractured humerus, decreased her stealing and redirected her interest toward doll play. About two weeks after hospitalization began, the mother accidentally mentioned that she was very concerned about a new problem in the family. Her twelve-year-old son was found smoking marijuana.

Other groupings for diagnosis and classification occur around *families that are in constant marital conflict with the children reacting* to, and influenced by, the parents' squabbles; there are often families in which the disturbed marital relationship intensely involves one particular child so that a threesome is formed. In this instance the removal of the child from the home is followed by an attempt by both parents and the child to recreate the pathological triad with new people.

Another group that can be identified are those who share a *common fantasy or belief* in which the hope for happiness in this world or salvation in the next depends on the family's cooperating in intense common ventures such as prayer, repeated stressful challenges, never admitting to sorrows or by thinking of doing good for others to such an extent that they deny their own individual needs. Families whose religious principles conflict with medical authority create special difficulties for their hospitalized children. For example, if they were to agree to certain medical or surgical treatments, their beliefs would be violated. Special difficulties are mistrust, fear and withdrawal in the child, along with clinging to the parents. The staff should try to persuade them of the child's best medical interests, though the parents' right to their own beliefs must be respected. When parents become vehement in their rejection of applied science, this may cause staff resentment, which further augments the child's anxiety.

Where there is close rapport with parents and respect for their beliefs, the child may begin to trust the staff. Such a child needs much support to develop a sense of security in the hospital. In chronic illness, parents should be informed of the expectation for future hospitalizations so that whatever consent they give for treatment can be subsequently applied. This obviates the necessity for repetitive discussion. When parents continue to refuse medical intervention, consultation with a medical–legal expert is helpful to determine the child's rights to adequate treatment. Court action may be involved because these parents cannot compromise their beliefs but will surrender to overwhelming secular authority. Outside resources should be used, such as the clergy of their denomination. Every attempt should be made to avoid recourse to litigation.

> Marion had visited with her divorced father for many weekends and vacations. When he died, 16-year-old Marion was told, and agreed to, a dictum that for the guests at the funeral she would not cry and that she would make certain that everyone who had come to the home be made comfortable. The ideal to be attained was stiff-upper-lip suffering and self-sacrifice. It was not a surprise that when she

needed to undergo chemotherapy that led to loss of her hair, Marion claimed not to mind so long as her visitors thought that the reddish-brown color of her hair was pleasing.

Another type of family belief involved Nick, a nine-year-old child with kidney failure necessitating constant kidney dialysis until a kidney transplant could be found. He said that he was sure that, as one of the hundreds of thousands chosen, if he should die, he would join his grandparents and live the life of the elect in heaven. When Nick's problems affected his medical care by his refusal to assist in cooperating with dialysis, it was necessary to bring in the whole family as a group to discuss for the course of a few weeks how he needed to live in this world for a longer time and move into the next world only after he had had a full life here.

Delia at 15 was recovering from an appendectomy when abdominal swelling was noted. Her family began around-the-clock vigils of chanting and praying. They wouldn't allow a reexploration after having consulted their minister, who told them that surgery had failed and only God would heal. As she became lethargic several days later, they consented to surgery, where their prayers were "answered" by removal of a sponge that had been left inside her.

The family that uses *magical-thinking* to deal with stress may see sickness as an omen of bad things to come, as a signal of God's displeasure or fate. Fundamentally suspicious of the majority culture, this family's thinking heightens the child's fear (especially of death) in the hospital and increases his mistrust of outsiders, as represented by medical and nursing staff. The child craves emblems and objects to protect him from further damage. His mother's scarf or his father's keys can give him much comfort. The infrequency of abstract thinking may be noticed. The child may pray to certain secret protectors for safety. The staff needs to be particularly careful that these families do not hear snippets of frightening medical talk.

Parents in these families are often docile and childlike. They ask for detailed instructions, which are followed reverentially. Whatever is said must be clear. These parents do best when they can call on the doctor to answer questions. Conditional statements such as "if the fever goes up two degrees, give more aspirin" only tend to confuse the parents.

> One such family told their also-literal-minded 19-year-old diabetic that if he felt shaky at college he should go to the student health center immediately. Martin did just that, and once inside the door asked a floor-washing custodian for directions to a doctor. He was sent several miles away to the personal quack of the custodian.

The staff needs to be vigilant, since a too literal interpretation of directions may be counterproductive. Also, when speaking with the child, simple direct language that avoids complex abstractions is best. One or two professionals should communicate all information to the family, as even slight vocabulary differences between professionals will seem to represent hidden dangers against which they have to guard.

The staff should be pleased when they hear that they are included in daily prayers. This shows that the staff is thought of as friends; on the other hand, this may indicate that the family believes the staff needs "outside" help.

Many families that come to the office of the mental health team are groupable under the title *panpathological*. When the overall function of the family is generally poorly defined and unintegrated, with ambiguous communication patterns so that the individuals in these families have either underdeveloped roles or are chaotic, fluctuating, and not integrated, or they are integrated but pathologically organized, these families are identified as panpathological.

Of the panpathological families it is possible to describe unintegrated subgroups. The first is identified as the *emotional* family, which is recognized by its histrionics and observable mood swings. In the hospital, family members mill about the corridors and reception areas, implying to the child that his condition must be serious. The parents themselves, under pressure by grandparents and relatives, are unable to shield their child from the alarming interactions with the extended family. Because the nuclear family has been splintered, an atmosphere of crisis takes over. Gossip goes on, and a worried pall hangs over everyone. Frequently, the occasion is used for mutal closeness and conviviality instead of being used to give support to the child. Bedside and corridor vigils are common, as are efforts to bring in home-cooked meals. Food becomes a major symbol for showing love for the child and hostility toward the staff.

The family's efforts to insulate him can only be interpreted by the child as their distrust of the hospital environment. This severely limits the child's adaptation. It takes firmness and patience for the staff to deal with these well-meaning, though disrupting, people. Reliance on hospital rules helps to set limits. Lengthy explanations of medical procedures or mental health needs of children are usually of no avail. Visiting hours for the extended family need to be curbed. The parents need much support toward keeping the nuclear family functioning as a unit despite the rest of their extended family. To this end, a good relationship with a staff person is crucial to this nuclear family. Often contact with these parents reveals that they both revere and fear one particular family figure who is directing the others and that they are usually grateful for any assistance in managing this individual.

Progress with this family is shown by a greater sense of calm, less frenetic handling of the child by relatives, a diminishing number of visitors and a certain relaxation in the child.

Another subgroup is the pathologically integrated family, an example of which is the *deceptive family*. This family makes untrue statements to the child regarding his illness. Commonly, information about the hospitalization is withheld; such important events as the timing of the trip to the hospital, the length of stay, and what will be done medically are either not given to the child or are lied about. Treatment is usually presented as if it were an amusement park experience. These attitudes affect the child and his family relationships severely. There may develop feelings of unease, confusion and betrayal, along with loss of the ability to trust any adults. Parents' reactions are complex. They think that concealing facts will diminish the pain for the child and may also seek to spare themselves awareness of the truth. These parents often make impossible promises as to the outcome of treatment while failing to discuss with the child what he expects from this trip to the hospital: to the child hospitalization might mean changing size, or acquiring the ability to hit home runs or being able to see better. The disappointments based on distorted knowledge subsequent to surgery occur just at the time the child needs security the most—during the painful early convalescence.

These deceptive family patterns can be inadvertently supported when the staff purposely avoids intervening in the dynamics, knowing how unpleasant the encounter may be. Emboldened by the staff's silence, the family may try to enlist the staff in tricking the child. At times these families even deceive themselves.

Another family constellation subgroup is one that could be called the *punitive-depriving* one. Threatened or actual physical abuse is a favored method of discipline. Children are made to tow the line and to submit. The mother's fear of spoiling the child is seen by her reluctance to hold and comfort him. The father is either hostile or withdrawn, and often uses alcohol. These children do nothing right except keep out of the way of grown-ups. Parents see the staff as indulgent and permissive and anticipate discipline problems when the child returns home. They are jealous that, while in the hospital, the child will become attached to a caring person who is kind and generous.

Sickness, to these parents, implies some new calamity, which they meet with anger. The child is accustomed to the idea that illness is caused by personal actions and is a punishment for badness. Because he is so overcontrolled and harassed by rules at home, the child becomes confused and filled with anxiety when he goes into the different and less structured situation of the hospital. The child, convinced that he is being punished, does not understand leniency and expects a surprise attack at any time. This dynamic was well described by Shengold.

Before a plan is made to help these families, the dynamics of their behavior should be made known to the staff. The parents are doing to their children what their parents did to them. The mothers, accustomed to hardship, are long-suffering and have low self-esteem. They were taught to expect a bleak existence. The fathers were infantilized and overcontrolled by mothers who were angry at men and uncomfortable with the manly assertiveness in their sons. Because they were not cherished and accepted as children, these men and women cannot offer tender forms of love to their offspring.

There are helpful and effective ways to assist these families while they are in the hospital setting.

On arrival, these children require clear, simple information as to what is expected, and consistent assignment to one staff person. This health care professional should offer a low-key verbal relationship because these children suspect adults who are overly warm. The mother needs to be indulged and respected; she might then allow similar kindness to be offered to her child. The staff needs to ask the mother what she does for pleasure and to encourage her to have a more fulfilled life. This will make her less jealous and less resentful when her child is treated as an individual. Improvement in both mother and child is signaled by increasing expressivity, joking, rebelliousness and candor. The main peril of carrying out the hospital plan can be initial staff hostility, which frequently develops when the rejecting and dehumanizing behavior of these parents is first observed. The staff, in their efforts to rescue these waiflike children, may be rude and judgmental, unnecessarily insulting the parents, who need more pity than punishment.

The final subgroup of the panpathological family is often found in the *culture of poverty* family, characterized by a fatalistic, present-oriented, authoritarian outlook. Male and female roles are rigidly defined. One finds a distrust of outsiders whose behavior is considered unpredictable and is judged on its immediate impact. Low self-esteem leads these families to have little belief in their own capacities.[17, 18] Generally, there is limited verbal communication, a passive attitude toward mastering new experiences, and ignorance of body physiology. The mother is chief caretaker, with the father often absent. When present, he can be harsh in his interactions within the family. Both parents usually have volatile tempers.

High marital conflict and frequent family breakdown are present, along with a low educational level and alienation among family members. There is a defeatist attitude toward the future. Generally, families of a lower social class have the mode of child rearing of overpowering the small person, who can either submit, rebel or withdraw. Without clear-cut authority, these people become anxious and defensively hostile. (See chart, page 146.) They are not accustomed to a democratic, inclusive form of treatment.

Children in this environment behave impulsively without regard for the deeper responsibility of their actions. They often project blame onto others rather than seeing what role they themselves play in the situation; thus a main objective for them is to keep from getting caught. When these children annoy their parents, they suffer ridicule and capriciously harsh discipline. Their parents rely on physical rather than verbal control of behavior and alternatively

(*Text continues on p. 148.*)

CHILD-REARING AND FAMILY LIFE PATTERNS REPORTED TO BE MORE CHARACTERISTIC OF FAMILIES OF CHILDREN WHO ARE EMOTIONALLY HEALTHY COMPARED WITH RELEVANT PATTERNS REPORTED TO BE MORE CHARACTERISTIC OF VERY POOR FAMILIES

EMOTIONALLY HEALTHY CHILDREN	POVERTY LIFE STYLES
1. Respect for child as individual whose behavior is caused by a multiple of factors. Acceptance of own role in events that occur.	1. Misbehavior regarded as such in terms of concrete pragmatic outcomes; reasons for behavior not considered. Projection of blame on others.
2. Commitment to slow development of child from infancy to maturity; stresses and pressures of each stage accepted by parent because of perceived worth of ultimate goal of raising "happy," successful son or daughter.	2. Lack of goal commitment and of belief in long-range success; a main object for parent and child is to "keep out of trouble"; orientation toward fatalism, impulse gratification, and sense of alienation.
3. Relative sense of competence in handling child's behavior.	3. Sense of powerlessness in handling children's behavior, as well as in other areas.
4. Discipline chiefly verbal, mild, reasonable, consistent, based on needs of child and family and of society; more emphasis on rewarding good behavior than on punishing bad behavior.	4. Discipline harsh, inconsistent, physical, makes use of ridicule; punishment based on whether child's behavior does or does not annoy parent.
5. Open, free, verbal communication between parent and child; control largely verbal.	5. Limited verbal communication; control largely physical.

6. Democratic rather than autocratic or laissez-faire methods of rearing, with both parents in egalitarian but not necessarily interchangeable roles. Companionship between parents and children.

7. Parents view selves as generally competent adults and are generally satisfied with themselves and their situation.

8. Intimate, expressive, warm relationship between parent and child, allowing for gradually increasing independence. Sense of continuing parental responsibility.

9. Free verbal communication about sex, acceptance of child's sex needs, channeling of sex drive through "healthy" psychological defenses, acceptance of slow growth toward impulse control and sex satisfaction in marriage; sex education by both father and mother.

10. Acceptance of child's drive for aggression but channeling it into socially approved outlets.

11. In favor of new experiences; flexible.

12. Happiness of parental marriage.

6. Authoritarian rearing methods; mother chief child-care agent; father, when in home, mainly punitive figure. Little support and acceptance of child as an individual.

7. Low parental self-esteem, sense of defeat.

8. Large families; more impulsive, narcissistic parent behavior. Orientation to "excitement." Abrupt, early yielding of independence.

9. Repressive, punitive attitude about sex, sex questioning, and experimentation. Sex viewed as exploitative relationship.

10. Alternating encouragement and restriction of aggression, primarily related to consequences of aggression for parents.

11. Distrust of new experiences. Constricted life, rigidity.

12. High rates of marital conflict and family breakdown.

Chilman, C. S.: Growing Up Poor. Washington, D.C., U.S. Department of Health, Education, and Welfare, 1966.

encourage and discourage assertiveness in their children. Because of previous disappointments and identification with role models who avoid the unexpected, these children are reluctant to encounter new experiences. Instead, they become anxious and aggressive when confronted by the novel. In fact, the continuous exposure to violent changes in atmosphere prevents an adaptive tolerance for anxiety. Turbulence can be integrated only in small doses. Consequently, these children panic easily, as is shown by their hyperactivity.

The staff needs to understand that their (usually) middle-class values are inappropriate in the management of these families. Wherever hospital personnel are verbal, future-oriented, and permissive, these children will rapidly become unruly and disruptive. Conversely, to use an authoritarian power-oriented approach only perpetuates their maladaptive style.

The professional who at the outset is able to be sensibly authoritarian is usually the one best able to instruct these families as well as to allay their fears. Lengthy discussions, talk of possible eventualities and discussion of the genetic implications of illness are not effective for these families. The earliest sign of change in these families may be their increasing verbalization and lessening of pessimism about the future. Early improvement in the child is shown by more purposeful behavior—that is, greater attention span and frustration tolerance.

In time the parents' domination of the children lessens. This lessening of domination can be instigated by the staff in various ways so that the child is seen as an individual whose behavior is motivated by multiple factors. Parents can observe how the staff interact with the child and can be told about the child's unique and praiseworthy characteristics. They can learn other methods of discipline[19] —particularly by observation—the best being to give praise for what is desired behavior and to disregard what is undesirable. The next best method of discipline is through the child's identification with positive parental attitudes and actions.

The *ambitious, overprotective* family indulges the child and makes him feel entitled to the gratification of every whim.[20] The parents, often self-sacrificing, live for the future when the child will bring credit to them. The child, as the standard-bearer of the family, embodies all their hopes for a better, more perfect image of themselves. Though this family appears to be child-centered, as the child is "given everything," it really is achievement oriented. In the hospital, the parents show a confusion of their own needs with those of the child by wanting a quick cure so the child can resume the "horse race" of life. This attitude leads them to frequent checking on the staff to assure themselves that their future investment is safe. There is latent hostility toward the child for being ill and interfering with their plans for his attainments.

The best management of this family is to begin by impressing them with staff competence, and letting them know that everyone is equally anxious and desirous of a quick cure. Praise should be given for how well the family has coped with the illness. Limits then need to be set for the parents and their frequently overindulged children; their anxiety will not abate until they understand the necessity of hospital regulations and realize the trustworthiness of the staff.

Careful explanations about diagnostic and therapeutic procedures are helpful, provided parents listen and do not use the knowledge to compete with professionals in the treatment of their child. Compliments for the staff signal a change in attitude and a lower anxiety. However, the staff must be cautious and not accept compliments; instead, they should turn them around and tell the parents, "You're so gracious; but really, you've had the hardest part of the job—the longest and most taxing." To accept a compliment without returning the courtesy can mislead, because parents may be merely polite, really hoping for the staff to recognize their efforts.

Children from these families are often openly aggressive and demanding and see themselves as the equals of adults. The parents' behavior toward the staff only reinforces the child's negative, petulant, testy attitudes. Eventually, there is a confrontation in which someone from the staff tells the child that in the hospital he must live by the regulations, though once at home, he can return to his usual bossiness. Amazingly, this is usually sufficient to curb the more obnoxious actions. If the child persists in his selfishness, variations of the GOLDEN RULE can be tried—"If you treat people this way, they will do the same to you"; or, "How can you expect consideration and warmth when you don't give them?" In addition, when these children show the least change toward being more pleasant, this improvement should be quickly, though casually, acknowledged.

A special category needs consideration: *accident- and abuse-*

prone families. They often cope with stress and lack of interpersonal support by use of frequent hospital emergency visits. Illness and neglect occur more often and with greater severity. Whether an injury is accidental or abusive may be an academic distinction in the emergency room, at the acute phase. Later on, the determination of causes requires that health practitioners learn how to define an injury.[21, 22]

These families show a disturbance in the marital relationship that undoes family cohesiveness, an attitude that the parents have a tenuous ability to effectively discipline the child, that there are meager support arrangements outside the family, that illness, accident, body injury have "created" a way for the family to organize and to establish a meaningful contact with each other and with helpful outsiders.[23]

The most concealed, controversial and chronic form of child abuse is sexual abuse. Mothers usually give a story of sexual abuse in their own childhoods. Incest correlates with later drug dependency, prostitution and feminine sexual incapacity.[24, 25, 26]

The *best-adapted* family is one that uses mild, firm, consistent discipline, is rational, evidence oriented and objective. It looks to future goals, is self-confident, trustful and enjoys new experience. Democratic and egalitarian, this family uses extensive verbal communication, valuing complexity and abstractions. Human behavior is seen as developmental in nature and having many causes.[27] There is high self-esteem, a belief in one's own coping capacity and an active attitude. Each child is seen as separate and unique and is given consistent support and gradual training for independence.

The marriage is harmonious, with both parents having achieved occupational and educational success. There is an intimate, expressive, warm relationship between parent and child; sexual and aggressive drives are accepted and channeled toward approved outlets and impulse control. Where there is a single-parent family, the caretaker (usually) is able to provide a supportive, nurturing atmosphere with frequent availability of significant others.

The hospitalized child from this family will not be immune to fears or regressive behaviors but, after the age of four, will be well able to adapt to stresses, provided that there are adequate mother substitutes and a secure, warm environment.

These children are inquisitive and imaginative. Conversations adequate for their age, play and instruction will fortify them for what is to be done to their bodies. The hospitalization becomes a challenge to be met and conquered, thus adding to their sense of competence and confidence.

What often distinguishes these families is their ability to preserve the usual relationship despite the separation and anxiety caused by illness. In fact, the relationship may gain added depth for their having experienced together a serious health crisis.

THE FAMILY DIAGNOSTIC INTERVIEW

Although family diagnosis is usually the prerogative of the psychiatrist and social worker, other pediatric professionals who practice in areas where these resource people are not available may find the techniques of the family diagnostic interview worthwhile.[28] Indeed, when extensive facilities are lacking or special consultants unavailable, anyone working with children will find this skill a necessity.

Much of the original work for family diagnosis was done with very disturbed patients and their families. Familiarity with its techniques and dynamics can benefit all professionals.[29, 30] These findings indicated the presence of severe disturbances in communication: the double bind and pseudomutual modes* of interaction leading to perplexity. These were found particularly in families having a schizophrenic patient. However, these pathologic patterns can exist to a lesser degree in any family. Abnormal communication patterns may exist in any of the previously mentioned family types.

To conduct a productive family diagnosis, all members of the family group need to be present. This would include nonrelatives if they play a significant role, or would exclude close relations if they are uninvolved. Family therapy is indicated in many instances.

A family diagnostic interview offers many possibilities.[31] The

---

*Pseudomutuality is the type of communication in a family where expression of conflict is not permitted and children are not differentiated from the parents and each other.
Double bind is a type of communication from an important person in the form of two messages, one denying the other. The child is forced to respond to a contradiction or incongruity.
Perplexity is the mental state resulting from being placed in pseudomutual or double-bind situations.

first one is to get an idea of family functioning as it actually is, rather than how the different members of the family report it to be. "One look is worth a thousand words" can save hospital personnel a great deal of speculation and error.

> Nancy, a pretty, dark-haired 12-year-old who came from a distant upstate town, was being prepared for revision of an optic muscle paralysis. She was uncommunicative and held herself apart from the three other girls in her room. The staff program was designed to help her socialize, presuming that she was highly selective in her friendships. After the surgery, though the bandages had been removed from her eyes, she continued to be isolated but polite.
>
> On the occasion of her family's visit, the liaison psychiatrist met with them, and the level of hostility was surprising, considering the previously held expectation that the family would be delighted with the postsurgical result. Nancy's sister criticized her for not keeping up with her schoolwork. Her mother wondered if eye muscles didn't have recurring problems, and her father was annoyed at the hospital costs overriding his insurance coverage.
>
> Nancy could not acknowledge these painful family communications to her favorite nurse. Instead, she reported that the session had been pleasant. Nancy's eyes narrowed when the nurse asked her what she thought of her sister's comment. It took several more meetings for her to confide that she would have preferred the family to share her relief at being out of surgery, but that was as far as she would comment. It was therefore decided that Nancy and the family be recommended for family therapy in their hometown to prevent her further withdrawal from peer relationships and to diminish the family's contribution to her sense of the abrasiveness of all relationships.

Not every family is as clear in their differences as Nancy's. One would want to find out why Nancy has been scapegoated, who she represents symbolically to the parents, whether the role she plays makes it possible for the parents to stay closer together and whether her ability to tolerate hostile messages serves as a release and support for family emotions. The family diagnostic interview could have gone further and delved into how each was communicating hostile thoughts while not permitting Nancy to be an individual. Or the family could have been encouraged to think about what they had in common—namely, how each one had strong emotions evoked by the surgery and how a significant event in one member of the family could trigger diverse emotions. This particular approach would be used to test the potentiality of the family's pulling together.

Additional diagnostic techniques would be used to see:

(1) If family members could support each other's needs and talk freely about themselves (rather than being obliged to show their "concern" for Nancy).

(2) If there was a coalition between the three visiting members on one side and the patient on the other.

Professionals who work with families for long periods describe varying combinations: father–daughter, father–son, mother–daughter, etc., and generational alliances that are used for different and various purposes.

Finally, when sufficient knowledge is obtained from observation and mild exploration, the staff can know whether family patterns are receptive to change and new experience by observing how a family reacts to a few straightforward suggestions. Any recommendations for family therapy should, therefore, include not only the diagnostic assessment of patterns but also the potentiality for improvement. In the case of Nancy, the hostility was considered so great that it could not be brought into the open. It was recommended that the family therapist in their town explore the negative emotions and the willingness of Nancy to offer herself as a sacrifice.

If the family as a group is facing some task that requires coping (for instance, deprivation and loss, birth or addition of a new member, illness and loss of physical powers), this would emerge during a conference. Then certain commonly found family interactional patterns should be noted such as:

the family that expresses intimacy through fighting. One family regularly created scenes in the public areas of the hospital while awaiting emergency treatment for their asthmatic son.

the family that utilizes the occasion of a neutral leader to say things that they are too frightened to say to each other.

the family that scapegoats—for example, one person is assigned a "sick" role.

the family that uses family myths—for instance, one family believed that the father was a tyrant until they saw that he was merely carrying out the orders of the grandmother.

the family that expects individual needs to be gratified without stating those needs openly.

the family that uses "push-pull" patterns, in which one member regularly provokes another to having a certain reaction.

Findings from family conferences reflect their uniqueness. From the diagnostic interview the family interactional pattern becomes clear. These interactions, added to the type of family (described previously as emotional, magical, etc.), the size of family and its development as a unit, will encompass the major part of a child's world. In general, for professionals there is a shift in vision from formerly seeing only the patient to now seeing that child in his usual milieu. One look at the way a child is treated by different family members is worth hours of close interview of the individuals separately.

How a child, given his unique amalgam of personal traits and experience, attempts to influence his surroundings and responds to the reactions he has set in motion is finally receiving the attention it deserves.

Before closing our thinking about families, some general considerations must be mentioned. For the privileged, hospitalization may be an exposure to an awareness that all persons are more similar than not in facing the larger issues of birth, sickness, caring and loss. For the deprived and conflicted, leaving their families can be a tonic, an opportunity to see peers and adults as kindly, helpful and fair; stimulating, yet capable of disciplining; easygoing but organized.

In some instances, returning home can cause something of a "culture shock" unless there is preparation of both patient and family for the coming-home experience. Brothers and sisters of patients often have not been allowed to visit in the hospital and may have grown accustomed to the absence, or have taken defensive postures as a way of not experiencing too much guilt for hidden wishes that the patient stay away or hidden resentment that the patient has taken so much of the parents' time.

Finally, one should be cognizant of the fact that the development of professional staff occurs in settings where intimate contact with other ways of living has a vividness and impact. Intensive academic training may alienate the student and recent graduate from his and her own family, and certainly from families of different origins. In becoming professional, there is frequently a removal from a family setting, not only because of student life but also because the student often surpasses his family's educational achievement. That this can lead the professional to be hypercritical of the family as an organization is a relatively common defense mechanism.

REFERENCES

1. Spiegel, J. P.: Cultural strain, family role patterns and intrapsychic conflict. *In* Howells, J. G.: Theory and Practice of Family Psychiatry. New York, Brunner/Mazel, 1971.
2. Erikson, E. H.: Childhood and Society, 2nd ed., pp. 277–325. New York, W. W. Norton, 1963.
3. Report of the Joint Commission on Mental Health of Children: Crisis in Child Mental Health, pp. 264–65. New York, Harper & Row, 1969.
4. Hollingshead, A., and Redlich, F.: Social Class and Mental Illness, Chapters 4 and 7. New York, Wiley & Sons, 1958.
5. Parke, R., and Collmer, C. W.: Child abuse: an interdisciplinary analysis. *In* Hetherington, E. M. (ed.): Review of Child Development Research, vol. 5. Chicago, University of Chicago Press, 1975.
6. Horowitz, I. L., and Liebowitz, L.: Social deviance and political marginality towards redefinition of the relation between sociology and politics. Social Problems 25:280–96, 1969.
7. National Academy of Sciences: Toward a National Policy for Children and Families. Washington, D.C., Government Printing Office, 1976.
8. Pelton, L. H.: Child abuse and neglect: the myth of classlessness. Amer. J. Orthopsychiat. 48(4):608–17, Oct. 1978.
9. Collins, A., and Pancoast, D.: Natural Helping Networks. Washington, D.C., National Association of Social Workers, 1976.
10. Gabarino, J., and Crouter, A.: Defining the community context for parent–child relations: The correlates of child maltreatment. Child Dev. 49:604–16, 1978.
11. Baughman, E.: Black Americans. New York, Academic Press, 1971.
12. Taylor, R. L.: Psychosocial development among black youth: a reexamination. Amer. J. Orthopsychiat. 46 (1), Jan. 1976,
13. Comer, J. P., and Poussaint, A. F.: Black Child Care: How to Bring up a Healthy Black Child in America. New York, Simon & Schuster, 1975.
14. Dohrenwend, B. and B.: Social Status and Psychological Disorder: A Casual Inquiry. New York, Wiley-Interscience, 1976.

15. Fandetti, D. V., and Gelfand, D. E.: Attitudes towards symptoms and services in the ethnic family and neighborhood. Amer. J. Orthopsychiat. 48 (3), July 1978.

16. Tseng, W. S., Arendorf, A. M., McDermott, J. F., Jr., Hansen, M., and Fukunaga, C. S.: Family diagnosis and classification. J. Amer. Acad. Child Psychiat. 15:15–35, 1976.

17. Reissman, F.: The Culturally Deprived Child, pp. 36–48. New York, Harper & Row, 1962.

18. Chilman, C. S.: Programs for disadvantaged parents, some major trends and related research. *In* Caldwell, B. M., and Ricciuti, H. N. (eds.): Review of Child Development Research, vol. III. Chicago, University of Chicago Press, 1973.

19. Becker, W. C.: Consequences of different kinds of parental discipline. *In* Hoffman, M. L., and Hoffman, L. W. (eds.): Review of Child Development Research, vol. 1. New York, Russell Sage Foundation, 1964.

20. Levy, D. M.: Maternal Overprotection, pp. 161–99. New York, W. W. Norton, 1966.

21. Gregg, G., and Elmer, E.: Infant injuries: accident or abuse? Pediatrics 44 (3): 434–39, 1969.

22. Elmer, E.: Studies of child abuse and infant accidents. *In* National Institute of Mental Health (eds.) Mental Health Program Report 5. Washington, D.C., Government Printing Office, 1971.

23. Plionis, E. M.: Family functioning and childhood accident occur-rence. Amer. J. Orthopsychiat. 47 (2):250–63, April 1977.

24. Giaretto, H.: Humanistic treatment of father-daughter incest. *In* Helfer, R., and Kempe, H. (eds.): Child Abuse and Neglect. Cambridge, Mass., Ballinger, 1976.

25. Summit, R., and Kyrso, J.: Sexual abuse of children: a clinical spectrum. Amer. J. Orthopsychiat. 48 (2):237–57, April 1978.

26. Pittman, F. S.: Incest. *In* Masserman, J. H. (ed.): Current Psychiatric Therapies (17), pp. 129–34, New York, Grune & Stratton, 1977.

27. Ackerman, N. W.: The Psychodynamics of Family Life: Diagnosis and Treatment of Family Relationships, pp. 3–25. New York, Basic Books, 1958.

28. Caplan, G.: An approach to the study of family mental health. *In* Galdston, I. (ed.): The Family, A Focal Point in Health Education. New York, International Universities Press, 1961.

29. Haley, J.: Family therapy. *In* Freedman, A. M., Kaplan, H. I., and Sadock, B. J. (eds.): Comprehensive Textbook of Psychiatry II, pp. 1181–1886. Baltimore, Williams & Wilkins, 1975.

30. McDermott, J. F., Jr.: The undeclared war between child and family therapy. J. Amer. Acad. Child Psychiat. 13:422–36, 1974.

31. Malone, C. A.: Family therapy in child psychiatry training. J. Amer. Acad. Child Psychiat. 13:436–58, 1974.

BIBLIOGRAPHY

Ackerman, N. W.: Treating the Troubled Family. New York, Basic Books, 1966.

Beiser, M.: Psychiatric epidemiology. *In* Nicholi, A. M., Jr. (ed.): The Harvard Guide to Modern Psychiatry. Cambridge, Mass., Harvard University Press, 1978.

Clausen, J. A.: Family structure, socialization and personality. *In* Hoffman, L. W., and Hoffman, M. L. (eds.): Review of Child Development Research, vol. 2. New York, Russell Sage Foundation, 1966.

Goldfarb, W., *et al.*: The concept of maternal perplexity. *In* Anthony, E. J., and Benedek, T. (eds.): Parenthood, Its Psychology and Psychopathology. Boston, Little, Brown, 1970.

Greenblatt, M., *et al.*: Poverty and mental health: implications for training. Psychiat. Res. Rep. Amer. Psychiat. Assn. 21:151, 1967.

Irelan, L. (ed.): Low-Income Life Styles. Washington, D.C., Dept. of Health, Education and Welfare, 1966.

Lidz, T.: The family. *In* The Person, rev. ed. p. 45. New York, Basic Books, 1976.

McDermott, J. F., *et al.*: Social class and mental illness in children: The diagnosis of organicity and mental retardation. J. Amer. Acad. Child Psychiat. 6:309, 1967.

McDonald, N. F., and Adams, P. L.: The psychotherapeutic workability of the poor. J. Amer. Acad. Child Psychiat. 6:663, 1967.

Report of the Joint Commission on Mental Health of Children: Crisis in Child Mental Health: Challenge for the 1970's. Chapter 2, Contemporary American society: its impact on the mental health of children and youth, and Chapter 4, Poverty and mental health. New York, Harper & Row, 1969.

Shengold, L.: Assault on a child's individuality: a kind of soul murder. The Psychoanalytic Quarterly 47 (3), 1978.

Speck, R. V., and Rueveni, U.: Treating the family in time of crisis. *In* Masserman, J. H. (ed.): Current Psychiatric Therapies, vol. 17. New York, Grune & Stratton, 1977.

Watzlawick, P.: A review of the double bind theory. *In* Howells, J. G. (ed.): Theory and Practice of Family Psychiatry. New York, Brunner/Mazel, 1971.

Wynne, L. C., *et al.*: Pseudo-mutuality in the family relations of schizophrenics. *In* Bell, N. W., and Vogel, E. F. (eds.): Modern Introduction to the Family, rev. ed. New York, Free Press, 1960.

5

Play in the Hospital

IMPORTANCE OF PLAY

Although play, along with all its functions, is not fully understood, it is known that it is crucial for the mental health and development of children. Erikson writes that "to play out is the most natural auto-therapeutic measure childhood affords. Whatever other roles play may have in the child's development . . . the child uses it to make up for defeats, sufferings and frustrations."[1]

Play is a natural phenomenon that leads to learning; it is often said that play is the work of the child. It is imaginative, yet is related to reality. Play also fosters and reflects the complexities in the style of emotional development. Through play, the young child expresses his feelings—fantasies, fears and conflicts—in an effort to cope with them, and in so doing he moves toward psychologically more mature behavior.

For many years play has been described as activity that involves reason, imagination and attention on one side and motivated feelings on the other. It is important to put these two together so that, when observing a child playing, one can see the status of his mental development interrelated with his emotional state.

The onset of the capacity to symbolize ends the very young child's egocentric concrete playing. Before the age of one-and-a-half to two years, after something is learned, the child repeats it often for the sheer pleasure of the mastery and the display to himself of his power to work with reality. Once symbolic functioning is developed, thought is representational, and an object, such as a simple piece of string, can mean many things to the child and be used in makebelieve. When this development is achieved, the young child has the ability to use play to reduce unpleasant feelings. At this stage he can also differentiate and integrate himself from other people and things in his environment. When such a child is in the hospital, it is important to remember that these processes are going on at the same time as are the effects of separation and the stress of a new environment.[2]

It is clear, also, that play—in Erikson's terms—creates model situations by experiment and planning. Play deals with emotional release by offering rich and significant channels for expression. It can function as a way of mastering fear and pain by affording the child the opportunity of being the person who gives the pain, thus alleviating the humiliation and helplessness of passively being the receiver. Whereas the young child is incapable of delay, symbolic functioning through play offers a way of delaying gratification.

Fig. 5–1. A child incorporates new experiences and roles into her play. (Photo by Sirgay Sanger)

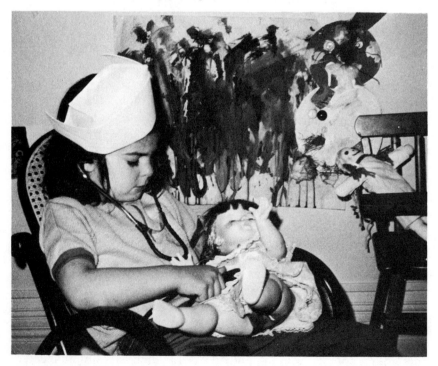

In the years between five and ten the reliance on rules in games and in play helps the child to control spontaneous impulses that might disrupt the atmosphere.³ At the same time, rules preserve the possibility of continued pleasurable social interchanges. After a number of years the reliance on rules for self-restraint and for structuring pleasures becomes internalized, and general codes of behavior including ethics and politeness become natural. It is with the arrival of this age that the greatest difficulty arises in trying to get children to express themselves, for expression implies breaking the rules and coming out with strong feelings that have been studiously controlled, suppressed and forgotten in the recent past.⁴

In the early adolescent years youngsters learn to become introspective about what they have learned and gradually find it easier and even appropriate to talk about deep desires and deep hurts. If one were to trace the history of the peekaboo game from the shallow joyousness of infancy through the skill of the hide-and-seek of childhood into the treasure hunt and sporting world of later childhood and finally to the seeking after and finding a love object, one can become aware of how play has different meanings throughout development.

Every child, healthy or disturbed, is constantly faced with experiences that cause resentments, deprivations and crises. Illness and hospitalization constitute a major stress in early development. They effect a profound change in the child's life-style; he faces separation from his parents and from the security of home routines. He also finds himself at the mercy of a hostile environment—a world of unfamiliar sights, sounds and smells, and of strange people who inflict pain. Tensions increase in this anxiety-provoking atmosphere, especially when facilities for maintaining normal activity are not available. Play restores, in part, normal aspects of living and prevents further disturbance. It also provides the child with the opportunity to reorganize his life; thus, it reduces anxiety and establishes a sense of perspective. When the opportunity for play is not available, destructive and unmanageable behavior is frequently the outcome.

Without suitable communication to enable the child to share his ideas during the actual period of stress, he may find methods that deal with his feelings in a pathological manner. These methods create difficulties in themselves, while the stress may go unrecognized and permanently unresolved.

> Ian was ultimately found to have been preoccupied with the fear that his younger and more charming brother would usurp his toys and family position during his hospital stay. This, unfortunately, he could not articulate. From the moment of his arrival, the staff observed that Ian was a sly, sad eight-year-old who managed to fill his night table with other children's possessions. He was reprimanded for doing so, and he became sadder and withdrawn. The only way he had of telling his problem—acting a caricature of what he feared his brother was doing at home—only brought him more abuse from the environment.

Helping Children Recognize Their Feelings

By reflective techniques, professionals help children recognize their intense feelings expressed in mood, words and play. Because of their 24-hour impact, hospital personnel are in an excellent position to help during a stressful period by not allowing feelings to be suppressed.

> Jerry was praised by the medical staff as a model patient during an exhaustive "workup" for diabetes. When a nurse from his unit arrived in the playroom to pick him up for another procedure, she found him putting the finishing touches on a painting and said to him, "This painting must have a story."
> Jerry: "Yea, but I can't tell it until I leave. It's a story about my floor—four."
> Nurse: "It's a story that can't be told until later?"
> Jerry: "Yea."
> Nurse: "How come? I won't be scared."
> Jerry: "Its about murders. That's all I have to say."
> Nurse: "Murders?"
> Jerry gave no answer. The nurse sat down, looking at the painting.
> Jerry said a moment later, "Yea . . . [in a whisper]

doctors' murders. See here [pointing to a purple figure] this means doctors. They're going to get it. I'll show them."
Nurse: "Some pretty awful things must have happened to make you so angry with them."
Jerry: "Yea, lots. They kept hurting me—poking and pinching—and they won't let me eat, and they keep me here. See this? [pointing to a ceiling light in the painting]. It's not a light. It's really a bomb, and it's going off two days after I leave. See this?" [pointing to a red figure]. This means nurses. They're not so bad. Some of them are pretty nice—except that they give needles."

Although he is suffering in silence, Jerry illustrates a child who feels rage toward powerful adults. Children who do not bother the staff may be overlooked. Social conformity is not necessarily an indication of good adjustment. In Jerry's case, closer scrutiny indicated long-standing difficulties with his mother, which he soon acknowledged by complaining of her unwillingness to care for him during this illness. The family required follow-up by social service on a long-term basis.

Helping Children Cope With a New Perception

Irving could not believe his eyes. He saw two body outlines, male and female, in the treatment room of the miniature hospital. He turned to his mother and said accusingly, "You mean to say you don't have a penis?" It was news to this five-year-old. His mother turned away in disgust, saying, "I don't know anything about these things; ask the nurse." The supportive hospital setting allowed him to pursue this novelty and learn more about this astounding revelation.

Helping Children Who Are Fearful of Abandonment

Cole, age three, delighted in playing with his own small dollhouse. Casual observation of him during morning care showed his preoccupation. He knocked on the front door, saying repeatedly, "Why won't anyone answer?" Finally, a small female figure from within spoke to him, "This is Amy. Don't you know you don't live here any more?" His nurse quickly picked up the toy figure and reopened the drama. "This is Amy again, Cole. I bet I fooled you. Sometimes I like to tease. Mamma says that you'll be coming home again soon and that you'll be well again. Then we can have fun. We all miss you." This timely intervention brought a large smile to Cole's face. He played this interchange over and over.

Helping Children Comprehend Threatening and Mysterious Occurrences in the Hospital

The staff on the unit complimented themselves on their cleverness in keeping the knowledge of Roger's death from all the other children. His body was taken away in the middle of the night. Both the nurses and the doctors reasoned that there was no need to deal with such a delicate problem because no one witnessed the event and no one asked about Roger. They were chagrined to learn that the children undertook to solve the riddle themselves because the adults were obviously deceitful. Several boys between the ages of five and ten had constructed a coffin out of large building blocks and were playing mortician. Each boy carefully took turns lying in the box, arranging his head in a comfortable elevated position, crossing his arms and having a sheet gently placed over him.

Even a young child can playfully reenact a new event and become more comfortable.

Mitzi, 11 months, cried a great deal when a nose culture was taken. After the procedure, her nurse tried to distract her by placing her crib by the window so that she could look out. In this location, the baby was able to reach the supply shelf. She grabbed a handful of applicators and immediately began stuffing them into her doll's nostrils.

Helping Children to Clarify
Distortions Received From Parents

Maury waited for his mother to leave before calling his nurse.

Maury: "Hey, can we do an operation now before my mother gets back? She gets very upset when I operate. You be the nurse, and I'll call you up to tell you what I want. [Pretends to call from the nurses' station of the play hospital.] Hello Ms. K, this is Doctor M. I have a young boy here who needs to have a kidney transplant right away."
Ms. K.: "What is a kidney transplant?"
Maury: "This large green tube like a beanstalk is put into a big hole in the belly."
Ms. K: "That's a new and unusual operation. Sounds like something the gardener uses outside this window. We don't do it on people. Let's talk about the green tube later. Meanwhile, what are the patient's name and age?"
Maury: "Oh, you know. It's Maury. He's five."
Ms. K: "Maury? I know a Maury. There's nothing wrong with his kidneys, Doctor. He had a bladder repair [for exstrophy of the bladder], and he's doing very well now. His boy does not need more surgery."
Maury: "Are you sure? How come his mother said, "The next thing I hear, you'll be needing a kidney transplant?"

Maury had been exposed to his mother's alarming and confusing words. His hospitalization for long periods allowed the staff to form relationships that served to clarify his illness and buffer him against the confusion at home. He went on to inform his mother and siblings of the true nature of his hospitalization, insisting that his mother hear the facts. When she doubted them, he arranged a conference between her and a house officer. Relief of this child's anxiety mobilized him to take productive action to help his mother learn about his health status.

DIAGNOSTIC USE OF PLAY

Play is an important diagnostic instrument. It increases our knowledge of the child's mental life—of his deeper reactions to events. In the hospital setting, play reflects the child's meaning of being away from home and the effects of medical routines and personnel on him. It can highlight areas of misinterpretation that require further intervention for the integration of experiences.

What Can Be Learned From Chance Observation

Following circumcision, Howie, age five, was asked by a recreation worker what kind of operation he was doing on his doll. He replied that he was cutting off the penis so that he could give it a new one.

Four-year-old Lew was serenely stringing beads. Occasionally, he looked about the playroom; then, suddenly, he dashed into an adjoining room in which the play hospital was located. Working against time, he toppled the furniture, threw doctor and nurse dolls into the wastebasket and destroyed the most fragile equipment. Within ten seconds, he returned to his seat and resumed work, quite unaware that he had been observed.

Lucy, age six, was found playing doctor and saying to her doll, "If you don't hold still, I'm going to stick you ten times."

A staff that is alert to the importance of play can make observations such as those of Howie, Lew and Lucy several times a day. These observations may require immediate intervention, but usually they can be postponed until they are discussed at the mental health team conferences.

What Can Be Learned With More Deliberate Attention to the Subtleties of Play

Closer observation of play indicates a child's developmental level (see Chapter 2). Other characteristics the staff will learn to look for are *regression in the presence of frustration* and *reversibility of the regression.* For example, when told he could not leave his bed, Arnold, age five, began to throw his food at the informant. When told what the reason was for being in bed, he became cooperative and curious about the x-ray picture he would be having. Another child may not have stopped so readily. The regressive behavior—food throwing—was short lived. He resumed socially acceptable behavior promptly. Play can reveal many of these regressive and reversible reactions.

However, a reaction that appears ominous in overt behavior may show a more benign perspective in play. For example, nine-year-old Ben was told on Monday he would have a bone marrow biopsy on Wednesday. The procedure was postponed twice. By the end of the week he was overheard whispering to his roommate that the staff were not to be trusted and were trying to keep the children guessing as to their future. In the playroom, he played a cowboy who was very angry at being cheated by the gambler. It emerged that Ben saw the doctor as a person who was untrustworthy. His seemingly pathological suspiciousness disappeared when the delay was discussed.

The following examples illustrate children's views of the many events that occur while they are hospitalized and how first appearances can be deceptive.

Craig, age seven, required elaborate preparation before heart surgery because he also had a blood disorder. The postoperative period was amazingly uneventful except that the child developed an intense fear of having his finger pricked daily for blood work. His reactions were discussed with the lab technician, who was told how to play with the child. She asked him why his friend across the hall was afraid of needles; Craig did not know. The next time blood was drawn, the technician asked John, the friend, to visit at Craig's bedside, where John pretended to use a syringe on a stuffed kangaroo. Seeing this, Craig said to him, "You can't take blood that way. Don't you know he has to have a transfusion after each test? Losing too much blood can kill you!"

Cyrena, age 12, asked her nurse to use the miniature equipment used to prepare her for open-heart surgery. She asked many questions but gave no clue to her preoccupation until the end of the session. The child played beautifully. She had the parents sweetly waving good-bye and a nurse accompanying the tiny patient to the treatment room. She revealed that she had a detailed knowledge of the heart. The nurse was startled when, from the doorway, she saw Cyrena pull a sheet over the doll's head and say, "That's it, she's dead!"

How the Children View the Staff

Because of his lengthy hospitalization, the staff made arrangements for Peter, age nine, to go down to the pediatric lobby in order to visit his younger siblings. Just before one visit, he prepared an album about his hospital experiences so that his brothers and sisters would know what he was experiencing. His favorite drawing showed a patient in the process of a kidney biopsy. He used it as a visual aid to illustrate his story to the family. "Well," he said, "some people think they know it all. I tried to tell the doctor that I couldn't hold still in that position, but she said I was being silly. I said it was cold; she said it was just right. O.K. for her; she was dressed up to her ears in a gown, cap and mask, and there I was, cold and practically naked. She said I wouldn't feel any pain; I said I did. She said she'd get it (the specimen) the first time; I know she didn't. So who the hell would know better?"

The mental health team was alerted by the child's accurate perception of a serious problem in a staff member. This doctor was known for her "no-nonsense" approach to procedures. Efforts were made to show the doctor how the child's use of the words "cold" and "naked" was symbolic of the effect of her perfunctory approach. She did not agree with this criticism and said that she had an excellent rapport with Peter.

Matt, age eight, who had leukemia, was encouraged to paint pictures of his hospital experiences. After a period of isolation (when his resistance to infection was low), he produced a series of paintings that he distributed to members of the pediatric staff. The repetitive theme of the paintings showed a very small boy shackled to a large treatment table. Two doctors stood by, making attacking gestures with syringes and needles larger than the boy's body.

A more vivid demonstration of the way play reveals children's views of the staff was exemplified by large posters. These posters were thinly veiled, hostile manifestations of the children's feelings.

> The older boys on the ward mischievously tacked up signs expressing their feelings regarding treatments and the nursing staff. Kevin, age ten, wrote, "Wanted. Nurse _____ who is unfair to children. Forty dollars reward." Then he drew her likeness in profile and full face.

> Edward, age 12, posted a sign on his door to keep intruders away. It said, "Beware of Mad Dogs. Will get anyone with needles."

This approach is the closest many children get toward expressing their anger and fear; however, it does not go far enough. The staff can take advantage of these clues to channel covert aspects of hostility into workable verbalization.

A useful technique for this is to have relevant staff apologize for painful treatments. An apology can have various reactions. One effect is to encourage brashness with those children who are preoccupied with power struggles in their relationships. The child sees this kind of apology as weakness in the staff; thus, the child thinks he can be rude. The other effect is to offer the child an example of an adult who compromises. If the child is looking for a grown-up with whom to identify, he will suppress further hostility in order to emulate this model. Therefore, if alerted to the reactions, an adult who apologizes can assay whether the patient is early phallic (competitive) or late phallic (concerned with gender identification). (See Chapter 2.)

> Daryl, age five, was recovering from circumcision. He painted a picture and told the story of a bomber that passed over his house and destroyed everything in sight. He said that it took three days for the sun to come out again. On that third day, he had received sympathy and an explanation for his condition.

The circumcision had defeated Daryl's competitive spirit and caused him to feel vanquished. Only after Daryl had checked out the environment did he feel strong enough to reveal his sunshine.

Manny, age eight, was so nasty that he alienated most of the staff with his laughing and provocative actions. After the incision and drainage of a large abscess, he painted a picture of Batman and Robin in a Batmobile, rushing to a cave entrance in order to get away from black raindrops. First, Manny wanted to show this painting to his favorite nurse, but then he decided not to. He said his roommate would understand his picture better and painted another one in its place. This picture was a large flowerpot with several bright flowers and small green raindrops surrounding them. When the nurse asked him for a story, he said, "What's the matter with you? Can't you see? It's a pot with dirt. These are flowers and the rain is making things come up good."

Manny shows the progression from early phallic preoccupation—picturing Batman hiding in a cave to avoid danger—to the boldly visible late phallic exuberance—picturing large, bright flowers in a pot. This mirrored a change in staff attitudes from punitive, repressive control toward more supportive, individualized care. The evidence obtained from the paintings helped the mental health team to continue in the latter direction against strong pressures to be vindictive.

Determining the Basis of a Problem

While Dossie was recovering from surgery for the reimplantation of a ureter, her mother complained that the child was chronically constipated. She asked the pediatrician to investigate the problem during Dossie's hospitalization. Observations made by the nurses indicated that a severe conflict existed between the mother and the three-year-old. As a result, diagnostic medical studies were postponed until more information could be obtained. It was characteristic of this mother to create situations that were frustrating for the child. When visiting her daughter, she spent much time playing with the small babies on the unit. She could not understand Dossie's jealousy and rage because none of this behavior had occurred at home; Dossie had an eight-month-old sibling.

Further observations were made in the play hospital, where Dossie collected several infant dolls from the nursery and deposited them on the operating table, in the toilet bowl and in wastebaskets. As Dossie continued, the nurse remarked that she played with babies a great deal. "Yes," she said. "I like babies—except when they cry or when they are held." This was the natural opening for the nurse to discuss with Dossie her negative feelings toward her sibling, and to encourage her to demand her mother's attention. Within seconds Dossie ran out to the bathroom and had a normal bowel movement. She returned quite relaxed and announced that she wanted to play again. This time she concentrated on doctor dolls and placed several doctors around the bed of a little-girl doll. When she was asked what the doctors were doing, she said, "They're scaring the BM out."

Additional sessions produced similar material followed by trips to the bathroom. Consequently, Dossie no longer needed diagnostic testing. Instead, her mother was referred to a social worker, who arranged counseling to ameliorate her frustration. Dossie increasingly used words to signify her anger; thus, she limited the attack, in the form of constipation, that she had formerly used against her mother. This case illustrates the deep oppositional struggle that can occur between a parent and child (see Chapter 2).

Evaluating the Effectiveness of Preoperative Teaching

Although Abe, age five, received thorough preparation for heart surgery, his play later revealed that his preoccupations were not touched on. He explained to his father who was watching him manipulate his teaching doll, "This kid has three holes in his heart, and he's a dead duck."

Cory, age four, had been carefully prepared for a tonsillectomy. It was clear that he did not retain the information for long. In playing with his teaching doll postoperatively, he kept mentioning, "Don't take off the boy's pants." Hearing this, his nurse remembered that Cory had objected violently to being completely undressed, except for a johnny shirt, prior to surgery. This indicated that additional teaching was required, and that the arbitrary policy of removing all undergarments before any operation only reinforced the child's fantasy of having other parts of the

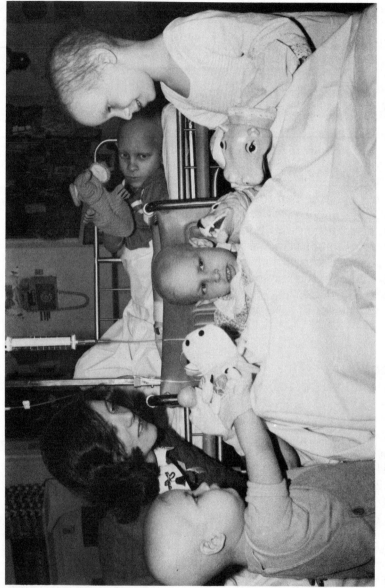

Fig. 5–2. A puppet play group led by a pediatric nurse oncologist discusses what it is like to be in the hospital. Group sessions inform children that others have similar feelings. (Photo by Terry Hanna)

body operated on. The policy was immediately changed
with the cooperation of the operating room staff.

The Usefulness of Play in Groups

"In group play . . . children assign to themselves roles which are
an expression or an extension of their basic problems. In such roles,
one either plays out the awareness of what he is, or a hopeful
phantasy of what he would like to be. . . . In a group such phantasies
are reinforced and find easy and natural means of coming through in
a variety of play forms and activity channels."[5]

The sight of others pretending and freely showing their concerns serves as a stimulus and gives the less playful child permission
to do the same thing. This child finds companionship and some
sympathy in his difficulty; however, he is not allowed to feel sorry
for himself. Group sessions also inform children that others have
similar feelings.

Fig. 5–3.   Group play consists of both imaginary and real stimuli. (From Play
School Association, "Play in the Hospital," Campus Films)

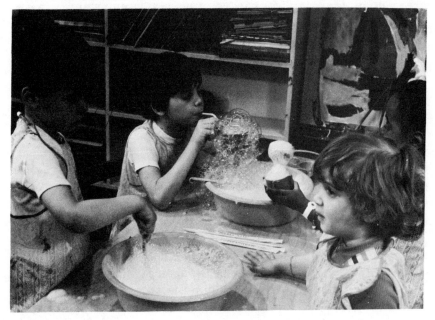

A group often takes up issues that would not be seen in individual play, such as sibling competition for the adult's attention.

If the group is sufficiently cohesive, it establishes values that impose certain restraints on unsociable behavior. Seeing how others cope, especially if they are younger and sicker, is an impressive learning experience. Group interaction may speed the possibility of positive affectionate role playing; on the other hand, it can be frightening to see how some children fail to cope. Any upset could be profitably used by recreation workers and other staff in later conversation and play with an individual child.

Group play consists of both imaginary and real stimuli. The child who can allow only one stimulus or the other is quickly revealed. Staff need to watch the content and style of the child's play. The highly imaginative child may be out of touch with others. The excessively practical child may be dully anchored to concrete events. The well-adjusted child needs and allows both stimuli.

TECHNIQUES OF PLAY

Initially it is important to get clues to a child's more obvious preoccupations. Some knowledge of his real circumstances makes possible individualized play approaches. Chance remarks picked up from the staff are helpful, such as, "After all Josh has been through, his only objection is to the daily finger pricks," or "How odd for Ms. D to go on vacation while her child is hospitalized," or "Every time I pass Maury, he tries to get me to play doctor games with him."

There are general rules that can be applied whenever effective play is to be initiated:

- Reflect only what the child expresses.
- Supply materials that stimulate play.
- Allow enough time without interruption.
- Permit a child to play at his own pace.
- Determine when it is appropriate to go beyond the child's expression.
- Play for the child who cannot play for himself.
- Allow direct play for the emotionally strong child. Be familiar with some artistic material as a medium of expression.
- Use knowledge of child growth and development as a guide to professional clinical judgment.

Reflecting Only What the Child Expresses

It is axiomatic that the creation of a play situation is based on a secure atmosphere. Unfamiliar words and ideas threaten a child, leading to the inhibition of his spontaneity.

While Connie was hospitalized, her mother took the opportunity to go on vacation; however, this was never directly mentioned by the child. Play with cutouts of Orphan Annie and Sandy revealed her true feelings. In one episode, Orphan Annie, after having abandoned Sandy, her canine friend, returned from the North Pole and picked him up at the kennel. Sandy whimpered and scolded her mercilessly. The nurse asked Connie what the dog was saying. Connie insisted that he had hated being left. The nurse sympathized with Sandy by saying that it wasn't pleasant being left behind with no one to play with and being all alone in a little box with only strangers around; he had a right to be angry. However, Connie did not agree, saying, "But he's only a dog."

It was obvious that Connie was not ready to admit her anger; therefore, the nurse did not go beyond the child's expression. The nurse had confidence that eventually Connie would be candid and would admit her anger as she felt more secure in her relationship with the nurse.

Supplying Materials for Play

Any toys and materials that children use are immediately invested with imaginative qualities. These concrete objects then become suitable vehicles for carrying out structured fantasies about the child's most current preoccupations. The clarity of the themes will vary depending on the degree of anxiety generated. Too much anxiety and the child will conceal the problem, try to change the subject or stop playing altogether. These actions are efforts by the child to cope with this anxiety-provoking theme, though the external manifestation appears to be different. The staff should not be misled: a child will remain preoccupied with the main challenge to his safety until it is met in some way.

In his play, Teddy continually wanted objects to fall off, such as the smokestacks on ships and the wings of planes. This obvious castration fear appeared to vanish when he stopped his aeronautical drawings and rushed to the window to exclaim about the missing screens. However, his first observation of missing screens was merely a continuation of the same fear.

The child who is in the grip of a specific conflict will return to it constantly. Nonetheless, he will use many disguises until he finds one that gives him sufficient distance to cope with the danger in order to achieve a happier solution.

For Teddy, the use of toy planes, boats and other transportation toys resulted in monotonous play. Even the windows of the elegant playhouse seemed unproductive of discussion. Only when he asked for another tongue depressor did he become animated—filling in an empty space in a wooden bridge he was building with tongue depressors. It was the closest he could comfortably get to castration anxiety. From this point he was able to gradually approach this anxiety by way of fallen screens, fallen wings and finally fallen "things."

This case shows that the play materials did not fit this boy's needs until he was allowed to choose his own media.

Veronica set up a bed, croupette and a bedside stand. She brought in a medicine dropper and cup on a tray, placing them on the table. As she opened the croupette, she said to the two dolls, "I'm putting you two in bed together. You'll be happier that way. Now I have to put this flap back so I can get to you two with triple measles. Now, now, don't cry, this medicine is good for you. It tastes just like cookies, and you know you only get good cookies in the hospital, not like at home."

This play sequence was made possible by the use of materials attractive and relevant to the child's experiences in the hospital. Real cookies were made available for play. Eventually, the staff realized that the cookies symbolized "starving" for affection at home. On interview with the parents, the social worker confirmed this play diagnosis.

Allowing the Child to Proceed at His Own Pace

A child cannot be rushed into approaching frightening ideas and changes in body functions.

> Five-year-old Millie completely rejected preoperative teaching for an ileo-conduit. She pulled off the play equipment—IV, drainage bags, and dressings—from the teaching doll and appeared to ignore any mention of impending surgery. Postoperatively, she was withdrawn, refused to look at the operative site and denied that she knew what had happened to her. An indirect approach was used with her because direct teaching upset her greatly. A box of equipment—tubes, small bottles, dressings, and pediatric urine collectors (PUC to represent "Ostomy" bags)—was left at her bedside without comment. On the next day, the nurse observed that the PUC was attached to the doll's head. She made no mention of this. On the following day the PUC moved to the right arm, and on the third day it moved to the chest. On the fourth day, it appeared on the abdomen. Concomitantly, Millie was able to look at the operative site and to talk about the procedure directly.

Going Beyond the Child's Expressions

In selected cases it is permissible to say things in play beyond what the child is expressing superficially. This gives the anxious child a chance to see that someone else can talk about a frightening topic and continue to be friendly. It gives security to find a companion for sharing fears.

> Patsy, age eight, suffered traumatic injury to one eye, followed by a severe infection that led to blindness in that eye. She was encouraged to reenact the treatments she experienced on her patient doll—injections, IVs, warm soaks and changing of dressings—as a way of stimulating discussion about the accident and its consequences. In

playing the part of the doll, her nurse expressed concern for the outcome of treatment—of how her sight would be affected. However, Patsy denied the loss of her vision and told the nurse that she could see through the bandage.

Because of impending surgery, a time limitation made it necessary to accelerate her play, so that she could face what she was trying to avoid. It was important for her nurse to let Patsy know that there was no sight through the bandage and that the staff was concerned about her vision. She needed to realize that the doctors could not promise a good treatment result, though they hoped for the best in treating the infection.

On the day before surgery, the idea of enucleation had to be broached with her. The pediatrician and mental health nurse first discussed this with the mother, who asked the staff to tell Patsy about the enucleation. These parents were thought to use deception when under stress; therefore, the doctor and nurse who knew Patsy best decided on a joint approach.

The doctor was to take the strong position about the reality; the nurse was to offer comfort and solace. Both doctor and nurse respected this youngster's dignity and bravery in the face of a mutilating experience.

Nurse: "You've probably been thinking a lot about the conversations we've had all week, and you might have some worries about what we've said."
Patsy nods her head.
Nurse: "What do you do when unpleasant thoughts come to your head?"
Patsy: "I put them under the pillow."
Nurse: "And they don't go away, do they?"
Patsy nods.
Nurse: "That's why we have to talk about them. Sometimes they're easier to take when you share them with someone else. Do you have an idea why the doctor is with me today?"
Patsy shakes her head as if she knows but doesn't want to hear.
Doctor: "Patsy, we've done everything possible to clear up the infection, but we couldn't do enough. You know we've been worried about your eye, and we have just come to the conclusion that there is nothing more we can do to make it better and to save the sight in your eye."

Nurse [observing tears in Patsy's eye]: "It makes you feel like crying, doesn't it?"
Patsy begins to cry.
Nurse: "You've got a lot to cry about. It's okay to cry." The nurse stayed with Patsy until her mother arrived to offer comfort.

Playing for a Child Who Cannot Play for Himself

Liam, age two-and-a-half, was extensively burned over his entire body; as a result, he was completely immobilized. All he had for coping with the problem was an extraordinary capacity for speech and an inquisitive mind.

The staff in the Intensive Care Unit requested the help of the nursing mental health consultant for the emotional aspects of his care. Liam was calling himself a bad boy and refusing to talk about the accident.

Play with this child was a challenge, complicated by the facts that he was unable to participate directly and that those playing with him had to use aseptic techniques such as wearing cap, gown, mask and gloves. Initially, stories were used as a way of establishing rapport. It was hoped that later he might be able to explore the theme of blame and guilt.

A modified version of the three bears in which the facts of Liam's own hospitalization were inserted served the purpose: Goldilocks, a very curious child, investigated the bears' home, trying out everything, including Baby Bear's own chair. Because she was too large for it, she broke the chair, but fixed it so it did not look broken. On Baby Bear's return, he sat on his favorite chair, fell and hurt himself very badly. He did not know that it was broken; it was not his fault. Mama and Papa Bear rushed him to the hospital in Police Chief Bear's private car so that the doctors and nurses could care for him.

Once Baby Bear got to the hospital, he needed to have the bumps and sores on his body cleaned. He also needed medicines and bandages to make him feel better, and he needed extra food and medicines through a little tube in his arm. (This was shown to a little teddy bear because he was curious and wanted to know what was going on.)

As this story was told, treatment was demonstrated and explained to Liam on a doll, with play equipment sterilized for this occasion. Because he could not use his body except for his eyes and mouth, he watched while the figure was animated for him.

The bear story continued: Once Baby Bear was treated at the hospital, a doctor asked him how he had gotten hurt. Baby Bear said that he was a bad bear, but of course that was not true. If he had known that the chair was broken, he would not have sat in it; and if Mama and Papa Bear knew that he was in danger, they would have come to help him. The accident was not their fault either.

After listening to the story attentively, Liam asked, "How did I get on the stove?"

The question was turned back to him, "I don't know. How did you get up there?"

He was then willing to tell, "I climbed up there and got burned." He was assured that it was not his fault; he did not know that the stove was hot. He just wanted to find out what it was all about because he was a curious boy—and usually curiosity is a safe thing to follow. Liam smiled and asked to have his Snoopy dog brought near. This request indicated that he was once more interested in his transitional object as he had been before the accident.

On one occasion Liam said that his father looked like a baker in his isolation gown and cap. He was asked what bakers did, and he responded that they made cookies. Liam was told that he too could make cookies in the playroom when he was better. He declined, saying, "I can't because I got burned." He was told that there were safe ways to make cookies without getting burned again.

There are a number of children who because of their illness or physical defects cannot use their bodies in play. For these children the staff must assume the didactic process and initiate the play activity. In this way, the child will select with his eyes or with words what issues he is grappling with. In Liam's case his intense curiosity was used to reexperience his accident and to support and recommence his developmental growth. He became quite happy and in touch with his family and visitors despite his immobility.

Even though he died several weeks later, the staff and family felt that all these efforts were worthwhile because Liam was his usual delightful self, right to the end.

Playing With an Emotionally Strong Child

Some children can tolerate thematic expression that is quite close to a painful reality.

> Several boys wearing leg bags for urinary drainage were gathered around the water trough. Will picked up a large syringe and accidentally discovered that it had three streams of water. He was delighted, and he showed the syringe to the other boys repeatedly. Will, hospitalized for repair of hypospadias, had that number of streams when he voided. In this case, no complex intervention in play was required. Instead, the large syringe was given to Will for the next few days. He tried a variety of colored liquids in his experiments. When the doctors came to his bed on rounds, he played a practical joke by suddenly showing his sprayer syringe in all its glory.

> Hanna stood before the mirror in the playroom and put on a long dress and floppy hat. She then packed a suitcase and took Eileen, a younger child, with her. Both girls sat on a bench in front of the elevator. Hanna explained that she was waiting for a bus to take her and the little girl home. A recreation worker talked to Hanna about her reasonable wish to go home. It was a great relief for her to hear from an adult that home was a place everyone wanted to be.

Using Art Materials

Art materials are particularly suitable for expressing internal emotions and thoughts. The child must be free to work on his own without direction from adults and without comment on the artistic merit of the production. Each child uses supplies in his own way. Adults need to be completely nonjudgmental and to discard preconceived notions on the nature of art. Painting should be treated as

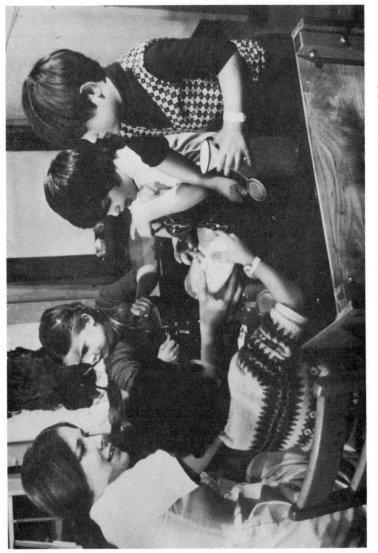

Fig. 5–4. Group water play for fun and relaxation, using simple materials. (Photo by Steve Campus)

symbolic of child's thoughts, not as an entity in itself. Asking simple questions of the child after the work is completed draws out the story to an even fuller extent. With older children it is more productive to talk about the theme that the painting illustrates.

Among ten-year-old Beckie's paintings before surgery for revision of a cleft lip repair were scenes in which two trees were at opposite ends of the paper. The significance of these productions became clear when she resumed her artwork postoperatively. In her first drawing she united the branch of one tree with the other, linking them with an arc similar to the instrument used on her lip to prevent tension on the suture line.

Before surgery, Pearl, age eight, painted a picture of Egypt with pyramids and palms. She explained that she was studying this in school. On the day after surgery for cleft lip repair, she painted a mess of blacks and reds. Two days later she began to reorganize and started again on Egyptian themes. Thus, as long as she could think of the possibility of a complete repair of the anomaly, she thought of Egypt, which symbolized to her a beautiful place. The horrible blacks and reds without definition represented her view of the inside of her mouth.

At a mental health team conference, Pearl's paintings were discussed and psychotherapy was recommended. It appeared as if she would never be satisfied with the surgical result; she had to learn that even with an excellent repair, she would not obtain the exotic, perfect atmosphere of the Egypt that was pictured in her mind. In addition, an effort would have to be made to reconcile the digust she felt (the mess of black and red) toward the preoperative oral cavity.

Lil, age 11, previously had had numerous surgical procedures for a congenital deformity of the leg. On her second postoperative day, she drew a picture of a leg in a cast and a hand with a wedding band close to it. She asked the child life worker, after handing her the picture, "Are you married, Ms. W?"

Ms. W pointed to the picture and said, "Here's someone who is married. Could you tell me about her?"

Lil said the figure in the drawing had found somebody

nice and cute and had married him. She said, "Do you think I'll get married? My cousin didn't get married because her boyfriend had very little hair."

Ms. W asked, "Do you think your leg would make someone change his mind about marrying you?" Lil was thoughtful, but did not reply, so Ms. went on, "I don't know what happened with your cousin, but usually people get married because they have deep feelings for one another, not because of the kind of hair or shape of the leg." (Lil's development showed that at age 11 she had an adolescent's concern about heterosexual possibilities.

It took more than a week to convey this message. After a while her drawings were of entire figures rather than isolated parts of the body.

How to Play When There Are No Clues About a Child's Preoperative Concerns

When little is known about a child's inner anxieties, effective play should be related to the chronological level of the child. Before age five, the concerns commonly held by children are abandonment, pain and mutilation, invasion of body orifices and loss of control over their usual routines. Stories about these themes could be about people who shut their eyes, children who cover their ears, children who are left at doorsteps or things that are missing or change their appearance.

Themes of mastery start early and continue throughout childhood—for example, pleasure in newness of function and knowledge. These can be expressed in stories about exploring big houses and the hospital, meeting strangers who turn out to be nice, jumping into water and finding it good, and trying new foods and finding them delicious.

For five- to ten-year-olds, play can be initiated with the following themes: making things that last, acquiring a skill better than that of others, pleasing adults other than parents, being ashamed or losing face, carrying out the usual patterns of living with friends, sports, hobbies and role model activities in the hospital. Other themes might occur in stories that tell of triumph over danger.

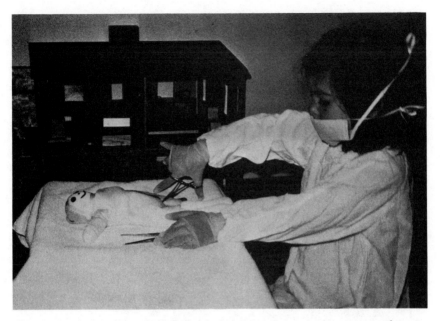

Fig. 5–5.   Each child used supplies in her own way to reenact events that are stressful and to cope with feelings. (photo by Sirgay Sanger)

The 11- to 16-year-olds usually dread returning to a dependent position with illness, regard their peer group as the final word on social success and worry about their occupational choice.

Some commercially available books present, in an attractive way, one or two developmental tasks. These are depicted by characters or animals with whom the child can identify—neither too close nor too distant from the challenge the child faces. The chief protagonist is sufficiently recognizable to capture the imagination.

The Appendix contains examples of numerous books that can be used to help children cope with hospitalization and feelings. They have held up clinically for hundreds of readings.

MASTERY THROUGH PLAY

In the process of growth and development, early egocentricity alters continuously in the direction of sociability. Concomitantly, there is a diminution of magical ideas of self-importance as arduously gained skills become the basis for a sense of real importance. For many children, this process is an injury to the self-esteem because they are reminded of their small size, awkwardness and needs for help in growing up. For them, hospitalization will reinforce a sense of impotence and helplessness.

These feelings may be expressed and at times surmounted by playing out stories of powerful and lowly characters. Bible stories such as the story of Samson and some of Aesop's fables contain many passive to active plots. The child will attempt to master situations in which he is a helpless victim by turning passive experiences into active ones.[6] This kind of play should be encouraged.

It is important to ensure the survival of puppets, dolls or animals that the child treats cruelly or murderously because in power reversal the player may go too far. Children feel secure when they are stopped from excessive destruction of equipment; however, when they are engaged in violent nondestructive acts, the play should be

Fig. 5-6.   When play becomes highly aggressive, but nondestructive, it should
be allowed to take its course. At the same time, a child can be
helped to put feelings into words so that he moves gradually toward
verbalizing rather than acting out aggression. (From Staff
Development Filmstrip Series: "Needle Play," Campus Films)

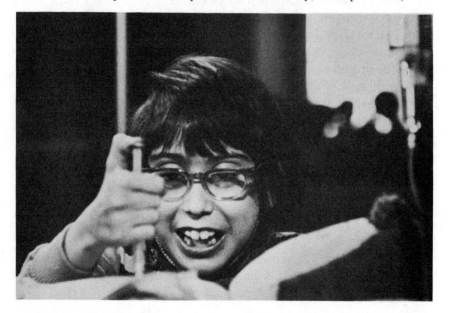

allowed to continue, and words should be used as a moderating force. This action is permissible, as children learn in this way to gradually modulate aggression by verbal expression instead of by physical expression. Furthermore, only a severely disturbed child would fail to differentiate the animate from the inanimate and would use the violent play against people.

Several boys were playing after transfusion clinic. Together they started to put several IV's into a large toy bear's body. Before long they were violently attacking the bear, urging each other on.

Grant underwent a kidney transplant at age seven. His hospitalization was particularly long and complicated. Of all the procedures he required, injections were the hardest for him to bear. There was much play with needles as a way of dealing with the difficulty. This soon led to his building the "Grant Animal Clinic." Each stuffed animal he acquired—snake, tiger, skunk and dog—became the new patient whose ailments required extensive treatment with injections. Doctor Grant possessed amazing powers to cure, and before long he had an extensive practice requiring the services of a nurse, whom he ordered about. "Make an appointment for him in three months; that treatment really did the job." His nurse, in turn, complimented him on being able to save even the sickest victims.

Dan, age five, and others were playing doctors' rounds. They surrounded a nurse in the playroom and proceeded to examine her with stethoscopes and tongue depressors. David, age seven, said, "I think this patient has to stay in bed for ten days and we'll give her more medicine."
Everyone agreed except Dan. He said, "Three days. I'm chief here and what I say goes. I've been on rounds before."

Elsie frequently placed her dolls on a stretcher and practiced taking them back and forth from her room to the corridor leading to the operating room. For this five-year-old, going to the operating room was a familiar trip because she required repeated skin grafting. On one occasion just prior to surgery, she asked her nurse to take her and the dolls for a ride on the stretcher in the same area. She appeared to gain strength from the practice sessions by building up a tolerance for the anxiety the operations provoked.

Edward, age eight, was distressed to learn about heart surgery and to see the miniature teaching equipment. "I don't know how I am going to stand it," he said. And then, as and afterthought, "I know what I'll do. I'll ask my father to make toys like this for me."

ORGANIZED PLAY PROGRAMS

Recreation Staff and Therapeutic Play

Therapeutic play programs[7, 8, 9] are an achievement of full-time professional child life or recreational workers. Extensive education in child development as well as clinical experience with both well and sick children are the basic qualifications. Judgments need to be made continuously on children's coping ability under stress. Such professionals require a variety of techniques and skills for evaluating and managing behavioral problems in a hospital setting. Good preparation is essential for perceiving what a child is thinking and feeling and for answering a child's needs as they emerge in play.

Recreational workers perceived by children as having a nonmedical role are readily accepted by children as supportive adults. They facilitate the expression of fears and anxiety and hasten the process of adaptation.

For most children, to sit down with an adult and to talk on a meaningful level about imaginative issues is a unique experience. The closeness that a child feels opens up vistas for warmth and acceptance by a powerful larger person that can only lead to increasing optimism about growing up.

Volunteers and students of all disciplines are valuable assistants to full-time workers in direct proportion to the amount of orientation and supervision they receive. Of special note are foster grandparents. However, their effectiveness is often limited by the lack of constant staff support. This is made difficult by the fact that most of these people are part-time workers. Nevertheless, with their participation, it is often possible to expand a program by supplying extensive support and companionship for children during treatments, prolonged separation from parents, periods of isolation, and serious illness that prevents attendance in the playroom, as well as those with no visitors.

Pediatric patients can deal with the traumas of hospitalization most effectively in a play area designed specifically for this purpose. Neutral, familiar and dissimilar from the general hospital territory with its threatening equipment, the playroom is geared to helping the process of mastery. Here children interact with each other and are given free reign to manipulate the environment to the extent their illnesses permit. Given the opportunity, children will seek solutions to situations that perplex them and find suitable outlets for the fear and anger generated by disruptive experiences.

The interaction of recreation, social work, nursing and medical staffs allows for a continuous exchange of information concerning the full range of the child's 24-hour activities. This contact leads to a continuity of approach and management. Participation of medical personnel in the play program may be reassuring to children because it implies that play is valued and enjoyed by staff, who may not have the time to be regularly present in the play area. The children particularly need to know that physicians and nurses are not always associated with pain.

> Debbie, age 12, observed a nurse surrounded by several children, each carrying out different types of needle play. She looked puzzled and finally asked, "What do you do, do you give needles?"
>
> Nurse: "Sometimes I do, but I'd rather teach children how to do it so they won't be so frightened."'
> Debbie: "Well, then, are you a nurse or are you . . ." (unable to finish question).
> Nurse: "Or what, Debbie?"
> Debbie: "A child helper?"

On the other hand, because the presence of medical personnel in the play area may be very threatening if the children feel that their arrival indicates that a treatment will occur on the premises, this entrance into the territory of the child must be made delicately. Children must be able to regard the playrooms, as well as their bedrooms, as safety zones where they may relax without this fear.

Play Materials

The organized play area should afford optimal conditions for free play. "In general, play activities are chosen that allow for a variety of approaches, that are unstructured, that can be used by a wide age range, by both boys and girls, by many children at the same time. It is also important to choose those which will stimulate and challenge but which do not impose arbitrary demands of completion in a given form."[10]

Pounding boards, play dough made by children, water play, finger paint, and painting are excellent for diversion, entertainment and expression of feelings. In addition, the professional knows how to use these activities to create stories and themes when children choose not to use puppets. Play in which children have available miniature beds, stretchers and wheelchairs stimulates realistic role taking. Blocks, dolls, a dollhouse, and a kitchen corner are ideal for preschoolers. Group play is stimulated by supplying several items of a kind and arranging equipment in clusters. The play staff can encourage play around episodes and fears that are significant. The hospital corner with real and toy equipment (dolls representing all personnel of the pediatric department, patient dolls, nurses' caps, stethoscopes, doctor bag containing syringes, alcohol wipes, bandages, tourniquets, dressings and equipment used in physical examination) is helpful in assisting both preschool and school-age children dramatize the experiences in which they have had little control. The miniature hospital (containing nurses' station, nursery, semi-private and multibed wards, bathroom, x-ray room, treatment and anesthesia rooms) stimulates imaginative play where intense feelings are given expression. The child becomes the manipulator instead of the helpless victim, thus turning passive experiences into action ones—the silent into the divulged in the process of mastery.

Many hospitals do not recognize the importance of sending children confined to beds of any size, stryker frames, wheelchairs, or stretchers to the play area. Even the quite debilitated can join some of the activities as a group member or with a few peers. Just the factor of being present beside a group activity, even when not involved, is reassuring to an incapacitated child. To leave a child behind and exclude him while others go off to play is obviously unfair and unprofessional.

(Text continues on p. 194.)

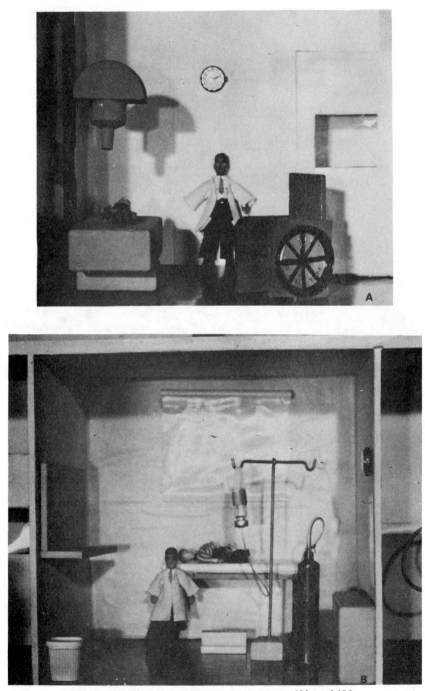

Fig. 5–7. *Illustration continues on pages 192 and 193.*

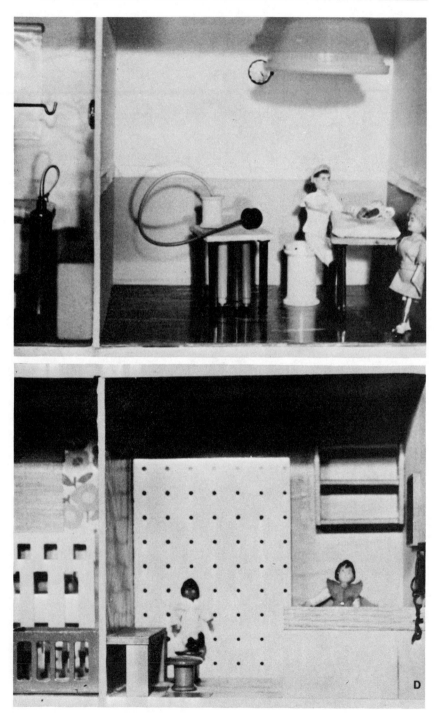

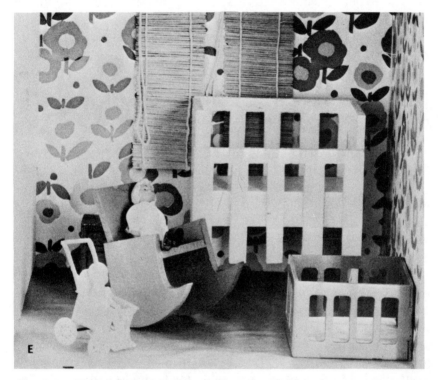

Fig. 5–7. The miniature hospital stimulates imaginative play where intensive feelings are given expression. (A) X-ray room. (B) Treatment room. (C) Anesthesia room. (D) Nurses' station. (E) Baby room.

Social, occupational and educational aspects of play are also planned. Arts, crafts and music are part of the well-equipped playroom and can easily synchronize with the school program.

The best assurance that play needs will be met is through organized recreational programs. In institutions where they are not yet developed, the burden for play activities rests heavily with the nursing staff, who have the greatest responsibility for the management of the child's daily activities. However, this frequently means that play, of necessity, becomes secondary to physical care and is unlikely to achieve the importance it deserves in the care of the hospitalized child.

Handling Feelings of Hostility and Aggression

Major physical hurt and loss of close relationships, both experienced in hospitalization, engender anger and anxiety. This will be shown in a multitude of ways. Especially vulnerable are children who already have disturbed relationships with the mother or significant parent, or those children who have been subject to family conflict. In situations where play is not a regular feature of the child's hospital life, the management of hostility and aggression may be a major problem. Destruction of property, kicking, biting, bullying and uncooperativeness are frequently manifestations. Children are disturbed in direct relationship to their instability prior to hospitalization.

Professionals need to know that not all children act out aggressive feelings, and that resentment emerges under permissive conditions. Where tight controls are maintained, children are not free to reveal themselves. It is more usual for a child to express negative feelings in an atmosphere of security. An appropriate balance between freedom and rules must be striven for.

Before pediatric personnel can deal with children's hostility constructively, its existence must be expected. Feelings are not resolved by denial and avoidance. The learning of nondestructive avenues of expression requires the guidance of understanding adults. Children who are permitted to dramatize and verbalize hostility can try new solutions to formerly unacceptable manifestations and thus achieve greater potential for adaptation.

Under no circumstances should the aggression of children be met with counteraggression from professionals. Firmness in limit-setting is appropriate where a child needs controls, but open hostility from the staff means that they perceive the child as dangerous. It also means that they do not understand normal behavior patterns in children. This reaction in turn creates further misbehavior or withdrawal on the part of the child.

There are as many opportunities to handle aggression on the pediatric units as there are in the play areas. Medical personnel are in strategic positions to take care of problems on the spot—for instance, when Bill does not eat his dinner because his mother failed to show up during visiting hours; when Carol beats her doll after medication is forced on her; when Victor does not speak to his pediatrician because he was not discharged as anticipated.

> Several boys ranging from four to seven years ganged up on the nurse passing medications. As she entered their room, they squirted her with carefully aimed syringes. She was startled at first but managed to maintain her composure. Expecting her to meet their aggression with the same, they began to flee until they realized she did not intend to retaliate. Instead, she surprised them by expressing sympathy for their feelings. "I suppose you're really angry with me for all the needles I've been giving you. I don't blame you." Her statement stimulated a barrage of feeling and opened discussions on why each was receiving intramuscular injections. She helped them to examine their reactions consciously.

The nature of aggression forces it to be recognized one way or another; this is true in family settings as well. However, the development of affection—the ability to love—is rarely, if ever, promoted in any setting. Why this is so may stem from the more threatening quality aggression has for its objects and the power it lends to the aggressor if not checked. Affection and tenderness can easily go unnoticed. The offerer of positive feelings is vulnerable to rejection and therefore is reticent.

As part of a therapeutic play program, evocation of hostility is therefore only half of the work. The staff must become attuned to the whisperings of tenderness, generosity and warmth that the children will make. Role playing, particularly the nurturant aspects of nurs-

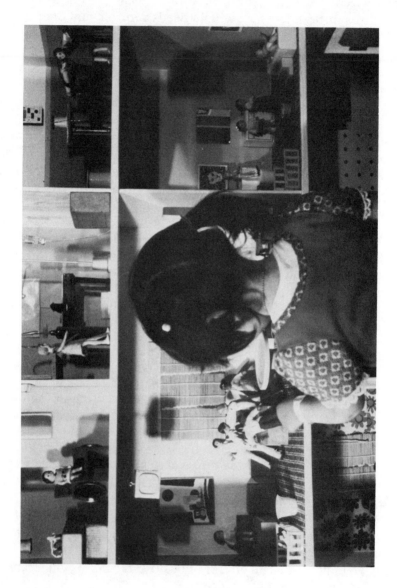

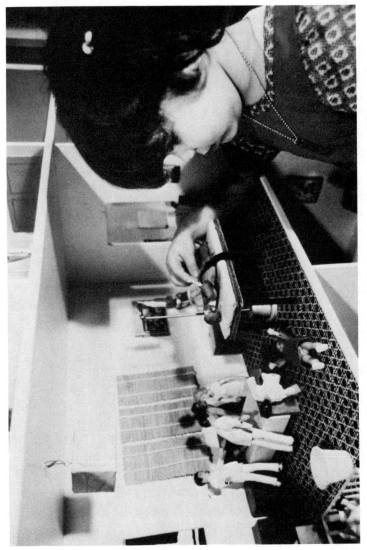

Fig. 5–8. The miniature hospital's realistic equipment helps the child become the manipulator instead of the victim, as with this young girl playing "making rounds." Soon she has the surgeon doll (in cap and mask) neatly strapped to a treatment table. (Photos by Steve Campus)

ing and doctoring, needs prominence once the hostility is evoked. To show the child how to be gentle toward a puppet or an animal shows him that grown-ups value these capacities that he can easily call forth in himself. A most skilled play session will leave the child aggressive in demanding and giving love. Such a program goes beyond the minimization of trauma and containment of children—it initiates and augments growth toward humaneness.

An individual's ability to encourage the expression of feeling in others depends to a great extent on the tolerance of such feelings in himself. Staff members who cannot tolerate overt positive and negative feelings will find it difficult to allow them in children; with such people children would learn to conceal their reactions or develop guilt regarding them.

A pediatric nurse reported that she found it necessary to stop a child's needle play because of the intensity of his reactions. "Adam jabbed the doll's head, abdomen and back repeatedly. The look of hatred on his face scared me. He wouldn't play nicely so I had to take away the equipment."

Needle Play

Injections, part of the treatment of almost all pediatric patients, are universally feared. The importance of therapeutic play in this area cannot be overstressed. The illustrations at the end of this discussion visually and graphically reveal just how important it is. (Figure 5–9: A–F). A child will interpret any sharp object stuck into his body as a brutal attack by a more powerful person.

Ideally, needle play follows immediately after and in between the experience of having an injection (of all types). Most children get started with very little help, but the nurse, doctor or technician must be willing to supply equipment, **supervision** and support in order to make this a therapeutic interaction. Whenever a real needle is used, adult supervision is mandatory.

Having equipment easily available in a dramatic play equipment area on the units allows for spur-of-the-moment action. Necessary props for IM, IV, and fingertip needle play are stuffed dolls or animals, alcohol wipes, clean syringes and needles, 30 cc. water

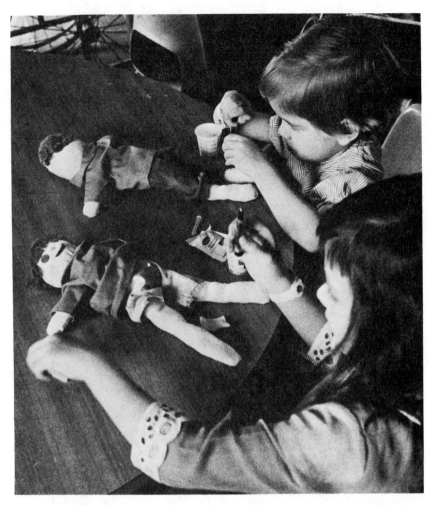

Fig. 5–9.   One way to encourage a fearful child is to allow group needle play.
(Photo by Hilary Smith)

vials labeled for dramatic play, miniature IV sets made with discarded IV tubing, clamps and small bottles, medicine cups, small
tourniquets, tongue blades (for arm boards), blood tubes, adhesive
tape and Band-Aids. Older children prefer withdrawing fluid from
vials while younger children are more adept at drawing water into a
syringe from a widemouthed container. Some patients may not want
to give an injection to a favorite doll, but they accept substitutes
easily.

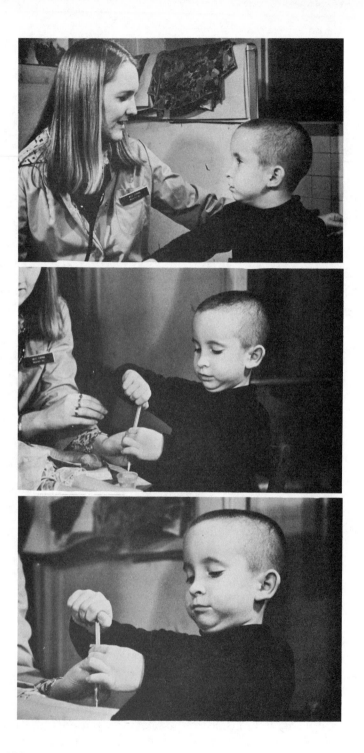

200

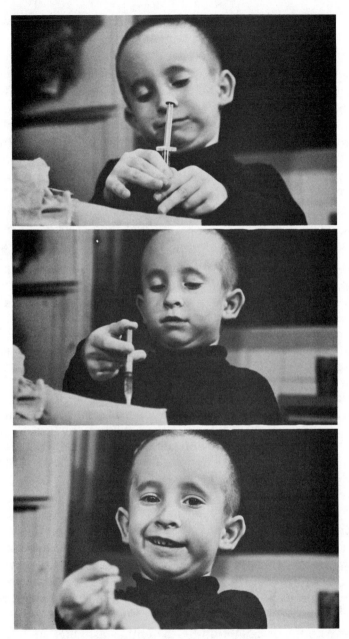

Fig. 5-10. As a way of involving this reluctant child in needle play, a play
therapist first plays for him; then pretends that it is too
difficult for her to do alone. She asks for help in drawing up the
water; later to push in the needle. Before long, the child is working on
his own and expressing pride in his mastery. His face
reveals everything. (From Staff Development Filmstrip
Series: "Needle Play," Campus Films)

201

To get started, a staff member may demonstrate the method of giving an injection. A child's attention is engaged by drawing up the solution and squirting a bit into the air. This demonstration is usually fascinating to the child and helps him to discover the nonpainful aspects of injection. Then strict attention to the actual technique involves him in the procedure and makes him less fearful of the tools. While administering the injection, making appropriate expressions of distress for the doll teaches the child that crying and protests are permitted and that the giver realizes that needles hurt. A staff member playing the part of both the doll and nurse (or doctor) may ask why needles are necessary and then respond to his own questions in order to bring out some of the child's fantasies:

> Doll: "Ow, that hurts. Why do I have to get these awful shots?"
> Nurse: "I know it hurts. Help me by holding still so that I can finish quickly. I don't blame you for not liking it."
> Doll: "Don't do it. I'll be good."
> Nurse: "Oh, you don't know why you're getting this needle. You think you're being punished? Do you know what's in this syringe and what the medicine does?"
> Doll: [Tearfully]'No, I don't."
> Nurse: "This medicine will make you a bit sleepy before your operation just as I told you. Some children think they are being punished—but we don't do things like that here. When we don't like what children are doing, we tell them so and also what we expect. We never give needles to punish."

When a child refuses to participate, it is wise to tell him that he does not have to until he wants to and to continue to play for him as a way of holding his interest. If he remains hesitant, pretend that it is too difficult to do it alone. Ask the child to place his hand on yours to help you draw up the water, later to push in the needle. Before long he should be working on his own with support. Another way to encourage a fearful child is to allow group dramatic play. It is a rare patient who is not caught up by the enthusiasm and confidence of peers. Allowing the child to keep a disposable syringe (without a needle) and other safe equipment permits him to practice afterward without staff supervision. Just because a child appears comfortable with a group or parents does not mean that this is true when he is alone. Therefore, after needle play of any sort he needs to be checked to make sure he understands and integrates the experience. The older child of seven on can have proportionately less play and more scientific explanation as to the usefulness of putting medicine directly into the body or taking blood samples out.

Parental approval of needle play ensures that the child can participate comfortably. Frequently there is a fear that this play will stir up feelings and make the child violent. Explaining that the technique is a way of helping the child overcome his fears by making him familiar with the instrument and giving him an acceptable way to handle feelings may decrease parent resistance. However, when disapproval continues, it means that the child most likely will be unable to continue in his parent's presence. (See Chapter 3).

In summary, play is an effective means by which a puzzling and sometimes painful real world can be approached. When he can deal with things that are small or inanimate, the child masters situations that to him may be otherwise overwhelming. By miniaturizing and experimenting with the dangers from the external world of the hospital and the internal world of his imagination, play strengthens the ego to more confidently adapt to and solve future challenges.

In the Appendix are listed useful materials to help health care professionals use play most productively and therapeutically.

REFERENCES

1. Erikson, E. H.: Studies in the interpretation of play. Genetic Psychology Monographs 22:561, 1940.
2. Whiteside, M. F., Busch, F., and Horner, T.: From egocentric to cooperative play in young children. J. Amer. Acad. Child Psychiat. 15–2 pp. 294–313, 1976.
3. Erikson, E. H.: Childhood and Society. New York, W. W. Norton, 1950.
4. Adams, M. A.: A hospital play program. Amer. J. Orthopsychiat. 46 (3), July 1976.
5. Slavson, S.: Play group therapy for young children. The Nervous Child 7:320, 1948.
6. Freud, A.: Normality and Pathology in Childhood, p. 136. New York, International Universities Press, 1965.
7. Blumgart, E., and Korsh, B. M.: Pediatric recreation. An approach to meeting the emotional needs of hospitalized children. Pediatrics 34:133, 1964.
8. Plank, E. N.: Working with Children in Hospitals ed. 2. Cleveland, The Press of Case Western Reserve University, 1971.
9. Tisza, V. B., et al.: The use of a play program by hospitalized children. J. Amer. Acad. Child Psychiat. 19:515, 1970.
10. Brooks, M.: Play for hospitalized children. Young Children 24:224, 1969.

BIBLIOGRAPHY

Adams, M.: A hospital play program: helping children with serious illness. Amer. J. Orthopsychiat. 46:416, 1976.

Aldis, O.: Play Fighting. New York, Academic Press, 1975.

Avedon, E. M., and Sutton-Smith, B.: The Study of Games. New York, Wiley & Sons, 1971.

Axline, V. M.: Play Therapy. Boston, Houghton Mifflin, 1974.

Azarnoff, P.: Mediating the traumas of serious illness and hospitalization in childhood. Child. Today 3:12, 1974.

———: Centers of learning in a pediatric clinic playroom. JACCH 4:33, 1975.

———, and Flegal, S.: A Pediatric Play Program: Developing a Therapeutic Play Program for Children in Medical Settings. Springfield, Ill., Charles C Thomas, 1975.

Bateson, G.: A theory of play and fantasy. Psychiat. Res., Report 2, 1955.

Bopp, J. (ed.): Guidelines for the Development of Hospital Programs for the Personnel Conducting Programs of Therapeutic Play for Pediatric Patients. ACCH, 3615 Wisconsin Ave., Wash., D.C. 20016.

Bruner, J. S., Jolly, A., and Sylvia, K.: Play—Its Role in Development and Evolution. New York, Basic Books, 1976.

Burns, R. C., and Kaufman, S. H.: Kinetic Family Drawings. New York, Brunner/Mazel, 1970.

Butler, A. *et al.* Play as Development. Columbus, Ohio, Merrill, 1978.

Caplan, F. and T.: The Power of Play. New York, Doubleday, 1973.

Cleverdon, D. *et al.*: Play in a Hospital: Why and How. Play Schools, 1971.

Dileo, J. H.: Children's Drawings as Diagnostic Aids. New York, Brunner/Mazel, 1973.

Erikson, H. H.: Toys and Reasons. New York, W. W. Norton, 1977.

Feigelson, C. I.: Play in child analysis. Psychoanalytic Study of the Child 29, 1974.

Feitelson, D., and Ross, G. S.: The neglected factor—Play. Human Dev. 16, 1973.

Flandorf, U. S.: Books to Help Children Adjust to a Hospital Situation. Chicago, American Library Association, 1967.

Frank, L. K.: Play in personality development. Amer. J. Orthopsychiat. 25:576, 1955.

Freud, A.: Research at the Hampstead Child-Therapy Clinic and Other Papers 1956–1965. London, Hogarth with the Institute of Psychoanalysis, 1970.

Furman, R. A., and Katan, A.: The Therapeutic Nursery School. New York, Universities Press, 1969. International.

Gardner, R. A.: Therapeutic Communication with Children: The Mutual Storytelling Technique. New York, Science House, 1971.

Ginott, H. G.: Group Psychotherapy with Children: The Theory and Practice of Play-Therapy. New York, McGraw-Hill, 1961.

Goodenough-Pitcher, E., and Prelinger, E.: Children Tell Stories: An Analysis of Fantasy. New York, International University Press, 1969.

Harvey, S., and Hales-Tooke, A. (eds.): Play in Hospital. London, Faber & Faber, 1972.

Head, J. A., and Newson, E.: Toys and handicap. Action, Autumn 1971.

Herron, R. E., and Sutton-Smith, B. (eds.): Child's Play. New York, Wiley & Sons, 1971.

Holt, J.: Rx: play P.R.N. in pediatric nursing. Nurs. Forum 9:288, 1970.

Kramer, E.: Art as Therapy with Children. New York, Schocken Books, 1971.

Landsman, E.: The function of a play

program in pediatrics. Pediatric Annals 1:64, 1972.

Let's Play Hospital. Children's Hospital at Stanford, 520 Willow Road, Palo Alto, Calif.

Lowe, M.: Trends in the development of representational play in the infants from one to three years: an observational study. J. Child Psychol. and Psychiat. 16, 1975.

Lowenfeld, M.: Play in Childhood. New York, Wiley & Sons, 1967.

Millar, S.: The Psychology of Play. Baltimore, Penguin, 1968.

Murphy, D.: The therapeutic value of children's literature. Nurs. Forum 2:141, 1972.

Opie, I. and P. Children's Games in Street and Playground. Oxford, Oxford University Press, 1969.

Piaget, J.: Play, Dreams and Imitation in Childhood. New York, W. W. Norton, 1962.

Piers, M. (ed.): Play and Development: A Symposium. New York, The Norton Press, 1972.

Play in the Hospital. Play Schools Association Film Library, Campus Films, Scarsdale, N.Y.

Read, K.: The Nursery School: Human Relationships and Learning, 6th ed. Philadelphia, W. B. Saunders, 1976.

Redl, F., and Wineman, D.: The Aggressive Child. New York, Free Press, 1957.

Reilly, M.: Play as Exploratory Learning: Studies of Curiosity Behavior. New York, Sage, 1974.

Robbins, A., and Sibley, L. B.: Creative Art Therapy. New York, Brunner/Mazel, 1976.

Robertson, J.: Young Children in Hospital, 2nd ed. London, Tavistock, 1970.

Schaefer, C. Therapeutic Use of Child's Play. New York, Jason Aronson, 1977.

Sheridan, M.: Spontaneous Play in Early Childhood. New York, Humanities, 1977.

Singer, J. L. (ed.): The Child's World of Makebelieve: Experimental Studies of Imaginative Play. New York, Academic Press, 1973.

Sutton-Smith, B.: The Folkgames of Children. Austin, University of Texas Press (for the American Folklore Society), 1972.

Tizard, B., and Harvey, D. (ed.): Biology of Play. Clinics in Developmental Medicine No. 62. Spastics International Medical Publications. Philadelphia, J. B. Lippincott, 1977.

Winnicott, D. W.: Playing and Reality New York, Basic Books, 1971.

6

Preparing Children and Parents for Diagnostic and Surgical Procedures or Teaching About Illness

PART 1. Guidelines for working with
    A. Newborns
    B. Infants
    C. Toddlers and Young Threes
    D. Older Threes to Seven-Year-Olds
    E. Seven- to 13-Year-Olds
    F. Adolescents

PART 2. Guidelines for Initiating Teaching About Illness, or Diagnostic and Surgical Procedures

PART 3. Preparation of a Child for/or Teaching About:
    A. Tonsillectomy
    B. Herniorrhaphy
    C. Eye Surgery (Strabismus)
    D. A Closed Kidney Biopsy
    E. Urologic Surgery (Repair of Bladder-Neck Obstruction and Reimplantation of One Ureter)
    F. Cardiac Catheterization
    G. Cardiac Surgery (Repair of Ventricular Septal Defect)
    H. Brain Surgery
    I. Amputation (Hip Disarticulation for Treatment of Malignancy
    J. Leukemia

PART 4. General Instructions for All Patients on the Day Before Treatment

PART 5. Instructions for All Patients on the Day of Surgery

PART 6. Helping the Child to Cope with Feelings Related to Hospitalization and Treatment: Postprocedural Period

Models for preparing children and parents for commonly encountered diagnostic and surgical procedures, or for teaching about illness, are presented on the following pages. Although these models were developed for use in specific hospitals and would therefore require some modification for use in other institutions, they are relevant to a multitude of situations.

The material is divided into six parts and is arranged to keep repetition to a minimum. In the first section are described developmental guidelines for working with six different age groups. The second section describes guidelines used in teaching children about illness and diagnostic or surgical procedures. In the third section are found specific procedure examples. These will also serve as useful models for similar or any other procedures. Sections four through six describe instructional processes before, during and post procedures or surgery.

PART 1. A
GUIDELINES FOR WORKING WITH NEWBORNS

DIRECTIONS	COMMENTS
For Delivery Room	
1. Allow father to be present during labor and to witness birth.	The presence of father during the birth serves as a powerful catalyst to bonding and initiates early infant–father interaction.[1]
2. Delay administration of medication to infant's eyes (approximately one hour) to avoid interference with the neonate's alert state.	The prolonged alert state (approximately 45 to 60 minutes) has been confirmed by numerous investigators. See Wolff, Desmond, Sander, Brazelton.

PART 1. A (Continued)
GUIDELINES FOR WORKING WITH NEWBORNS

DIRECTIONS	COMMENTS
3. Allow for interaction of baby and parents during the newborn's alert state immediately after birth.	In the alert state the neonate can see and demonstrates an innate form preference for eyes and mouth,[2] when sedation of mother during labor and hospital routines do not interfere.
	Complex and mutually satisfying interaction between mother and infant leading to attachment can be elicited soon after birth. The neonate is an active participant in this process: He visually searches for the mother over an arc of 180 degrees;[3] he listens and moves rhythmically in response to adult speech;[4] he vocalizes, smiles and sucks—all behaviors calculated to trigger responses from the object of attachment (mother).[5, 6]
	Reciprocal attachment behavior in the mother is demonstrated by her gazing into the newborn's eyes, exploring his body, touching, talking to, cuddling and nursing the baby—behaviors that in turn trigger the neonate's responses.[7]
4. Encourage prolonged contact of infant and parents during the first hours after birth, and rooming-in to facilitate bonding and competence in infant care.	Parental attachment is intensified with close, early and extended contact and physical caretaking of the infant in the neonatal period. Klaus and Kennell offer strong evidence for a "sensitive period," specifically the first few minutes and hours after birth, during which bonding flourishes.[8]
	By the fifth day of life the neonate can distinguish his mother's breast pad by odor. Odor is thought to play a part in the attachment process.

PART 1. A (Continued)
GUIDELINES FOR WORKING WITH NEWBORNS

DIRECTIONS	COMMENTS
	With rooming-in the mother has greater control of the environment and the opportunity to get to know her small infant. She is usually quite receptive to suggestions for handling and responding to the child's needs.

For Nursery Care

DIRECTIONS	COMMENTS
1. Assign one staff member to assist mother in care of newborn and to interact with parents.	Newborns have been found to distinguish between equally competent caretakers at ten days of age.
2. Establish calm, quiet comforting environment: a. subdued lighting b. soundproofing c. maintenance of constant warmth	From the moment of birth, the newborn is acutely aware of his surroundings. This includes sight, hearing, touch and temperature.
d. sure, gentle handling with tactile stimulation (closeness, holding, rocking and pacifiers when distressed)	The startle reflex of some newborns reveals those who have heightened sensitivities. An immediate response to alleviate distress is partly responsible for establishing basic trust. (See Chapter 2.)
3. Permit routines to be determined by the newborn: a. feeding b. diapering c. bathing d. sleeping e. examining	Each newborn is unique. It is inhumane to force artificial schedules based on the conveninece of hospital shifts. Newborns will begin their own vegetative cycles if allowed to do so. These are noted in the first few weeks only by special measurements. However, unless the individual infant is allowed this freedom, later clnically apparent patterns are either made chaotic or permanently rigid. In particular, sleep cycles can be disrupted for months after too much time is spent in a brightly lit nursery.

PART 1. A (Continued)
GUIDELINES FOR WORKING WITH NEWBORNS

DIRECTIONS	COMMENTS
	Examinations, if timed when the newborn is awake, interfere least with the carefully established environment of security.
4. Explain to parents the rationale behind the nursery policies and teach infant care.	By instruction and example, parents will incorporate these tenets. They also have the leisure and freedom from the larger family to discuss doubts with their doctor or nurse.
5. Develop classes for parents during hospitalization and follow-up periodically throughout the first year.	This will stimulate discussion of different infant care practices and family-cultural attitudes and will give a unique opportunity for the application of concepts of preventive psychiatry and the early detection of disturbed parental–infant relationships.

For Premature or Sick Neonates

1. Allow parents to see and touch infant immediately after birth and maintain frequent physical and visual contact in the first week of life.	Early infant–mother separation and/or illness of the newborn interferes with bonding and the learning of maternal tasks and may permanently disrupt effective mothering. This is demonstrated by the increased incidence of failure-to-thrive syndrome, disturbed mother–child relationships, accidents and child abuse among children who were hospitalized during the neonatal period or who were adopted.[9]

For Premature Infants

1. Permit visiting in the premature nursery after parents have been instructed in gowning, hand washing techniques and policies of unit.	Prepare parents for appearance of infant and accompany them during initial visits until they feel comfortable in infant's presence.

PART 1. A (Continued)
GUIDELINES FOR WORKING WITH NEWBORNS

DIRECTIONS	COMMENTS
2. Designate primary caretakers (physician, nurse and social worker).	Contact with primary caretakers in person or by telephone increases the parents' trust in staff and attachment to infant.
3. Supply periodic auditory stimulation by use of tape recordings of mother's voice and soothing music.	Chapman's study demonstrated that auditory stimulation was beneficial in reducing gross motor activity in both premature and full-term neonates and in promoting quiet sleep patterns for short gestation infants.
	Musical stimulation was effective in decreasing weight loss by conserving energy.
	Both music and speech contributed to the acceleration of limb acitivity patterns, while only auditory speech stimulation advanced infants' development of laterality and adaptation to new experiences.[10]
4. Supply vestibular stimulation.	Neal and Litt demonstrated that a specific motor pattern accelerated general maturation, increased weight and visual and motor function.[11]
	Weight gain and rate of development are the criteria for determining the duration of hospitalization for short gestation infants.

PART 1. B
GUIDELINES FOR WORKING WITH INFANTS

DIRECTIONS	COMMENTS
1. See guidelines for working with newborns for directions and comments that can be applied to the care of infants.	

PART 1. B (Continued)
GUIDELINES FOR WORKING WITH INFANTS

DIRECTIONS	COMMENTS
2. Assign one staff member and a relief person to care for child and to work with mother.	Most of the staff's support is given to the mother so that she can continue mothering responsibilities under stress.
3. Interview parents for information on infant's routines. Incorporate what is appropriate into hospital schedule, allowing for flexibility.	The staff should inquire about eating habits, home routine and methods of comforting baby, so that the infant develops trust that needs will be met in a new environment.

During interview it is possible to pick up areas where parents need assistance with infant care. |
4. Provide opportunity for parents to express feelings regarding the baby's illness and hospital experiences.	When parents are stifled, under stress they frequently find outlets by making the staff scapegoats or in becoming irritated with the child or each other.
5. Prepare parents for all tests and treatments scheduled for infant.	
6. Be alert to manifestations of separation anxiety and its management.	Recent studies indicate that infants of less than two months can already distinguish between parents and strangers.[12]
7. Encourage rooming-in.	Even those under three months of age will show distress on separation. By six months, separation will produce signs of mourning in infants with close ties to the mother.
8. Encourage mother to participate in the infant's care as much as possible.	It is important for a mother to feel comfortable with her sick child. Continuous contact and the learning of routine procedures facilitate this.

When rooming-in is not feasible, emphasize the importance of a regular visiting pattern. The closer the child is to the toddler age group, the more imperative the mother's presence becomes, because this is the time of the |

PART 1. B (Continued)
GUIDELINES FOR WORKING WITH INFANTS

DIRECTIONS	COMMENTS
	normal separation-individuation phase, which requires the mother's presence for success.
9. Play peekaboo with infant.	From repeated experiences, the infant begins to learn that objects out of sight continue to exist.
10. Be alert to manifestations of stranger anxiety and its management. a. Allow parent participation in care. b. Make initial contacts with infant in mother's presence to reduce fear. c. Work in vicinity of infant and approach slowly until he regards you as a safe person. d. Keep the number of caretakers at a minimum.	By eight months of age, through continued contact with parents, the infant develops a schema for their faces, forms and voices. For infants who have had uninterrupted contact with parents, a schema for them will develop earlier. Exposure to a variety of strangers results in a more generalized perception of the human face, form and voice. Stranger anxiety indicates that the infant has observed a discrepancy from the familiar schema, and this produces a fear response.[13]
11. Maintain eye-to-eye contact while interacting with infant, especially during feeding. Teach parents the significance of this measure.	The significance of eye contact in the establishment of bonding cannot be overstated.[14, 15] Eye-to-eye contact serves another important function. The infant begins to develop a self-image from the attitudes and responses he evokes in the mother (caretaker). When the mother's face is responsive, he gets a reflection of himself. Thus, the mother's face serves as a mirror.[16]
12. Provide infant with tactile and sensory stimulation. a. Supply singing, talking, music, mobiles, infant seats and swings, strollers, carriages,	

PART 1. B (Continued)
GUIDELINES FOR WORKING WITH INFANTS

DIRECTIONS	COMMENTS
rockers, cuddling, security objects from home, hand toys.	
b. Include water play and food play.	
c. Change scenery frequently.	Babies can be positioned alternately from head to foot of crib; placed by window or door; or in various areas of ward.
d. Imitate infant's vocalizations.	This serves to increase his vocalizations.
e. Suspend mobile approximately 12 inches from infant's face to ensure visibility. Attach a string from mobile to infant's wrist or ankle.	Infant will soon learn to control movement of mobile.
	Hospitalized babies who receive social stimulation demonstrate ability to develop attachments to family members faster than those who have not been adequately stimulated.[17]
13. Be alert for infants requiring additional stimulation and nurturing care (the unhappy baby). See tactile and sensory stimulation.	Frequent crying, restlessness, withdrawal, self-rocking, head banging, depression, insomnia and frequent gastrointestinal upsets are some indications of insufficient gratification of needs.
14. Provide comfort measures for distressed infants:	Babies cannot be spoiled by being made comfortable.
a. human contact	
b. high-pitched voice	The infant whose needs are met consistently will demonstrate the ability to wait for attention by three months of age. He develops the expectation for gratification (trust) because of prompt responsiveness on the part of his mother.
c. vestibular stimulation, such as rapid rocking in supine position (on back, face upward) or being held upright over caretaker's shoulder.	
d. pacifier, when NPO	
e. demand feedings	

PART 1. B (Continued)
GUIDELINES FOR WORKING WITH INFANTS

DIRECTIONS	COMMENTS
f. recording fo parents' voices played back periodically	This is especially helpful for long-term hospitalization.
15. Provide opportunities for development of motor skills.	For example, help in walking, or the provision of a clean, safe, warm space for crawling.
16. Techniques of Infant Feeding for Staff and Parent Teaching	
a. Include mother in feeding routine. Encourage continuation of breast feeding.	
b. Allow demand feeding.	This may entail change in routine, such as feeding before bath. Infant will soon establish his own predictable schedule.
c. Dilute solids to a soupy consistency for young babies.	
d. Assume comfortable position, preferably in rocker with arm support. This will prevent tension buildup in caretaker's arm.	
e. Cradle infant close to body. Assume **en face** position (infant turned toward caretaker so that eye contact is maintained).	See functions of eye contact.
f. When infant is very hungry, allow short sucking period to calm him before giving solids.	
g. Supply tactile and sensory stimulation.	This includes cuddling, singing and talking. The infant will incorporate attitudes of the caretaker and aspects of the environment along with the food.
h. Maintain perpendicular position of bottle so that nipple is filled with milk continuously.	

PART 1. B (Continued)
GUIDELINES FOR WORKING WITH INFANTS

DIRECTIONS	COMMENTS
i. To bubble infant, wait to remove nipple from infant's mouth until he has stopped sucking.	Some infants become fearful that nipple will not return. Good experiences teach otherwise.
j. Provide adequate sucking time— approximately 25 to 30 minutes per feeding.	Sucking relieves tension and aids breathing and digestion. Babies who finish feedings quickly because of strong sucking need harder nipples with small holes to prolong the process. Breast-fed infants obtain most of the milk within the first five minutes, but are motivated to continue sucking because of the small amount of milk that continues to flow.
	At least 120 minutes of sucking daily prevents thumb- and finger-sucking.[18]
k. Provide pacifier after feeding or when infant is fasting before treatment.	Pacifiers are used principally to ensure adequate sucking gratification, not as a substitute for maternal care.
	For infants, continuity of maternal care (on which emotional, social and intellectual growth is dependent) is of paramount importance. In the absence of a constant mother figure, arrange for a mother substitute. Staff needs to take responsibility for maintaining constancy of care.
	The relationship the infant develops with the mother or other early caretaker will influence the quality of all future relationships the child establishes. Early caretaking attitudes toward the infant will produce similar responses from the child toward others.

Turn to Part 2 for further guidelines that can be applied to infants.

PART 1. C
GUIDELINES FOR WORKING WITH TODDLERS AND YOUNG THREES

DIRECTIONS	COMMENTS
1. Assign one person to care for child and to work with mother.	Much of the staff's support should be given to the mother so that she can continue mothering responsibilities under stress.
2. Interview parents for information on child's habits and routines. Incorporate what is appropriate into hospital schedule.	Provide potty-chair when child is trained and is able to maintain already learned skills during illness; if mother wishes a two- or three-year-old to have pacifier or bottles, do not attempt to change his habits in the hospital. Allow night-light if used at home.
	Provide family-type dining facilities.
	For long-term hospitalization, new routines and training can be introduced gradually as child's medical condition and parents allow.
	Staff responsibilities for directing growth and development increase with lengthy illness or in the absence of parents.
3. Provide opportunities for parents to express feelings regarding child's illness and hospital experiences.	
4. See comments and directions re: stranger and separation anxiety in Guidelines for Working with Infants.	The toddler group experiences the greatest amount of regression due to separation. Attachment to mother is very strong and the child's capacity for verbal expression is not yet well established. His chief preoccupations are abandonment and individuation.
5. Be attuned to manifestations of separation anxiety and its management. a. Encourage rooming-in and participation in child's care.	The closer the relationship to the mother, the more intense the distress on separation and the evidence of mourning. See pp. 90–94.

PART 1. C (<u>Continued</u>)
GUIDELINES FOR WORKING WITH TODDLERS AND YOUNG THREES

DIRECTIONS	COMMENTS
b. Arrange for a mother substitute when a constant mothering figure is not available.	Nondistressed behavior on the part of the toddler after separation is an indication of lack of social attachment.
c. Allow use of transitional objects.	Because the infant or toddler does not always have his mother at his disposal, he begins to make intimate attachments to other objects (transitional objects), such as stuffed animals, blanket or other objects that become security objects because they substitute for mother.
d. Play hide-and-seek (a variation of peekaboo) with toddler.	With repeated experiences, he learns that objects out of sight continue to exist.
e. Give parents permission to leave their child and help in separating from him. Instruct them to indicate when they will return in relation to the child's activities, because time is not understood by this age group.	Many parents experience guilt when the child protests their leaving, and need extra support at these times. Some try "sneaking out" to avoid scenes. They must understand that such action impairs the child's trust in them. Clinging needs to be interpreted as separation anxiety, which subsides when parents set up a pattern of reappearance and keep promises made to the child.
f. Intervene if parents leave without notice.	
g. Ask parents to leave personal articles with child to assure him of their return.	
h. Assist parents in leaving immediately after announcing their departure. Stay with the child to help him over the difficult period.	
i. Ask parents to bring in familiar toys and family photos. Make up stories involving pleasant home activities. Encourage parents to do the same.	Repeat effective stories again and again. This provides for stability when everything else appears to be changing for the child. Avoid stories with separation themes, unless they end with a reunion (for example, "King Midas and the Golden Touch"); they increase feelings of abandonment.

PART 1. C (Underline: Continued)
GUIDELINES FOR WORKING WITH TODDLERS AND YOUNG THREES

DIRECTIONS	COMMENTS
	Avoid fairy tales and analogies because this age group cannot distinguish fact from fiction, or make comparisons. If child reveals fantasies, help him to end them happily.
6. Develop a toddler play program: provide intellectual, social and motor stimulation.	Indoor and outdoor play with nursery school atmosphere: story periods, music and musical instruments, mud, sand and water play, building blocks and boxes, dolls, pull toys and telephones.
7. When a treatment or surgery is scheduled: a. Tell the toddler about it just before carrying it out. Verbal toddlers can be told the day before or early in the morning when surgery is to occur later in the day. Three-year-olds are told the day before or earlier if extensive preparation is required. b. Be truthful about hurting. c. Give permission to object to a painful procedure, but be positive about what you are doing. d. If there is no choice, do not imply there is by asking the child if you may proceed. e. Delete body outline for child (use for parents) and avoid giving information about the inside of the body since it is not understood by this age group. f. Depersonalize teaching. g. Deal with "illness as punishment" theme common in toddlers.	Telling about an event which then occurs builds confidence that the staff mean what they say. Talk about a doll who has a problem (symptoms) instead of the child, and how the doctor and nurse will care for it. Pretend that the doll thinks he has

PART 1. C (Continued)
GUIDELINES FOR WORKING WITH TODDLERS AND YOUNG THREES

DIRECTIONS	COMMENTS
	been hospitalized because of being bad. Reassure the doll that he is not to blame and indicate again the reason for treatment. Be explicit about the body part affected. Show on doll. Attach appliances, bandages, IVs (whatever applies) to doll to help toddler visualize what is to be expected.
h. Allow toddler to play with safe equipment used in his treatment.	The child should have the use of stethoscopes, reflex hammer, tongue blades, syringes without needles, dolls with appropriate attachments for a particular procedure.
	Turning passive experiences into active ones helps to master the anxiety associated with treatment.
8. Refrain from talking about a young child within his hearing. Assume that he understands.	A young child's capacity to understand far exceeds his capacity to verbalize. His interpretations are literal. Choose words with care. See Egocentric thinking, page 41.
	For the toddler and young three-year-old hospitalization is less of a devastating event when medical personnel understand the need for (1) continuity of the mother–child relationship, (2) the incorporation of familiar routines and rituals (when they are not in conflict with medical goals), (3) structure and limit setting, and (4) mastery and control.
9. Turn to Part 2 for further guidelines that can be applied to toddlers and young threes.	

PART 1. D
GUIDELINES FOR WORKING WITH OLDER THREES- TO SEVEN-YEAR-OLDS

DIRECTIONS	COMMENTS
1. Assign one nurse to the child as consistently as possible. Designate a relief person.	
2. For three- and four-year-olds, encourage rooming-in, participation in child care and willingness to leave child periodically in staff's care.	This tells the child that mother approves of hospital routines and helps the child integrate concepts of body care; also, that the pediatric staff are safe people.
3. Impress mother with the importance of a regular visiting pattern.	A pattern of visiting builds confidence in her return. From three to four years, ambivalence is characteristic, as is demonstrated in alternating behavior: expression of love and hate, defiance and compliance, clinging and independence.
4. For five-year olds, encourage participation in medical care and self-hygiene.	For this age, self-care has just been accomplished; thus, it is threatening to relinquish it to others. The child tends to be upset by smells and messiness, as he has just achieved bowel and bladder control and learned prohibitions against dirt. He needs to participate in cleaning up. Responsibility for self-care also includes the avoidance of unnecessary risks and the knowledge of safety equipment on the unit.
5. Observe for evidence of silent attachment to the staff. This positive sign from the child can be openly recognized and appropriately supported.	For three- to seven-year-olds, the staff needs to be aware of the development of oedipal attachments—that is, girls may become flirtatious or silent with male personnel. Boys may show sexual curiosity overtly or covertly toward female personnel. Boys and girls may compete with one another to win the favor of the secretly loved adult. To have a warm response from an esteemed and favored grown-up may further healthy identification and

PART 1. D (Continued)
GUIDELINES FOR WORKING WITH OLDER THREES- TO SEVEN-YEAR-OLDS

DIRECTIONS	COMMENTS
	build confidence the child this age needs to enter latency competitions: physically, socially and academically.
6. For teaching about illness or preparation for treatment: a. Use a body outline, doll and other visual aids in teaching.	This age group is capable of understanding the inside of the body; so a simple explanation of anatomy and physiology is given and drawn in on the outline.
	A doll is used to visualize external appearance post-procedure or surgery (tubes, bandages, intravenous equipment). Toys or models representing equipment used in the child's care increase comprehension and are conducive to dramatic play. This age group is challenging to teach; three- to seven-year-olds are highly imaginative and have developed communication skills that facilitate active participation in teaching.
	Encourage child's questions and compliment his inquisitiveness. Give him credit for understanding. Maximize initiative and mastery in order to increase the child's pride in himself.
b. Deal with the castration and mutilation fantasies common to this age group (phallic phase) by talking of damage and repair.	See example of restitutive play in the story of Robinson, page 341.
c. Reassure child repeatedly, whenever appropriate, that no one is to blame for his condition or hospitalization, and that the procedures are limited.	Although this is recommended in all teaching, it is especially important for three- to seven-year-olds, who are preoccupied with guilt and blame. The child tends to generalize and feels that all body parts are vulnerable.

PART 1. D (Continued)
GUIDELINES FOR WORKING WITH OLDER THREES- TO SEVEN-YEAR-OLDS

DIRECTIONS	COMMENTS
	Use playful repetition to clarify operative site or part of body involved as described on p. 17.
7. Provide a play program.	This group needs a nursery school environment for play, with plants, pets and clothing and props for imitating staff and community figures.
8. Turn to Part 2 for further guidelines that can be applied to three- to seven-year-olds.	

PART 1. E
GUIDELINES FOR WORKING WITH 7- TO 13-YEAR-OLDS

DIRECTIONS	COMMENTS
	The period of latency, between the ages of 6 and 12, begins with the resolution of the oedipal conflict. Following this event, there is a repression of much of the fantasy material normally associated with the mental life of three to six-year-olds—that is, the preoccupation with castration and mutilation. In well-adjusted children of this age group, the conclusion of the oedipal phase results also in identification with the parent of the same sex, the search for love objects outside of the family and the internalization of the conscience.
	The personality characteristics of latency period children are built on these outcomes. Because of the incorporation of parents' and society's values, they become self-directing, although strong external control may be

PART 1. E (Continued)
GUIDELINES FOR WORKING WITH 7- TO 13-YEAR-OLDS

DIRECTIONS	COMMENTS
	required occasionally to curb antisocial behavior when newly established controls break down.
	With sexual preoccupation diminished, energies are expended on roughhousing, sports, teasing, schoolwork and a fantasy life that is used to combat the injustices of life. Through these activities, the facade of emotional stability is maintained.[19]
1. Assign one person to care regularly for child. This person should maintain schedules, routines and rules consistently. Designate a relief person.	
2. Encourage a consistent visiting pattern with family, especially for the under-eight group. Allow sibling and peer visiting.	It is important to check first for young visitors' exposure to communicable disease.
3. Discourage rooming-in except during acute illness and initially in the event of regression, which is common in young latency children. Encourage relationships with peers and staff.	Adjustment to the hospital is easier for 6- to 13-year-olds than it is for younger children, because they are capable of reason and understand the concept of time. Therefore, separation anxiety is significantly reduced or nonexistent. They develop friendships with other patients and staff and enjoy the social aspects of the experience, provided preparation and support are adequate. Immature or regressed children of this group react to hospitalization much like those under six. They may fear abandonment, mutilation and monsters.
4. Encourage self-care and participation in treatment planning.	Familiar routines, preparation for treatment and self-care reduce the likelihood of regression.

PART 1. E (Continued)
GUIDELINES FOR WORKING WITH 7- TO 13-YEAR-OLDS

DIRECTIONS	COMMENTS
5. Develop daily routines to foster social, academic, motor and artistic skills, including school, recreation—indoor and outdoor—and opportunities for group friendships.	Mastery, achievement and excellence are important themes throughout this phase. Recognition and popularity are gained through the acquisition of skills. But more important, they become the basis for feelings of worthiness and self-esteem and help to shape lifelong attitudes toward work and productivity. In this, the role of school and teachers is highly influential in determining the course of children's lives.
	As children strive to become emotionally independent of adults, they turn to their peers for acceptance. Usually this group seeks its own sex as a way of reinforcing sexual identifications. The peer group signals the beginning of a real social life. In these relationships, children move from egocentricity—become anxious to please, learn to give as well as to take and observe the rules of group living.
6. In preparation for treatment: a. Determine whether a doll is to be used in teaching.	Some children ask for them while others are embarrassed to be be seen with dolls. If used, the doll can be called a dummy or teaching doll. When postoperative appearance is difficult to describe, visualization on a dummy is recommended.
b. Continue with the use of body outlines for explanation of anatomy and physiology and visualization of postoperative appearance.	
c. Teach child scientific terminology for body parts and medical procedures after learning his words for them.	Teaching for these children should consider their eagerness for new knowledge. Write new terminology on body outline.

PART 1. E (Continued)
GUIDELINES FOR WORKING WITH 7- TO 13-YEAR-OLDS

DIRECTIONS	COMMENTS
	Exposure to the hospital may possibly spark interest in medical careers, as vocational choices are frequently made during this period.
d. Be straightforward about telling the child that no other part of the body will be involved—only the operative area described.	If a child is immature for his age or preoccupied with mutilation, follow directions for the under-seven group.
e. Encourage questioning, expression of feelings and active participation in his teaching.	Although the teaching plan is similar to that of younger children, the response of 7- to 13-year-olds is usually more enthusiastic. In relating to this age level, we can take advantage of the characteristics already developed: the ability to reason, to make generalizations and to understand the concept of time. Teaching and management are easier because these children can verbalize feelings, comprehend cause and effect and have a scientific orientation.
f. Beware of reassuring a child about his condition before eliciting his notion of what is wrong and how it happened. First ask about experiences with illness and hospitalization, and of other members of his family and friends.	Fear of death is normal and common for latency. Frequently a child will ask directly if he is going to die, or tell stories of children who have had complicated illnesses. Do not change the subject. After determining the child's story, it is important to emphasize the differences and similarities between his problem and those of others. This can be most reassuring. Despite the reality-orientation of this group, one must be alert to misconceptions about illness. It is also helpful to express confidence in his doctor and in a staff that is well trained in the management of his problem and to mention the numbers of children successfully treated. Children can comprehend simple statistical probability. (See Chapter 2.)

PART 1. E (Continued)
GUIDELINES FOR WORKING WITH 7- TO 13-YEAR-OLDS

DIRECTIONS	COMMENTS
g. Allow child to keep safe, disposable hospital equipment used in his care.	This gratifies the latency child's need to collect and also provides the visual aids for telling about his experiences.
7. Turn to Part 2 for further guidelines that may be applied to 7- to 13-year-olds.	

PART 1. F
GUIDELINES FOR WORKING WITH ADOLESCENTS

DIRECTIONS	COMMENTS
1. Assign primary nurse and physician to care for the patient consistently. Designate relief persons.	Staff members assigned should not be close to period of adolescence. Mature, consistent but flexible individuals who have understanding of their behavior are ideal caretakers.
2. In preparation for surgery or treatment: a. Include patient in conferences with family and medical–nursing team to discuss plans for his treatment. b. Obtain his consent.	By midadolescence, the patient wants to be in on the planning and to retain control over what happens to his body although sometimes he prefers not to know when findings are too threatening. Thus, do not invariably give direct answers to questions before checking out the purpose of the question.
c. Plan teaching for periods when parents are absent. Make provision to see the parents at another time.	It is difficult for the adolescent to confide in his nurse or doctor in the presence of his parents. Respect his need for privacy.
d. Discover the words he uses for body parts. Then teach him scientific terms for gaps in his knowledge.	Medical terminology will be readily absorbed into his vocabulary.

PART 1. F (Continued)
GUIDELINES FOR WORKING WITH ADOLESCENTS

DIRECTIONS	COMMENTS
e. Encourage him to ask questions. Common sense and good humor are best approaches with this age group.	It will be easier for him to approach the staff when he has the verbal tools. Tell him that most patients think of questions later on and that he probably will also.
f. Be attuned to the adolescent's concern about physical imperfections, body manipulation and need for privacy.	Characteristically, the adolescent is preoccupied about physical changes and having a body that is different from that of others. He is curious about sex and may give the impression of knowing more or less than he actually does know. A trusting atmosphere may lead to sex education opportunities. The staff should be receptive and informative.
	Castration anxiety shows itself at this stage by concern about body size and secondary sexual development, and in a boy's hostility toward girls or a girl's denial of femininity.
	Private bathing facilities, proper draping and screening during procedures, talking to a doctor of the same sex about personal problems help the adolescent cope with acute feelings of embarrassment. Provide privacy for times of sexual arousal and sexual functioning in masturbation.
	The adolescent should have personal space that can be identified as his own. Should be allowed to wear own clothing.
g. Reassure the patient that his questions and your conversations are confidential.	The only time a confidence cannot be respected is when it places the patient in jeopardy. In such an instance, tell the patient this.

PART 1. F (Continued)
GUIDELINES FOR WORKING WITH ADOLESCENTS

DIRECTIONS	COMMENTS
h. Determine whether the teenager has done reading about his disease or condition. If the patient is concerned about genetic factors, arrange for genetic counseling.	
i. Use a body diagram to give a scientific explanation of the anatomy and physiology involved in his surgery or procedure.	Often medical personnel credit the adolescent with understanding that he does not have. His misconceptions need clarification. He may have vague ideas about body function that remain unclear because he is embarrassed to ask or does not have the ability to make his needs known. He may need help in doing so, but he is capable of abstract thinking and learning on a sophisticated level.
3. Provide for continuation of social activities and mature identifications. Encourage group meetings.	The child should have telephone facilities and opportunities to visit outside of the hospital when confinement is lengthy. Teen recreation program, peer relationships from the patient population and peer visiting should be allowed as liberally as possible. Encourage patients to assist with younger children and clerical activities.
4. Arrange for diet preferences (when medically sound) and accessible kitchen facilities.	Teenagers enjoy being able to prepare their own food and snacks. Reinforces independence.
5. Arrange for continuing education (hospital school or tutor) when illness is prolonged.	Intellectual talk may be a useful way to start a relationship.
6. Determine rules and regulations for teenagers on the unit or for an adolescent unit. Make information available to staff and patients, preferably in writing.	Policies must be flexible and respectful of individual and developing needs. However, rules designed to protect the rights of others must be consistently enforced.

Early Adolescence

Characteristically, during this phase there is a withdrawal of interest in the

PART 1. F (Continued)
GUIDELINES FOR WORKING WITH ADOLESCENTS

DIRECTIONS	COMMENTS
	original love objects as the adolescent makes initial attempts at emancipation from the family. The use of hostility, provocative behavior, questioning of traditional values, secretiveness and vacillation between dependent and independent attitudes (as measures for loosening ties) is strong and may be manifested also in relationships to authority figures (such as hospital personnel), as well as with parents. He may be antisocial or delinquent. Before new love relationships can be established, the adolescent experiences loneliness and depression resulting in much self-preoccupation. Self-focus increases with illness to the point, at times, of hypochondriasis.
7. Talk to the youngster about his body if he seems comfortable.	
8. It is useful for the staff to be more personal about how they chose their vocations.	A hospitalization at this time may influence the teenager to seriously consider a health career (formation of new ego ideal).
9. Beware of being drawn in on the child's anger toward the family. Empathize with difficulties and infatuations but avoid identifying (allowing self to take on the adolescent's hostilities and yearnings).	Middle Adolescence Alienation from parents prevails. The adolescent relies heavily on the peer group. Now he has acquired some sense of self and is capable of seeking out new love objects. Mourning and being in love are typical moods. Introspective daydreaming often helps to relieve feelings of isolation until a close tie is established with the opposite sex. Heterosexual love objects vary: they either strongly resemble or are completely different from the parent of the opposite sex. Although sudden attachments or hostilities to hospital personnel may appear to be unfounded, they are actually of much

PART 1. F (Continued)
GUIDELINES FOR WORKING WITH ADOLESCENTS

DIRECTIONS	COMMENTS

relevance to understanding the dynamics of behavior and in understanding the adolescent's vulnerability to rejection. Provision needs to be made for consistency in relationships to key people throughout hospitalization.

Intense feelings are common, as is intellectualization to avoid the same unmanageable feelings. There is the tendency to asceticism in order to bolster the denial of unacceptable feelings, such as the welcoming of tribulation and pain. Loneliness is countered by self-stimulation—masturbation, the taking of physical risks, the use of drugs. Consequently, the adolescent may be prone to addiction, especially if it is a fad of the peer group.

Late Adolescence

In this phase, the adolescent is capable of mature logical reflection. He evaluates his ideals, strengths, aspirations and thinks in terms of the future— of a life plan. The conflict between dependence and independence is resolved. He is emancipated from his parents and from the peer group as well. It is a period of consolidation, of acceptance and of coming to grips with feelings.

In the hospital, the adolescent girl reacts to illness by showing concern for appearance, by giving attention to the whole body. Treatment is viewed in terms of how it will affect relationships with boys and the reproductive process.

The adolescent boy shows concern about virility and prowess, and how

PART 1. F (Continued)
GUIDELINES FOR WORKING WITH ADOLESCENTS

DIRECTIONS	COMMENTS
	mutilation of the body will affect his abilities.
10. Be reasonably complimentary. The teenager deserves credit for being stoical in the face of the humiliation illness imposes.	The self-image is threatened for both sexes. They are future-oriented in relation to the opposite sex and vocational choice. They need all the support the staff can realistically give in these areas.
	A chronic or severe illness in adolescence may interfere with any or all of the major developmental goals for this period—emancipation from the family, heterosexual attachments, management of feelings, development of a personal code of behavior and preparation for a vocation.
	The chief defense mechanisms used during this period to cope with stress of illness, physical limitation or death are intellectualization, denial, projection, overcompensation and regression.
11. Turn to Part 2 for further guidelines that can be applied to adolescents.	

PART 2.
GUIDELINES FOR INITIATING TEACHING ABOUT ILLNESS, OR DIAGNOSTIC AND SURGICAL PROCEDURES

DIRECTIONS	COMMENTS
1. After referring to Part 1 for information on preparing a specific age group, you are ready to initiate teaching. Assign one person to carry out preparation and a relief person.	Consistency in relationships will facilitate the development of the child's trust in the teacher.
	For most hospitals, at present, the nursing staff is in the best position to follow through on teaching and dra-

PART 2. (Continued)
GUIDELINES FOR INITIATING TEACHING ABOUT ILLNESS, OR DIAGNOSTIC AND SURGICAL PROCEDURES

DIRECTIONS	COMMENTS
	matic play. It is practical to have this aspect of the program organized under one discipline. The participation of other professional staff and parents, however, is to be encouraged after a complete briefing on events and routines.
2. Consult with pediatrician or surgeon regarding the plan of treatment and the information given to the parents.	
3. Review the parents' understanding of what is going to take place and how they have explained it to their child. What terms were used? What symptoms did the child exhibit at home? How were they related to the child's condition? Has the child been hospitalized in the past? What questions is he asking? In addition, asking in what ways is the patient growing well, in what areas he needs help, his favorite types of play, what kind of discipline works and how often it is necessary all give a picture of the child and of parent/child interaction.	This information will indicate how much additional help the child and his parents will need and the direction the teaching should take.
4. Determine whether the parents are to participate in the teaching or whether they should be present. See Parent Participation, page 67.	When parents are cooperative and supportive to the child, their presence in teaching sessions is desirable. Otherwise, plan separate sessions for parents and child.
5. Plan to cover the entire teaching in approximately three sessions.	Even when time is limited, this allows the child to assimilate the material and to ask questions. Too much at one time overwhelms him and he is likely to "tune out." Moreover, focus is lost with

PART 2. (Continued)
GUIDELINES FOR INITIATING TEACHING ABOUT ILLNESS, OR DIAGNOSTIC AND SURGICAL PROCEDURES

DIRECTIONS	COMMENTS
	a greater number of sessions. Ideally, children are admitted a minimum of two days in advance of major surgery so that there is sufficient time for the child to overcome the anticipatory anxiety that is invariably part of the preparation process, and so adequate time is available for the staff to deal with the child's feelings.
	Thinking about the treatment or surgery and tolerating the anxiety are aids to coping with stress and preparing for danger.[20]
6. Make a sketchy outline of each session to be used as reference during preparation.	See Appendix ii for Work-sheet/Outline.
7. Decide appropriate explanation for age and emotional maturity and choose vocabulary suitable to child's intellectual understanding. Use neutral words like "opening," (or "incision" for children over six), "drainage" or "oozing" instead of "cut" and "bleed."	Neutral words are less likely to frighten the child and allow him to control going into more dangerous connotations or holding to harmless meanings.
8. Gather all visual aids and dramatic play materials to be used.	Having a supply of teaching aids and dramatic play materials prepared in advance in a designated place makes it easier to proceed—for example, body outlines, dolls, drainage tubing, model IV equipment, bandages, syringes and needles, anesthesia mask, model of croupette made out of plastic bag, and even models of frequently used machines.
	Also, having a scrapbook showing doctors and nurses at work, children being cooperative with treatment (going to operating room, waking up

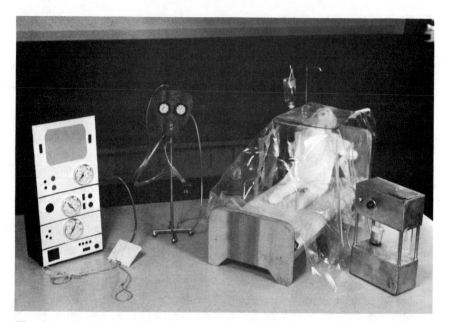

Fig. 6–1. Having a supply of visual aids and dramatic play materials makes it easier to proceed with preoperative teaching. (Photo by Steve Campus)

PART 2. (Continued)
GUIDELINES FOR INITIATING TEACHING ABOUT ILLNESS, OR DIAGNOSTIC AND SURGICAL PROCEDURES

DIRECTIONS	COMMENTS
	in recovery room, using equipment, etc.) is helpful in explaining events. Photos can be taken for this purpose or cut from medical or nursing journals.
9. Before giving the child any information, determine his understanding of the problem and the reason for hospitalization.	This frequently discloses fantasies that might be missed if teaching is started immediately. His answers will indicate the emphasis of your teaching and the kind of reassurances needed.
	When a child denies any knowledge, do not take this at face value. He may be using denial as a way of coping with event. Ask him instead, "How did you know that you needed to come to

PART 2. (Continued)
GUIDELINES FOR INITIATING TEACHING ABOUT ILLNESS, OR DIAGNOSTIC AND SURGICAL PROCEDURES

DIRECTIONS	COMMENTS
	the hospital? What did the doctor say? What did mother and father tell you?" If he still professes ignorance, try this approach. "I guess you must be wondering what it's all about. Naturally you can't know if your ideas are right, but tell me what things have come to your mind." Or, "You can't possibly know since you haven't been in this situation before. Are you the kind of person who lets things happen without asking? If I were you, I'd like to know. I don't like surprises."
	Another approach for a child under six would be to tell a story of an animal or child left in the repair shop to have something fixed.
10. Turn now to Part 3 for specific information on preparing a patient for a procedure or surgery.	

PART 3. A
PREPARATION OF A CHILD FOR TONSILLECTOMY

DIRECTIONS	COMMENTS AND EXAMPLES
1. Refer to Parts 1 and 2 before continuing.	
2. After determining the child's understanding of the need for hospitalization, as explained in Part 2, give him a simple explanation to reinforce his knowledge or to correct his misunderstanding. Introduce symptoms.	"Tonsils are two small lumps in the back of your throat (or mouth). When you were smaller, your tonsils helped to keep you from getting sick with sore throats, earaches and colds. But now your tonsils are not working well. In fact, they are causing trouble by giving you earaches, sore throats, and colds (whatever applies), and we

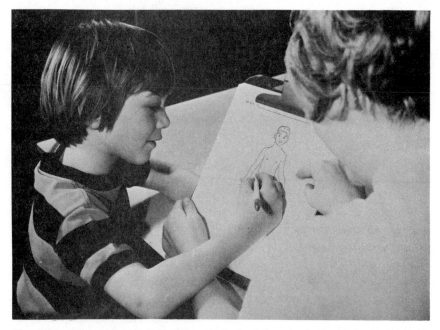

Fig. 6–2. An explanation of anatomy and physiology is given and drawn in on the body outline after determining the child's understanding of his illness. (Photo by Steve Campus)

PART 3. A (Continued)
PREPARATION OF A CHILD FOR TONSILLECTOMY

DIRECTIONS	COMMENTS AND EXAMPLES
	know that's no fun. Your doctor can help. Because you don't need your tonsils any more, they are going to be taken out. That's the reason you came to the hospital."
3. Ask the child what he thinks may have caused the problem.	This gives another opportunity to elicit fantasy material.
Reassure the child that no one is to blame for his condition. Make it clear that nothing he did or thought is responsible.	

PART 3. A (Continued)
PREPARATION OF A CHILD FOR TONSILLECTOMY

DIRECTIONS	COMMENTS AND EXAMPLES

4. Indicate postoperative expectations:
  a. sore throat
  b. ice collar
  c. medication
  d. positioning and emesis of old blood
  e. food and fluid restriction
	"When you wake up from your operation, your throat will feel quite sore. But we can make it feel better by putting an ice collar around your neck." (Show him an ice collar; open the top and indicate where the ice goes in. Allow him to try it on. Emphasize the coolness.) "And if it is necessary we can give medicine too."
	
	"You will be placed on your belly because it will be easier for you to spit up old blood and phlegm that way. There will probably be a bit of old blood in your nose too. This usually happens. We expect it."
	
	"In about two hours after returning to your room, you'll be ready to have something to drink. First we'll give you some cool ginger ale, because it will feel good. And later you may have some juices like apricot and pear. By tomorrow morning, you'll be ready for ice cream for breakfast, and that will feel good too. By then, you will be much better and you'll be able to go home. Your throat will still be sore, but every day it will feel better and soon you will feel fine again."

5. Ask child to show you the operative site on a body outline.	This frequently reveals confusion.
6. Reassure child that no other part of the body will be operated on.	Use playful repetition to clarify operative area for child under six. (See page 17. Older children may be told directly.)
7. Introduce needle play related to blood work already experienced.	This is introduced at the end of the session, because it is quite stimulating for the child. We want to be sure of his attention to the preceding material first.

PART 3. A (Continued)
PREPARATION OF A CHILD FOR TONSILLECTOMY

DIRECTIONS	COMMENTS AND EXAMPLES
	Allow needle play. See Needle Play, page 198.
8. Play up rewards—how much he will have to tell his family and friends about the hospital, the new things he has seen, the different people he has met.	This allows the memory of stressful procedures to be associated with bravery and the wish for good health.
9. Turn to Part 4.	

PART 3. B
PREPARATION OF A CHILD FOR HERNIORRHAPHY

DIRECTIONS	COMMENTS AND EXAMPLES
1. Refer to Parts 1 and 2 before continuing.	
2. After determining child's understanding or fantasy regarding illness and hospitalization, give him a simple explanation of the anatomy and physiology involved, introducing symptoms.	Toddlers to Young Threes: "The doctor is going to fix this bump. [Indicate are on child and doll.] He will do a little operation."
	Older Threes to Seven Group:
	"Have you heard about muscles? Show me one (biceps). Muscles are the parts of the body that allow you to move your arms and legs. Muscles also help to keep your back straight and your belly flat and firm. For some reason we don't know, your muscle here . . . [indicate on drawing] . . . isn't as strong as it needs to be. Many children are born this way, but your doctor knows how to make the muscle stronger and tighter so that the bump will no longer be there. To do this, he needs to do a small operation. The doctor will make a little opening here . . . [draw in on outline] . . . so that he can reach the muscle to be fixed."

PART 3. B (Continued)
PREPARATION OF A CHILD FOR HERNIORRHAPHY

DIRECTIONS	COMMENTS AND EXAMPLES
	Seven Years and Older:
	Include the description of muscles and in addition, the following:
	"For some reason we don't understand, before you were born, when the abdomen was being formed, part of the lining from inside the abdomen grew between the layers of muscles, forming two little sacs in the groin areas. The bulges on each side are caused by the intestines pressing between the layers of muscles that cover the abdomen.
	"If the intestines slip through the muscles and into the little sacs, it could cause trouble. So it has to be taken care of. Your doctor says that it's easy to fix. He's going to get rid of the sacs and then sew the muscles back into normal position."
	Boys can be told that the abdominal lining grew through the muscle layers and formed a sac(s) in the inguinal canal(s) and down into the scrotum.
	For umbilical hernia, the child can be told that part of the abdominal lining grew through the opening from which the umbilical cord passed. It formed a little sac around the navel. The bump comes from the intestines' slipping into the sac.
	Adolescents:
	Give the same explanation in sophisticated language.
3. Ask the child what he thinks may have caused the problem.	This gives another opportunity to elicit fantasy material.

PART 3. B (Continued)
PREPARATION OF A CHILD FOR HERNIORRHAPHY

DIRECTIONS	COMMENTS AND EXAMPLES
4. Reassure child that no one is to blame for his condition. Make it clear that nothing he has done or thought contributed to it.	This is especially important for the three to seven group because guilt regarding illness is a paramount feature.
5. Indicate postoperative appearance:	"After the doctor fixes the muscle, he sews the opening with little black stiches.
a. sutures or steri strips	Instead of stiches, steri strips may be used to close the skin. They're small pieces of tape placed side by side, like this.
b. bandage	[draw on outline or doll.] Over the spot he places a big bandage to keep the spot clean and to protect it."
c. intravenous infusion (not usually done for infants and toddlers)	[If appropriate] "You will also have a little tube in your arm that is attached to a bottle of sugar water. This is the way we feed children after an operation, until they are ready to eat again. This is to keep your stomach from getting upset."
6. Ascertain the child's understanding of your explanation by asking him simple questions and allowing him to place equipment on doll (bandage, IV) or to draw in answers on outline. Tell him he may ask questions at any time; in fact, many children do.	Use a doll for toddlers; a doll and outline for the three to seven group; an outline and visual aids for seven years and above. As the child permits, his own body may be used.
7. Reassure child that no other part of the body will be operated on.	Use playful repetition to clarify operative area for children under six. (See page 17.) Older children are told directly.
8. Introduce needle play related to blood work already experienced.	This is introduced at the end of the session, because it is quite stimulating for the child. We want to be sure of his at-

PART 3. B (Continued)
PREPARATION OF A CHILD FOR HERNIORRHAPHY

DIRECTIONS	COMMENTS AND EXAMPLES
	tention to the preceding material first. See Needle Play, page 198.
9. Play up rewards—how much he will have to tell his family and friends about the hospital, the new things he has seen, the many people he has met.	This allows the memory of stressful procedures to be associated with bravery and the wish for good health.
10. Turn to Part 4.	

PART 3. C
PREPARATION OF A CHILD FOR EYE SURGERY (STRABISMUS)

DIRECTIONS	COMMENTS AND EXAMPLES
1. Refer to Parts 1 and 2 before continuing.	
2. After determining the child's understanding of his condition and the reason for hospitalization, as explained in Part 2, give him a simple explanation to reinforce his ideas or to correct his misunderstanding. Introduce symptoms.	Toddlers to Young Threes: "The doctor is going to straighten your eyes." Older Threes to Seven Group: "Do you know about muscles?" [Point to arm and leg.] They are the parts of the body that allow you to move. Some muscles are large, like those in your arms and legs; there are small muscles too, like the ones that move your eyes. We know that the muscles of each eye are not working together; one eye turns in (or out) and the eyes don't line up together. And you say that you see double [if it applies]. The reason for this is that the muscles for each eye are not the same size. We don't know why this is true; some children are probably born that way. Your

PART 3. C (Continued)
PREPARATION OF A CHILD FOR EYE SURGERY
(STRABISMUS)

DIRECTIONS	COMMENTS AND EXAMPLES
	doctor knows how to fix the muscles so that they can work together."
	Seven Years and Older:
	In addition to above: "The unequal size and strength of the muscles cause a greater pull in one direction. This pull has happened to one eye (both eyes)."
3. Ask the child what he thinks may have caused the problem.	This gives another opportunity to elicit fantasy material.
4. Reassure child that no one is to blame for his condition. Make it clear that nothing he has done has contributed to it.	
5. Indicate the postoperative expectations:	Some surgeons will eliminate patches altogether.
a. bandages over one or both eyes	When both eyes are to be bandaged, it is important to arrange in advance for the continuous presence of a family member.

b. recognition of people by voice
   c. member of family or nurse will be nearby to read to him, feed him, play music, keep him safe and tell him what is going on.
   d. wrist restraints to help him remember to keep hands away from eyes (when he is not constantly attended or when he dozes)	

6. Ascertain the child's understanding of your explanation by asking simple questions and allowing him to place equipment on a doll. Indicate that you expect him to have questions and that he may ask at any time.	Familiarize the child with eye patches, restraints. Also play at recognizing voices and events in room with eyes closed.

PART 3. C <u>(Continued)</u>
PREPARATION OF A CHILD FOR EYE SURGERY (STRABISMUS)

DIRECTIONS	COMMENTS AND EXAMPLES
7. Reassure child that no other part of the body will be operated on.	Use playful repetition to clarify operative area for children under six; older children may be told directly. (See page 17.)
8. Introduce needle play regarding blood work already experienced.	This is introduced at the end of the session, because it is quite stimulating for the child. We want to be sure of his attention to the preceding material first. See Needle Play, page 198.
9. Play up rewards—how much he will have to tell his family and friends about his hospital experiences, the new things he has seen, and the new people he has met.	This allows the memory of stressful procedures to be associated with bravery and the wish for good health.
10. Turn to Part 4.	

PART 3. D
PREPARATION OF A CHILD FOR A CLOSED KIDNEY BIOPSY

DIRECTIONS	COMMENTS AND EXAMPLES
1. Refer to Parts 1 and 2 before continuing.	
2. After determining the child's fantasy regarding illness and hospitalization, as explained in Part 2, give a simple explanation of the anatomy and physiology of the urinary system, using a body outline for a child over three and a half.	Toddlers and Young Threes: "The doctor is going to do a test to find out how to make you feel better. This is the place where the test will be." (Point to area.) Continue to focus on the outside of the body and external events. Older Threes to Seven Group: "You haven't heard of the word 'kidney' before? Well, I'm not surprised; many boys and girls haven't. Let me draw them in on this picture of a boy (girl) I have brought for you. Kidneys

PART 3. D (Continued)
PREPARATION OF A CHILD FOR A CLOSED KIDNEY BIOPSY

DIRECTIONS	COMMENTS AND EXAMPLES
	are shaped like large beans, like this. [Draw kidneys in.] There are two of them. Can you guess what kidneys do? It's their job to make urine. What do you call urine—wee wee, sisy, tinkle? When urine is made, it passes along these tubes coming from the kidneys and goes into a part called the bladder, where it collects. The bladder looks like a balloon; when it's full of urine, its large. When you urinate (make wee wee) the urine comes out of the penis (or little opening between your legs), and the bladder empties."
	Seven Years and Older Group:
	Grown-up terms such as "ureters" and "urine" are used, and childish jargon and analogies are eliminated. In addition, a more scientific explanation is understood: "The work of the kidneys is to purify the blood by filtering (straining) the blood as it constantly passes through the kidneys. The kidneys hold back the parts of the blood that your body needs and allow water and waste products to pass off as urine. That's why your doctor does blood and urine tests—so he knows how well the kidneys are doing their job."
3. Introduce the child's symptoms and explain them in relation to the diagnostic procedure for the child over three and a half.	"You seem to understand how the kidneys work. Remember the reasons your doctor brought you to the hospital; for instance, fever, puffiness, elevated blood pressure. These things gave your doctor the idea that your kidneys are not working as well as they could. So the doctor wants to do a test to find out exactly what the problem is. To do this, he needs to look at a tiny part of the kidney under a micro-

PART 3. D (Continued)
PREPARATION OF A CHILD FOR A CLOSED KIDNEY BIOPSY

DIRECTIONS	COMMENTS AND EXAMPLES

	scope. (That's a machine that makes things look much bigger than they are.) Once the doctor knows how the kidneys are working, he can decide how to help you get well."
4. Ask the child what he thinks may have caused the problem.	This gives another opportunity to elicit fantasy material.
5. Reassure the child that no one is to blame for his problem; that nothing he did or thought is responsible.	

6. Explain kidney biopsy in terms of specific steps:
  a. place for test
  b. x-ray table
  c. blood pressure cuff
  d. intravenous infusion
	"You are probably wondering how this test is done. For this test, you will go to the x-ray room. Do you remember having an x-ray picture before? [Recall details; show picture of an x-ray machine.] You will be placed on the x-ray table, which has a camera overhead. All during the test a blood pressure cuff will be around one arm. On the other arm, the doctor will start an intravenous infusion—that's an IV; a small tube will be put into your arm and a bottle of sugar water will be attached to it. This tube will be in place for a few hours, even after you get back to your room."

e. personnel and attire	"Several people will be there with you; some you already know—your doctors, a nurse, and the man or woman who takes the pictures. They will be wearing caps, masks, gowns and gloves."
f. positioning	"You will be placed on the table like this—on your tummny with this small blanket roll under your belly. [Demonstrate with child on bed, placing the

PART 3. D (Continued)
PREPARATION OF A CHILD FOR A CLOSED KIDNEY BIOPSY

DIRECTIONS	COMMENTS AND EXAMPLES
	roll under the lower abdomen.] This is done to raise your hips and to make it easier for the doctor to find the right spot to do the test. Where did I say the kidneys are?"
g. draping and skin preparation	"Once you are in position, one doctor puts on gloves and cleans your skin with a special medicine on one side only and then places towels around the spot where the test is going to be done. The reason for this is to make sure everything stays clean."
h. local anesthesia	"To make sure that you do not feel the test, the doctor will put some medicine into your skin with a tiny needle. You will know this, it will feel like a pinch, but you will feel nothing after that except pressure."
i. obtaining a specimen	"Right after this the doctor is ready to take a small piece of kidney—just a tiny amount, like a grain of rice—with a special instrument that is used for this. You won't feel any hurt, but you may feel the doctor's hand pressing on your side. It's uncomfortable, but it's supposed to feel that way."
j. fluoroscopy	"While the test is going on, the x-ray man or lady will be taking pictures of your kidney. This is done to help the doctor find the best spot. In order to take these pictures, the room needs to be almost dark."
k. blood pressure readings	"While the doctors are doing the test, the nurse will be taking your blood pressure quite often. She will also be reminding you of what is going on. You may want to ask her questions."

PART 3. D (Continued)
PREPARATION OF A CHILD FOR A CLOSED KIDNEY BIOPSY

DIRECTIONS	COMMENTS AND EXAMPLES
l. bandage	"After the doctors take a tiny piece of kidney, the test is over. A small bandage will be placed over the spot to make sure it stays clean and protected."

End session here; resume after an interval.

7. Review material covered in previous session. Evaluate how much has been retained. Ask child if he has thought of any questions since you spoke to him.

8. Explain routine following the test.

"When the test is over, you will return to your own room and this is what you can expect:
a. bed rest on your back for about 24 hours (a whole day);
b. frequent taking of your blood pressure, temperature and pulse;
c. collection of all urine for 24 hours;
d. intravenous for a few hours;
e. regular meals."

9. Explain imminent events last:
a. fasting

"When you go to bed this evening, we will place a tag on your bed that says NOTHING BY MOUTH. Because you will be getting medicine before your test, we don't want you to have anything to eat or drink during the night and in the morning. This is so your stomach will not become upset."

b. preprocedure medication

"During the test it is important to stay in the position I described to you. [Remind child.] In order to help you do this and so you won't mind the test too much, we will give you some medicine to make you drowsy. It has to be given by a small needle. I'll show you how it is done on this doll later."

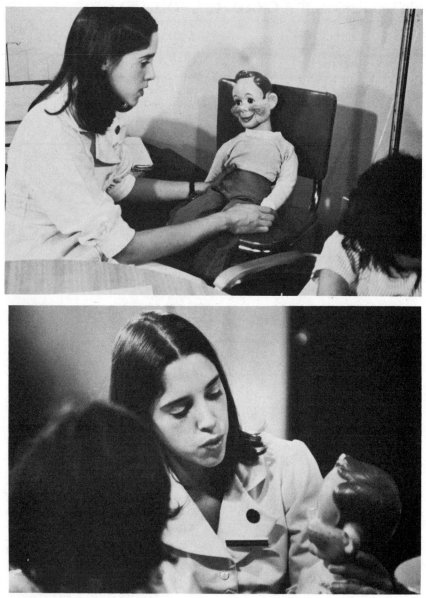

Fig. 6–3.   *Continued on opposite page.*

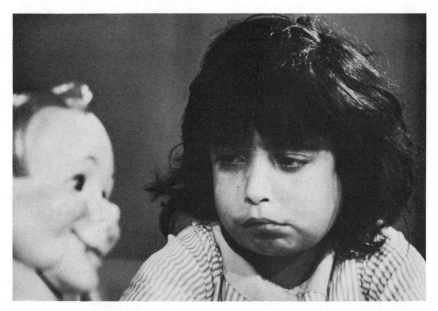

Fig. 6–3. It is helpful to depersonalize teaching when a child becomes excessively anxious or regresses during a preparation session. For this latency-age child who turns her back to the nurse, information is directed to her puppet until she feels comfortable enough to participate directly again. (From Staff Development Filmstrip Series: "Preparing a Child for Renal Transplant," Campus Films)

PART 3. D (Continued)
PREPARATION OF A CHILD FOR A CLOSED KIDNEY BIOPSY

DIRECTIONS	COMMENTS AND EXAMPLES
10. Reassure child that no other part of the body will be involved.	Use playful repetition to clarify operative area for children under six. (See page 17.) Older children may be told directly.
11. Ascertain child's understanding of your explanation by asking him simple questions in relation to the diagram or doll. Allow him to re-enact the procedure—attaching equipment, positioning doll, and taking a specimen.	Some children will not be able to verbalize answers but are able to playact or draw in answers on diagram.
12. Tell child that you will be with him during the procedure (if true) and that he will be taken in his bed (or stretcher) to the x-ray room.	This can be one of the most supportive measures we can provide. It can be managed when planned in advance.
13. Play up some of the rewards—that he will be seeing many new things and meeting many different people; that he will have a great deal to tell his family and friends about how big the x-ray machine was, how the doctors and nurses were dressed, how lights went on and off.	This allows the memory of stressful procedures to be associated with bravery and the wish for good health.
14. Introduce needle play around blood work already experienced. Demonstrate and allow practice.	This is introduced at the end of the session so that it does not distract from the preceding material. See Needle Play, page 198.
15. Next, turn to Part 5, omitting Part 4.	

PART 3. E
PREPARATION OF A CHILD FOR UROLOGIC SURGERY (REPAIR OF BLADDER–NECK OBSTRUCTION AND REIMPLANTATION OF ONE URETER)

DIRECTIONS	COMMENTS AND EXAMPLES
1. Refer to Parts 1 and 2 before continuing.	

PART 3. E (Continued)
PREPARATION OF A CHILD FOR UROLOGIC SURGERY (REPAIR OF BLADDER–NECK OBSTRUCTION AND REIMPLANTATION OF ONE URETER)

DIRECTIONS	COMMENTS AND EXAMPLES
2. After determining the child's fantasy regarding illness and hospitalization, as explained in Part 2, give him a simple explanation of the anatomy and physiology involved.	See explanation under Kidney Biopsy, page 245.
3. Introduce symptoms in relation to anatomy for those children above three and a half, using a body outline.	"You have already told me that you came to the hospital because of fevers and trouble making urine. There's a reason for this. I've told you how the kidneys, ureters (tubes) and bladder look and work. [Refer to drawing.] This is the way it's supposed to be, but for some reason we don't understand, yours looks like this. This part of the bladder has a very small opening, so the urine (wee wee) cannot pass out easily; and this ureter (tube) is attached to the bladder higher up than it should be (or has a narrow part). It makes it hard for the urine to flow out. This is why sometimes the urine backs up, presses on the kidney, hurts, or causes fever. We know this because of the tests you have had (IVP, cystogram) and by the way you have been feeling."
4. When symptoms are absent, modify the approach.	"Although you haven't felt sick, the doctor knows that your kidneys, ureters and bladder are not working as they should because of the tests he has done and the examination he gave you in his office (clinic). He took your blood pressure, made x-ray pictures and did urine tests. The doctor knows that if this problem is not taken care of now, you may be sick later on."

PART 3. E (Continued)
PREPARATION OF A CHILD FOR UROLOGIC SURGERY (REPAIR OF BLADDER–NECK OBSTRUCTION AND REIMPLANTATION OF ONE URETER)

DIRECTIONS	COMMENTS AND EXAMPLES
5. Ask the child what he thinks may have caused the problem.	This gives another opportunity to elicit fantasy material.
6. Reassure the child that no one is to blame for his condition, and that nothing he has done or thought contributed to it.	"We don't know why this is so. It's the way some people are born. No one's to blame. It's certainly not because of anything you have done. But your doctor knows how to fix the parts—to make both these parts bigger so that the urine can pass through without any trouble. That's why you are going to have an operation." Avoid specific details of the operative procedure. "The doctor will make an opening here so that he can reach the parts to be fixed." Draw in on diagram or doll.
7. Indicate postoperative appearance on drawing for child over three and a half. For child under three and a half, talk about external appearance on doll: a. urinary drainage tubing and collection bags	"After the doctor fixes the tube and bladder, he wants the parts to rest so that they will heal (get better) fast. To help do that, he puts in tubes in three parts. They are placed like this: one high in the ureter, one in the ureter lower down, and one in the bladder. [Draw in.] This means that the urine will drain off without touching the parts that have been fixed." "You won't be urinating (making wee wee) for a while. The urine will pass through the tubes into collection bags. [Draw in.] At first the urine looks dark, then it becomes pink and finally yellow again. Sometimes you may feel like passing urine, but you won't NEED to."
b. sutures c. bandage	"After the drainage tubes are in, the doctor closes the opening with little

PART 3. E (Continued)
PREPARATION OF A CHILD FOR UROLOGIC SURGERY
(REPAIR OF BLADDER–NECK OBSTRUCTION AND
REIMPLANTATION OF ONE URETER)

DIRECTIONS	COMMENTS AND EXAMPLES
	stitches and then places a large bandage over the spot. After the parts get better (heal), the doctor will take out the tubes, probably one at a time. Later he will take out stitches. We will show you how when it's about to happen."
d. intravenous infusion	"After your operation, you won't be eating or drinking right away. We don't want to upset your stomach. So, instead of feeding you, we will give you sugar water through a tube in your arm. [Draw in.] When you are ready to start eating again, we will start by giving you sips of water and juice first."
e. croupette or oxygen tent.	"Very often after operations, we place children in small plastic tents. You have probably seen them already. This helps them to breathe well and to keep cool. You will have one too." [Show child a croupette or model of one.]
8. Ascertain child's understanding of your explanation by asking simple questions regarding the drawing. Help him attach IV equipment, tubes, bandages to doll.	Some children will not be able to verbalize answers to questions but may be able to point to or draw in answers on a diagram or playact their understanding.
9. Reassure child that no other part of the body will be operated on.	Use playful repetition to clarify operative area for child under six. Older child may be told directly.
10. Play up rewards—that he will be seeing many new things and meeting different people; that he will have a great deal to tell his friends and family about the operation; that he will be able to explain it all with his diagram or doll.	This allows the memory of stressful procedures to be associated with bravery and the wish for good health.

PART 3. E (Continued)
PREPARATION OF A CHILD FOR UROLOGIC SURGERY (REPAIR OF BLADDER–NECK OBSTRUCTION AND REIMPLANTATION OF ONE URETER)

DIRECTIONS	COMMENTS AND EXAMPLES
11. Introduce needle play regarding blood work already experienced. Demonstrate and allow practice.	This is introduced at the end of the session so that it does not distract from the preceding material. See Needle Play, page 198.
12. Continue with Part 4 after an interval.	

PART 3. F
PREPARATION OF A CHILD FOR CARDIAC CATHETERIZATION

DIRECTIONS	COMMENTS
1. Refer to Parts 1 and 2 before continuing.	
2. After determining child's understanding of hospitalization, as explained in part 2, clarify or reinforce his understanding by discussing tests and visits to the cardiologist that may have occurred in the past—relating these to his present admission.	Most of these children have had either ECGs and chest x-ray pictures, or may remember the doctor listening to the chest and heart. Some may have overheard adults talking about them and consequently have more knowledge than parents believe.
3. If the child has symptoms, explain that they are indications that to the doctor that his heart may not be working as well as it could.	
4. Ask child what he thinks may have caused the problem.	This gives another opportunity to elicit fantasy material.
5. Reassure child that no one is responsible for his condition; that nothing he did or thought is responsible. Make it clear.	

PART 3. F (Continued)
PREPARATION OF A CHILD FOR CARDIAC CATHETERIZATION

DIRECTIONS	COMMENTS
6. If a child is asymptomatic, discuss with him how the doctor became aware that his heart might not be working as well as it should.	For example, tell the child that the doctor listened to his chest and heard a murmur. Allow him to use a stethoscope.
7. Explain to child that he needs to have a special test and pictures of his heart so that the doctor can discover what the problem is and also how to treat it.	
8. Explain that he will be taken to a special place called the cardiac catheterization room.	
9. Describe how people will be dressed.	
10. Explain that he will be lying on a movable table and that ECG leads will be placed on his arms and legs.	Recall other experiences with ECGs.
11. Tell child that his arms and legs will be loosely restrained.	"The loose ties around your arms and legs help you to remember to keep them in one place, so that you won't move about."
12. Explain that a nurse will insert a rectal thermometer and will leave it in place throughout the test, so that she will know his temperature.	
13. Explain that the doctor will wash the arm or groin and put some medicine into the skin with a small needle. It will feel like a pinch, but thereafter he will not feel any pain (hurt). After the medicine, the doctor will make a small opening and insert a tiny tube. Later he may use stitches to close the small opening. End session here. Resume after an interval.	Use a patient doll for toddlers, a doll and outline for three-and-a-half- to six-year-olds, and an outline and visual aids for older children to indicate the place where the tube will be inserted.

PART 3. F (Continued)
PREPARATION OF A CHILD FOR CARDIAC
CATHETERIZATION

DIRECTIONS	COMMENTS
14. Ask child simple questions to ascertain his understanding of the preceding material. Correct as necessary.	
15. Describe atmosphere: a. noise and talk	"One machine will be making a humming sound all during the test." "Some machines make clicking sounds." "People talk all the time—mostly about their work." "Sometimes the doctor will ask you questions." "Sometimes you will ask questions." "Sometimes the nurse will remind you of things you have been told." "You will hear doors opening and closing throughout the test."
b. lights	"After the doctor takes pictures of the heart, he needs to turn out the lights. It won't be completely dark. During the test lights are turned on and off."
16. Describe the angiogram—at least one is done for all patients.	"In this test, medicine . . . [avoid the word "dye"] . . . is put through the tube in your arm or groin; then many pictures are taken quickly. The clack-clack sounds you will hear are the pictures falling into a box. Children often wonder what is going on." "The nurse will tell you when it's about to happen. During this time all the people in the room will step out into the hallway." "You will know when the medicine is used because you will get a warm

PART 3. F (Continued)
PREPARATION OF A CHILD FOR CARDIAC CATHETERIZATION

DIRECTIONS	COMMENTS
	feeling in your chest that goes away quickly. It's supposed to feel like that. The special medicine allows the heart to show up on the film."
	"After these pictures are taken, everyone comes back into the room."
17. Describe the Hydrogen Test. If a septal defect is suspected, anticipate that this test will be done.	"The nurse will hold a mask over your nose and mouth for a second to give you a puff of air. You will hear a sound like sh, sh."
18. Describe the end of the test—suturing and dressing.	"When the tests are over, the doctor removes the tube from your arm or groin. He may need to put little stitches in to close the opening. Maybe they won't be needed. Then he will place a bandage over the spot."
19. Tell child that he will be transported to another room for one last set of pictures before returning to his room.	This is done if KUB x-ray pictures are needed to determine any GU anomalies since medication is already present in the system.
20. Describe routine for child after he returns to unit: a. bed rest for 4 hours or longer b. force fluids to help get rid of medicine c. T, BPs, apical pulses d. radial or pedal pulses e. regular dressing when vein has been used or pressure dressing when artery has been used End session here. Resume after an interval.	
21. Ask child simple questions to ascertain his understanding of the preceding material.	
22. Tell child about preparation for test:	

PART 3. F (Continued)
PREPARATION OF A CHILD FOR CARDIAC CATHETERIZATION

DIRECTIONS	COMMENTS
a. tag on bed the night before the test	"The NOTHING BY MOUTH tag means you won't be having anything to eat or drink after you go to bed; you won't have breakfast either. This is done to make sure your stomach will not be upset when you get medicines."
b. transportation to catheterization room—he will be taken in his bed or stretcher. (If you are to accompany him, tell him so; if not, tell him that a nurse will be with him during the procedure.)	
c. preprocedure medications. Demonstrate needle play and allow participation.	"Before your test, we will give you medicines so that you will become sleepy and won't mind the long test (approximately three hours). You may want to sleep most of the time; it's all right to do so." This information is given at the end of the session. Otherwise, the child may become excited so that previous information may not be heard. See Needle Play, page 198.
23. Remind child that after the small needle prick to insert tube, he will not feel any hurt. Convey to child that whoever hurts him is sorry though they may not have time to tell him so.	
24. Reassure child that no other part of the body will be tested or worked on.	Use playful repetition to clarify operative site for child under six. (See page 17.) Reassure older child directly.
25. Give permission to ask questions at any time and to discuss areas you might have missed, if any.	

PART 3. F (Continued)
PREPARATION OF A CHILD FOR CARDIAC CATHETERIZATION

DIRECTIONS	COMMENTS
26. Play up rewards—that he will be able to talk to his family and friends about this exciting event; that he will see new things and meet many people.	This allows the memory of stressful procedures to be associated with bravery and the wish for good health.
27. Ascertain the child's understanding of your explanations by asking him simple questions in relation to body outline or doll and allowing him to attach ECG leads, restraints, catheter to doll.	Some children will not be able to verbalize answers to questions but may be able to draw responses on the body outline or to point to appropriate areas.
28. Give another opportunity for needle play.	
29. Turn to Part 5, omitting Part 4.	

Note: General anesthesia is used only in cases of severe aortic stenosis when a left ventricular puncture is necessary. In such a case, prepare the child for anesthesia. See part 4.

PART 3. G
PREPARATION OF A CHILD FOR CARDIAC SURGERY (REPAIR OF VENTRICULAR SEPTAL DEFECT)

DIRECTIONS	COMMENTS AND EXAMPLES
1. Refer to Parts 1 and 2 before continuing.	
2. After determining the child's fantasy regarding illness and hospitalization, as explained in Part 2, give him a simple explanation of the anatomy and physiology of the cardiac system. Introduce symptoms and attempt to relate them to his problem. Use a body outline for the child over three and a half.	For Toddlers and Young Threes: "The doctor is going to fix your heart." Older Threes to Seven Group: "The heart is in the middle of your chest. Its job is to send blood around the body, taking food and nourishment to make you grow and stay strong. In your heart, you have a little hole that doesn't belong there. It makes more work for the heart. We

PART 3. G (Continued)
PREPARATION OF A CHILD FOR CARDIAC SURGERY
(REPAIR OF VENTRICULAR SEPTAL DEFECT)

DIRECTIONS	COMMENTS AND EXAMPLES
	don't know why; you were born that way. Your doctor knows how to sew up the hole so it will not cause you any trouble."
	Seven Years and Older: Give same explanation as for older threes to seven group. In addition, use model and/or diagram of the heart.
3. If symptoms are absent, modify the approach.	"Although you haven't felt sick, we know that if your heart isn't fixed, it will give you trouble later on. We are going to take care of it now, so that you will continue to grow well."
4. Ask the child what he thinks may have caused the problem.	This gives another opportunity to elicit fantasy material.
5. Reassure the child that no one is to blame for his condition. Make it clear that nothing he did or thought is responsible.	
6. Indicate operative site and post-operative appearance. a. incision	"This is where the doctor will make an opening in your chest (either lateral or midline). Then he can sew up the hole in your heart." Draw incision on body outline or doll.
b. chest tube, sutures and band-age	"After your operation, there will be a tube coming from your chest to drain off old blood and air. The tube will be connected to a bag by the bedside. In about a day or so, the doctor will remove this tube because you won't need it any more. There will also be little black stitches that are used to close the opening. A large bandage on top will keep everything safe and clean."

PART 3. G (Continued)
PREPARATION OF A CHILD FOR CARDIAC SURGERY (REPAIR OF VENTRICULAR SEPTAL DEFECT)

DIRECTIONS	COMMENTS AND EXAMPLES
c. pacemaker (if anticipated by catheterization data)	"You may find after the operation that a tiny wire has been placed under the skin where the doctor makes the opening. This wire is attached to a small box that looks like a pocket radio. It is used to regulate the heartbeat—to make sure that the heart beats as fast as it should. We won't be able to tell you now how long you will need this box, but we will let you know later." Show him a pacemaker.
d. Foley catheter	"The bladder is the place where urine (wee wee) stays. When the bladder is full, you feel like urinating (making wee wee) and the urine comes out of the penis (or the little opening between the legs). [Draw in bladder on outline.] After the operation you will have a small tube going into the bladder to drain off the urine so that we know how much urine is made. This means that you won't need to urinate. Before long, this tube will come out and you will urinate just as you do now." [Draw on body outline.]
e. nasogastric tube (if used)	"When you wake up, there will be a small tube going from your nose into your stomach (tummy). This will keep your stomach empty and it will also keep your stomach from being upset. It may be uncomfortable."
f. intravenous infusions, usually two; one may be a cutdown	"Because you won't be able to eat for a while, you will have a tube going into your arm and leg. Through the tubes we can give you sugar water and medicines until you are allowed to eat again."

PART 3. G (Continued)
PREPARATION OF A CHILD FOR CARDIAC SURGERY
(REPAIR OF VENTRICULAR SEPTAL DEFECT)

DIRECTIONS	COMMENTS AND EXAMPLES
g. ECG leads and monitors	"Do you remember having a picture of your heartbeat (electrocardiogram)? When the operation is over, the doctor and nurses will want to watch your heartbeat for a while; so you will be wearing those sponge rubber disks and wires on your arms and legs. However, instead of watching the heartbeat on a strip of paper, they will watch it on a TV screen, like this." Show patient a monitor.
h. endotracheal tube and Pressure/Volume Control Respirator	"When you wake up, there will be a tube in your mouth to help you breathe deeply. The tube will be held in place by tape so that you won't be able to talk to us, but we will talk to you and you will hear us. If you want to tell us something, your nurse will give you pencil and paper to write notes. [Younger children may point to pictures.] We know that having this tube in your throat will be uncomfortable, but you will be sleeping most of the first day and night. Usually the tube can be taken out the day after your operation."
7. Ask child simple questions to help him recall what you have told him and assist him in placing equipment on his doll (to visualize postoperative appearance) and to draw in responses on a body outline.	For complex surgery, the use of a doll is recommended, even for children over seven, but call it a dummy. Continue to use a body outline in conjunction with the doll for patients over three and a half.
8. Reassure child that no other part of the body will be operated on.	Use playful repetition to clarify operative area for the children under six. (See page 17.) Reassure older child directly.
9. Introduce needle play related to blood work already experienced. Demonstrate and allow participation. See Needle Play, page 198.	This is introduced at the end of a session because it is quite exciting for the child. Preceding material may not be heard otherwise.

PART 3. G (<u>Continued</u>)
PREPARATION OF A CHILD FOR CARDIAC SURGERY
(REPAIR OF VENTRICULAR SEPTAL DEFECT)

DIRECTIONS	COMMENTS AND EXAMPLES
10. Play up rewards. Tell the child that he will be able to talk to his family and friends about this exciting event—about the new things he will see and do, and the people he will meet. Tell him that everyone will be surprised to hear about his hospitalization. Indicate that he will be able to show them how it was done on his patient doll.	This allows the memory of stressful procedures to be associated with bravery and the wish for good health.
11. End session here. Resume after an interval. Order blow bottles or incentive spirometer so that they will be available for practice at the next teaching session.	
12. Ask the child simple questions to ascertain his understanding of the preceding material. Correct as necessary.	
13. Introduce the croupette for the under-four group.	"About a day or two after the operation, the tube that helps you to breathe deeply will be taken out of your mouth. When this happens, your nurse will place a plastic tent over your bed or a plastic piece around your face. A vaporizer will pump cool air and moisture into the tent to help you breathe well and to make you more comfortable. The room will look misty (foggy)."
14. Introduce mistifier.	Show the child a croupette or face tent.
15. Introduce blow bottles or incentive spirometer.	"We will want you to breathe deeply and to cough up mucus (phlegm), the way you do when you have a cold. This is hard to do all by yourself. So we give you help to do it." Allow ample time for practice. Tell child that he may be asked to blow up balloons or blow bubbles instead.

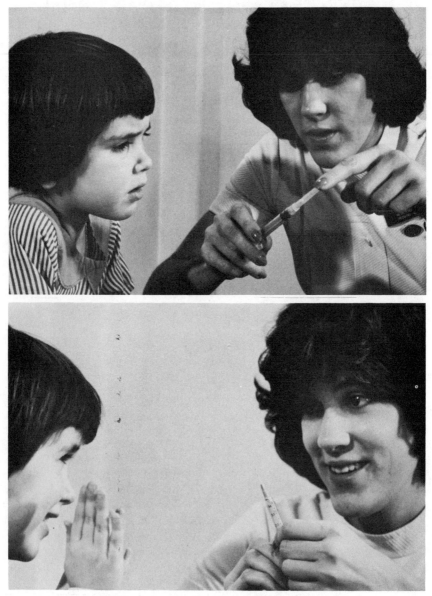

Fig. 6–4. *Continued on opposite page.*

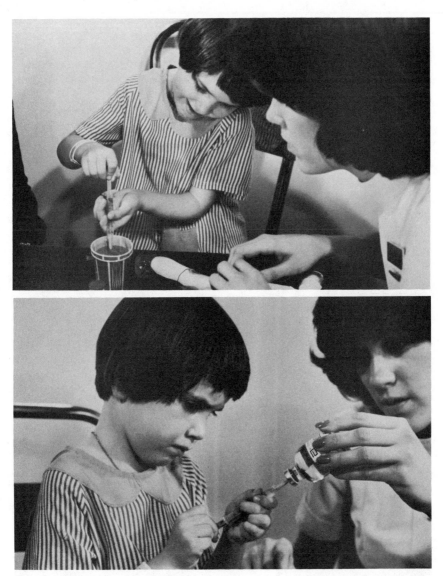

Fig. 6–4. Needle play is introduced at the close of a teaching session because it is an exciting experience. Preceding material may not be heard otherwise. Here a nurse demonstrates giving an injection to a dummy. The child's attention is engaged by the squirting of a bit of water into the air. This playful behavior is fascinating to the child and helps her to discover the painless aspects of injections. Then strict attention to the actual technique involves the child in the procedure and makes her less fearful of the equipment. Note the intensity of the child's involvement. (From Staff Development Filmstrip Series: "Needle Play," Campus Films)

PART 3. G (Continued)
PREPARATION OF A CHILD FOR CARDIAC SURGERY
(REPAIR OF VENTRICULAR SEPTAL DEFECT)

DIRECTIONS	COMMENTS AND EXAMPLES
16. Introduce suctioning.	"Sometimes it is very difficult to get up the mucus (phlegm). This little tube goes down into the throat and pulls it up. It isn't so pleasant, but afterward you will feel a lot better." Show him a suction machine or a model.
17. Explain turning and coughing, splinting, cupping, vibrating and deep breathing. Demonstrate with patient. This is difficult for the child to learn, but staff in the Intensive Care Unit must have his cooperation.	"Because we know that it will be hard for you to cough after your operation, there are other ways in which your nurse will help you. She will place a pillow on your chest or hold your chest with her hands, so that it won't hurt you so much," etc. Demonstrate this. Does

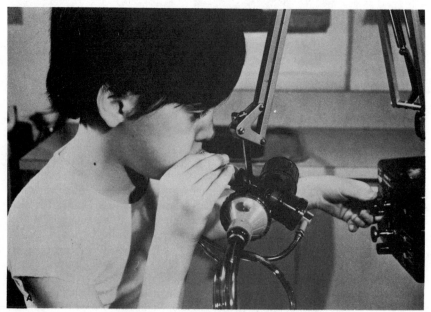

Fig. 6–5.   *Continued on opposite page.*

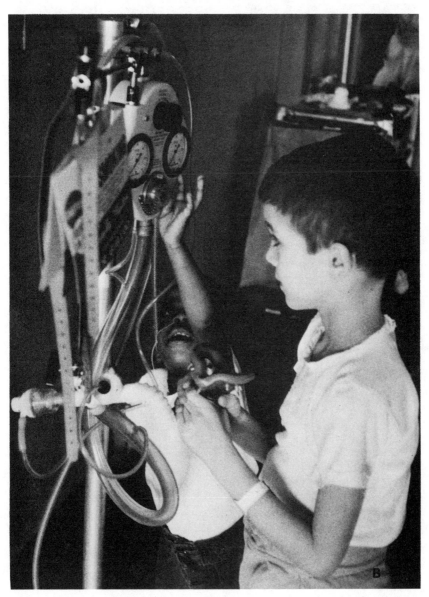

Fig. 6–5. When intricate and ominous equipment is introduced before it is actually needed, the child is more cooperative and less likely to become anxious. (Photos 6–4 A by Steve Campus, photo 6–4 B by Hilary Smith)

PART 3. G (Continued)
PREPARATION OF A CHILD FOR CARDIAC SURGERY (REPAIR OF VENTRICULAR SEPTAL DEFECT)

DIRECTIONS	COMMENTS AND EXAMPLES
	the patient understand what is expected by: 1) take a deep breath? 2) cough? 3) cough up the mucus?
Introduce Bennett or Bird respirator (if used).	IPPB is used in selected cases.
18. Explain to the child that he will feel some pain (hurt) but that the nurses and doctors know how to take care of it with medicine.	"You may find it hard to keep from getting angry, but the nurses and doctors will appreciate your help. They know it isn't easy."
19. Explain that the room where he will be staying after the operation is usually a very noisy place; there is a great deal of activity and many people will visit him there, sometimes all at once.	
20. Inform the child that he will be weighed daily (nude) on a stretcher scale. Show him the scale if this is a routine.	Some children will resist getting onto the stretcher scale, believing that they are going to the operating room again, if it is not explained in advance.
21. Place the child's teaching tools—doll, body outline and other play materials—in a bag and secure to end of bed so that staff in the ICU will have these articles to help them care for the child.	
22. Turn to Part 4.	

PART 3. H
PREPARATION OF A CHILD FOR BRAIN SURGERY

DIRECTIONS	COMMENTS AND EXAMPLES
1. Refer to Parts 1 and 2 before continuing.	

PART 3. H (Continued)
PREPARATION OF A CHILD FOR BRAIN SURGERY

DIRECTIONS	COMMENTS AND EXAMPLES
2. After determining the child's fantasy regarding hospitalization, illness, as explained in Part 2, and his concept of the brain, give a simple explanation of the anatomy and physiology involved. Introduce symptoms and refer to diagnostic testing.	Because many children react unfavorably to discussion of treatment of the brain, it is advantageous to refer to the affected areas as "nerve areas" and "inside the head."

<u>Toddlers and Young Threes:</u>
"The doctor knows how to make you feel better; to take away (whatever symptoms the child demonstrates). He is going to do an operation here . . . [indicate on doll] . . . to fix what is making you sick."

<u>Older Threes to Seven Group:</u>
"You've had a great many tests lately (body scanning, x-ray pictures, pneumoencephalogram, electroencephalogram, spinal tap). By doing these tests, your doctor has found out what has been making you sick—why you have had movement of the eyes, difficulty seeing, walking and standing, speech problems or headaches and vomiting" (whatever applies).

"The tests and the way you have been feeling tell your doctor that there is a small lump (growth) in your head that is pressing on some nerves (or a collection of fluid that is pressing on nerves). There are different kinds of nerves; some have to do with seeing, talking, hearing, smelling, swallowing. The growth he has found has been pressing on your _____ nerves. That's why your doctor has decided to do an operation to get rid of the growth (or fluid). This is where the operation is done, right here." Show on outline.

<u>Seven Years and Older:</u>
A variation of the above. "As the growth gets larger, it causes pressure and irritates the nerves that control

PART 3. H (Continued)
PREPARATION OF A CHILD FOR BRAIN SURGERY

DIRECTIONS	COMMENTS AND EXAMPLES
	sight, hearing, walking. Your problems tell us which nerves are affected. That's why your doctor has decided to remove the growth."
	When symptoms are due to obstruction to the flow fo cerebrospinal fluid— "The growth is blocking the movement of fluid that constantly flows around brain and spinal cord. [Draw on outline.] When this happens, pressure builds up and makes you feel uncomfortable and sick. That's why you have been irritable and tired, have been vomiting, have had difficulty with sight. [Say whatever applies.] The doctor can remove the growth that is causing the blockage. That's why you are having the operation."
3. Ask the child what he thinks may have caused the problem.	This gives another opportunity to elicit fantasy material.
4. Reassure him that nothing he did or thought is responsible, that no one is to blame.	
5. Explain area of incision and preparation of operative site.	For cerebral lesions the operative site is frontal behind the hairline; for cerebellar and brain stem lesions the incision is occipital.
	"In order to do the operation, a part of your head needs to be shaved— just the section where the doctor makes the opening." [Children over seven can be told that a bone wedge is removed so that the doctor can reach the affected part and that the bone is saved.] "After the hair grows in, the opening (incision) will no longer be noticeable. In the meantime, we

PART 3. H (Continued)
PREPARATION OF A CHILD FOR BRAIN SURGERY

DIRECTIONS	COMMENTS AND EXAMPLES
	can arrange your hair to cover the spot . . . [if hair is long enough] . . . or you may want to wear a scarf, a wig, or a cap."
6. Describe postoperative appearance and expectations:	
a. sutures	"When the operation is over, the doctor closes the opening with black stitches (or other materials) or the doctor replaces the bone to cover the spot so that it will be just as it was."
b. bandage	"Then he winds a large bandage around your head. It will be very large and feel like a pillow for resting your head. It might look like a turban or a helmet."
c. positioning of bed	"You might notice that your bed is turned around so that the head is at the foot. It will make it easier to take care of you this way."
d. positioning in bed and turning	"We will place you in bed according to the doctor's directions—flat and on your (unaffected) side—and we will turn you often."
e. suctioning	"Because it is quite hard to cough up mucus (phlegm) when you are flat in bed, we will help you do it. We have a little tube that goes down into the throat and pulls the mucus out. It's not too pleasant while it is being done. You might feel like gagging, but afterward you will feel a lot better. It will help you breathe easier. Whoever does this knows how hard it is to bear, and she is sorry there's no easier way." Show child a suction machine.

PART 3. H (Continued)
PREPARATION OF A CHILD FOR BRAIN SURGERY

DIRECTIONS	COMMENTS AND EXAMPLES
f. vital signs	"Your nurses will take your temperature, pulse and blood pressure often. This is supposed to happen. These things tell us what needs to be done for you; for example, you may feel very warm, and we will need to make you feel cooler."
g. croupette or oxygen tent	"One of the ways we use to make you feel cooler is to place you in a plastic tent after the operation. A vaporizer will pump cool air and moisture into the tent. This is also used to help you breathe better and to make you more comfortable. I'll show you what the tent is like."
h. intravenous infusion	"For a while after the operation, you won't feel like eating or drinking. We know how to take care of you so that you will get the food and water you need to keep strong. The doctor places a tube in your vein (of arm or leg); it is connected to a bottle of sugar water. Your arm or leg will be placed on a small board to help you keep it from moving about."
i. elbow restraints and side rails	"Sometimes it is hard to remember not to touch the bandage on the head or to keep your arm still. If it is necessary, we will place loose ties around your arms and legs to help you remember. [Do not imply punishment.] We will have side rails on your bed so that you will feel safe."
j. edema and discoloration (In cases of frontal incision, prepare the child and family for the likely possibility of head and facial edema—especially swelling of the eyelids—and	"Sometimes after this kind of operation there is swelling around the head, face and eyes. And the skin around the eyes may turn black-and-blue. This may not happen, but I'm telling you now so that you won't think it is unusual.

PART 3. H (Continued)
PREPARATION OF A CHILD FOR BRAIN SURGERY

DIRECTIONS	COMMENTS AND EXAMPLES
discoloration around the eyes —ecchymoses.)	If it does occur, it will disappear in a week or two. We can use ice around the face to make you feel more comfortable."
k. ventricular catheter	Explain the possibility of a ventricular catheter to the family. "Sometimes after surgery, a small tube (catheter) is placed within the brain for a few days to drain off excess fluid. This prevents the buildup of pressure. The fluid is collected in a bottle attached to the head of the bed. If it is used, you will see it right away. We don't know definitely now. We can tell your child postoperatively, if necessary."
l. tracheostomy (In cases of routine tracheostomy, prepare child in advance.)	In surgery involving the area of the brain stem, pressure on the respiratory center is anticipated. Some surgeons will routinely perform a tracheostomy. Tell the child and his family, "For this type of operation, we will do a procedure to make breathing easier. It is called a tracheostomy. A small opening is made into the windpipe (trachea). The opening can be seen on the neck. A tube will be inserted to keep the opening from blocking off. We will show you later how to hold your finger over the tube when you want to speak. If you forget to cover it, no sound will come out when you speak." Reintroduce suctioning.
7. Reassure child and family of the surgeon's and staff's skill in managing this type of problem; that it has been done many times.	This type of surgery is highly threatening to the child and family; they will need continuous support.

PART 3. H (Continued)
PREPARATION OF A CHILD FOR BRAIN SURGERY

DIRECTIONS	COMMENTS AND EXAMPLES
8. When a child appears stuporous or uncomprehending, caution family to refrain from discussing his condition in his presence. Direct them to explain activities and events as though he understands.	Frequently a child who is apparently comatose will hear and comprehend what is said although he gives no clue.
9. Set up signals for the nonverbal child to indicate yes and no, and to represent his needs. Inform staff and family of communication system.	
10. Reassure child that no other part of the body will be operated on.	Use playful repetition to clarify operative site for the child under 6. (See page 17.) Reassure older child directly.
11. Ask the child simple questions to ascertain his understanding of your teaching. Help him draw in answers on the body outline. Help young children attach equipment to a doll.	
12. Play up rewards—how much he will have to tell his family and friends about the hospital, about the new things he has seen, and about the different people he has met.	This allows the memory of stressful procedures to be associated with bravery and the wish for good health.
13. Turn to Part 4. Before continuing, determine whether preoperative sedation is to be used. Central nervous system depressants are ordinarily eliminated before brain surgery.	

Note: Because the performance of a ventriculogram requires the use of general anesthesia, surgery will follow directly when there is evidence of brain tumor. When surgery is dependent on the results of this diagnostic procedure, the family and child must be prepared in advance.

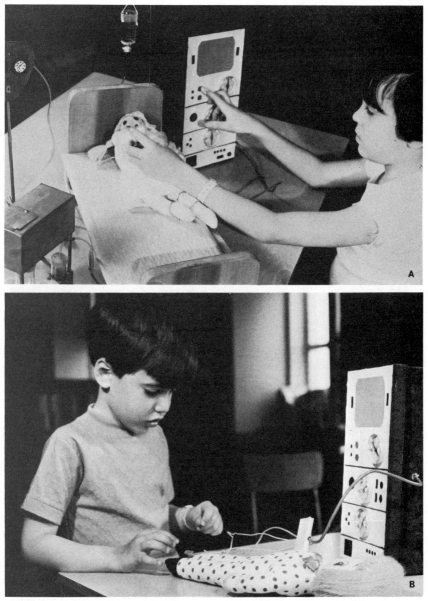

Fig. 6-6. The child learns that he will be required to cooperate with treatments that necessitate physical restraint and discomfort. Talking about how the puppets feel helps the child cope with the prolonged ordeal. (Photos by Steve Campus)

277

PART 3. I
PREPARATION OF A CHILD FOR AMPUTATION (HIP DISARTICULATION FOR TREATMENT OF MALIGNANCY)

DIRECTIONS	COMMENTS AND EXAMPLES
1. Accompany parents and physician when child is told about amputation. Be available to child and family.	It is important to be present in order to clarify information later and to be supportive to child/family. Wait at least two hours before beginning preparation. This will give child time to recover from the initial shock. Preparation is most effective when it is started 48 hours before surgery.
2. Consult with surgeon and physical therapist on rehabilitation plan.	
3. Refer to Parts 1 and 2 before continuing.	In addition to equipment needed, as listed in Part 2, include a second age-appropriate body outline on which you have obliterated the area to be amputated, using typing correction fluid. Eliminate this step for under three and a half group. For patients ages two to ten years (approximately), prepare a dummy with amputated part. Stitch area to prevent loss of stuffing.
After determining the child's understanding for hospitalization as explained in Part 2, give him a simple explanation to reinforce his knowledge or to correct misunderstanding. Introduce symptoms.	Draw in femur on first body outline and explain. For example, "I'm drawing in the bone that is affected—the femur. The tests you've had show a growth about here. The biopsy (examination of the growth) shows that this type (of growth, tumor, cells, or lump) will spread to other parts of the body and cause more trouble if it is not removed. Since the leg is already involved, it must be removed." AVOID telling patient he will die if tumor spreads. Child will remember this if metastasis occurs. Metastasis does not rule out treatment.
4. Ask child what he thinks may have caused his illness.	This gives another opportunity to elicit fantasy material.

PART 3. I (Continued)
PREPARATION OF A CHILD FOR AMPUTATION (HIP DISARTICULATION FOR TREATMENT OF MALIGNANCY)

DIRECTIONS	COMMENTS AND EXAMPLES
5. Reassure him that no one is to blame, that nothing he did or thought is responsible.	
6. Help child express his fears and concerns.	For example, "Many boys and girls have told me that they wonder what it will be like afterward. You probably have been wondering too. What have you thought about?" Expect tears and great emotional upset. Encourage talking at same time. Do not change the subject.
7. Tell child that his doctor has thought about the treatment he needs for a long time, and he is planning an amputation because it is the best kind of treatment for his problem.	Tell child that his doctor and nurses know how hard this is to accept.
8. Indicate postoperative expectations and appearance on body outline with obliterated limb.	
a. sutures	"After the leg is removed the doctor sews the area with many stitches." (Draw in on outline).
b. hemovac	"The doctor expects that there will be a great deal of swelling around the hip after the amputation. That's why he stitches in a small tube to help drain it. Fluid drains from the tube into the plastic box attached to it. The fluid is quite red; it's supposed to be." If patient asks if it's blood, tell him that it's old blood that needs to come out after the operation. (Draw in hemovac.)
c. large bandage	"You will feel a large bandage in place. It will help keep the area clean and comfortable." (Draw in.)

PART 3. I (Continued)
PREPARATION OF A CHILD FOR AMPUTATION (HIP DISARTICULATION FOR TREATMENT OF MALIGNANCY)

DIRECTIONS	COMMENTS AND EXAMPLES
d. foot of bed elevated	"You will notice that the foot of your bed is raised. We find that this helps keep down the swelling in the hip."
e. edema of scrotum and penis or vulva in girls	"It's not unusual to find that the areas around the hip become swollen also. This might happen to the scrotum and penis (vulva), too. It disappears in a few days."
f. Foley catheter	"After the operation, you may have a small tube in your bladder to drain off urine. You won't need to use the bedpan (or urinal) to urinate (do pee pee). It's more comfortable this way. When the tube is removed, you will urinate again."
g. IVs	"You won't feel like eating or drinking right away, so we give you the food you need from a bottle of sugar water attached to a tube that goes into your arm. You may have more than one IV."
h. trapeze	"A frame will be placed over your bed from which a short bar will be suspended. When this trapeze is in place, you will be able to use it to pull yourself up in bed or to turn from side to side."
i. phantom limb/pain	"After the operation, you may feel that the leg is still in place or that you have the sensation of pain in that area. It doesn't always happen, but you should know its not unusual."
9. Ascertain the child's understanding by asking simple questions related to body outline and inserted drawings. Indicate that you expect him to have questions and that he may ask at any time.	Young children are asked to answer questions by placing equipment such as hemovac, bandage and IVs on the doll with severed limb.

PART 3. I (Continued)
PREPARATION OF A CHILD FOR AMPUTATION (HIP DISARTICULATION FOR TREATMENT OF MALIGNANCY)

DIRECTIONS	COMMENTS AND EXAMPLES
10. Determine whether child knows what part of body will be operated on, especially for under-six group.	Reassure that no other part will be affected. Use playful repetition to clarify operative area for children under six. See page 17.
11. Introduce needle play for children under eight to ten years.	This is introduced at the end of the session to prevent distraction.
12. Ask child which of his friends and family he will tell about surgery.	If child declines to talk about his experiences, tell him he may change his mind later. Talking about his experiences helps to relieve anxiety and allows the memory of stressful events to be associated with bravery and the wish for good results.
13. Turn to Part 4.	

PART 3. J
TEACHING A CHILD ABOUT LEUKEMIA

DIRECTIONS	COMMENTS AND EXAMPLES
1. Refer to Parts 1 and 2 before continuing.	
2. Arrange a conference with parent(s) to discuss teaching of child, so that the material to be covered will not come as a surprise.	This will also give an opportunity to discuss the family's reaction to the illness and their coping ability; discipline for the sick child; and explanation of illness to siblings.
3. Begin teaching by reviewing with child his hospital experiences.	For 6- to 12-year-olds For example, "Your parents and I have been talking about the things that

Adapted from STAFF DEVELOPMENT SERIES: "Teaching a Child About Leukemia," (M. Petrillo). Campus Film Distributors

PART 3. J (Continued)
TEACHING A CHILD ABOUT LEUKEMIA

DIRECTIONS	COMMENTS AND EXAMPLES
	have been happening to you in the past few days. We think you need more explanations about your illness."
	"We explained the tests to you as we did them, but there is more to tell. Which tests do you remember?"
	Child may recall bone marrow aspiration, spinal tap and blood work. If not, ask parent or help child to talk about what he does remember.
4. Let child know that nursing/medical staff realize that it has been a busy and uncomfortable time for him.	"The important tests have been done. We can't say you won't have more later on, but for now, that's it. And you have been very cooperative about it all. We appreciate that. It isn't easy."
5. After determining the child's understanding of the illness, as explained in Part 2, give him a simple explanation of the problem.	"How did you know you were sick? Have you heard about someone else with a blood problem? Have you studied about blood in science class?"
	"Your doctor has already told you that you have a blood problem. The tests have proved this to be true. He explained it very carefully to your parents, and I'm giving you a full explanation today. I brought some pictures to help you understand."
6. Show child (and parents) drawings taken from medical journals or anatomy book: a. Bone with marrow.	"Here is a drawing of a bone. This section is called the marrow. It's the place where the blood is formed. Most children I know are surprised to hear that, and even adults may need to learn more about the body. People are especially curious when they're sick."

PART 3. J (Continued)
TEACHING A CHILD ABOUT LEUKEMIA

DIRECTIONS	COMMENTS AND EXAMPLES
	"Let me tell you more about the marrow. It makes different kinds of cells— white cells, red cells and platelets."
b. White cells. Explain physiology.	"The white ones are stained so that we can see them. Their job is to fight germs and keep us from getting infections. There is one type of white cell that is formed elsewhere, in the lymph tissue —that means in the nodes or bumps you saw on your body a few days ago —and some are formed in the spleen."
c. Red cells. Explain physiology.	"The red cells do much work too. Their job is to carry oxygen from the air you breathe to all parts of the body and to carry away wastes like carbon dioxide from the blood, and to get rid of it when you breathe out.
d. Platelets. Explain physiology.	"And the work of some of the cells, called platelets, is to clot the blood. When there is a scratch or an injury, these cells stop the bleeding by forming a clot over the injured part. Do you have any questions so far?"
7. Summarize the problem with bone marrow.	"This is your problem here in the bone marrow. Right now it isn't working properly. As a matter of fact, it is making many more white cells than you need, but they're not the right kind. This means that they are not doing the work they are intended to do. The white cells are the main problem, and because the bone marrow gets filled up with the wrong kind of cells, red cells and platelets can't be made either."
8. Allow patient to view cells under microscope.	For toddlers Eliminate discussion of marrow and cells. Focus instead on symptoms—

PART 3. J (Continued)
TEACHING A CHILD ABOUT LEUKEMIA

DIRECTIONS	COMMENTS AND EXAMPLES
	for example, "You're in the hospital because you have a blood problem. That's why you have a fever, bumps on your neck and so many black-and-blue spots (or whatever applies)."
	For three-and-a-half- to six-year-olds Show drawing of bone and cells made by marrow, with just a simple explanation of the work of each. Focus on obvious symptoms.
	For adolescents Adolescents require sophisticated language and scientific detail of essentially the same material as the six to twelve group.
9. Refrain from giving the diagnosis of leukemia to the child unless parents have already agreed. This is the prerogative of parents and physician.	Leukemia is described, but not named. Characteristically the under-ten group does not ask for labels. Most physicians and parents are comfortable with this explanation, as it makes it possible for the patient to ask questions and to discuss his illness openly. When parents refuse to divulge diagnosis, their wishes must be respected. But at the same time, they need support to achieve honest, open communication with the child. For adolescent patients, however, it is foolhardy to think that full disclosure is avoidable. The patient will know. Parents frequently need counseling to permit a straightforward approach in order to maintain the child's trust.
10. From age six through adolescence, continue the teaching, with an explanation of the symptoms, such as fever, infection,	"Because your white cells don't work properly, you have been having infections; and because the number of platelets is reduced, you've had

PART 3. J (Continued)
TEACHING A CHILD ABOUT LEUKEMIA

DIRECTIONS	COMMENTS AND EXAMPLES
bleeding, and fatigue, in relation to the underlying problem.	bleeding episodes. You know about the black-and-blue marks and the nosebleeds. And since there are fewer red cells to carry oxygen around the body, you have been tired and pale. The body has been trying to make up for this by speeding up your heart."
11. Ask child what he thinks may have caused the blood problem.	This gives another opportunity to elicit fantasy or misunderstanding.
12. Reassure patient that no one is to blame for his illness.	"We don't know what made you sick. It could be many different reasons. Although we don't have the answers, we know it wasn't anything you or your parents did or thought that caused it."
13. Conclude session with a discussion of treatment goals.	(If true) "You know that the treatments you're getting are beginning to work. Your bumps (nodes) are smaller, and you've stopped bleeding. What else?" (Involve child in discussion.)
	Mention whatever applies: Less fatigue, drop in temperature. Indicate that these are ways in which we know treatment is working.
	"Some of the improvement comes from the blood transfusions and some from the medications. You know how they are given in so many different ways—IVs, injections, and by mouth. Some of the medicines are used to fight infections until your bone marrow takes over the work again. Some chemicals are used to knock out the cells that are not working and to keep them from moving into healthy parts of the body and causing trouble elsewhere. Your doctor says he can keep treating you for a long time this way.

PART 3. J (Continued)
TEACHING A CHILD ABOUT LEUKEMIA

DIRECTIONS	COMMENTS AND EXAMPLES
	"The spinal test was done to discover if any of the unwanted cells were in the spinal fluid, and your doctor feels your belly every day to find out if any organs in the abdomen are involved."
14. Allow time for child and parents to ask questions; then ask simple questions to determine understanding.	
15. Schedule next teaching session for discussion of treatment protocol and side effects.	
16. Schedule needle play/hospital play for children under eight years (and older if indicated).	
17. Delete Parts 4 and 5 unless child requires anesthesia for a procedure. Turn to Part 6.	

PART 4
GENERAL INSTRUCTIONS FOR ALL PATIENTS ON THE DAY BEFORE TREATMENT

DIRECTIONS	COMMENTS AND EXAMPLES
Explain imminent events to child.	
1. Fasting after bedtime and in the morning.	"You will find a tag on your bed that says NOTHING BY MOUTH. It means that after bedtime you will not be getting anything to eat or drink. You won't have any breakfast either, so you may feel hungry and thirsty. We do this so that your stomach (tummy) will not be upset when we give you medicine before your operation."

PART 4. (Continued)
GENERAL INSTRUCTIONS FOR ALL PATIENTS ON THE DAY
BEFORE TREATMENT

DIRECTIONS	COMMENTS AND EXAMPLES
	If an intravenous feeding is anticipated, reintroduce it here. Explain that he will be fed again just as soon as he is able to tolerate it, and that he will be given fluids first.
2. Explain bath to make the skin very clean.	
3. Explain transportation to operating room in his own bed or on a stretcher. If you plan to accompany the child, tell him so.	This is one of the most supportive measures we can supply for the child. A familiar and supportive person who accompanies the child minimizes insecurity. When planned in advance, it can be managed.
4. Tell child that you know that children are usually lonely at these times and that they prefer their parents; but because parents cannot go along, you will be there to help as his mother or father would. Tell him parents will be waiting in his room (if true).	Take along a favorite toy. Secure it to the bed to prevent loss. In some hospitals, parents are allowed to accompany children to the operating room and to stay during anesthesia induction. Teaching should be modified accordingly.
5. Describe attire of anesthesia and operating room personnel.	"On the way, if you are not asleep, you'll probably see doctors and nurses in blue or green caps, masks and gowns. Sometimes nurses wear brightly printed caps. Did you ever see someone wearing a mask? Here they are used to keep others from catching colds. The mask covers the nose and mouth and keeps germs from spreading in case people who work in the OR sneeze or cough."
	Most young children associate masks with "bad guys" or games, so it is important to explain their use.
	Give the child a disposable mask to play with and to show his friends.

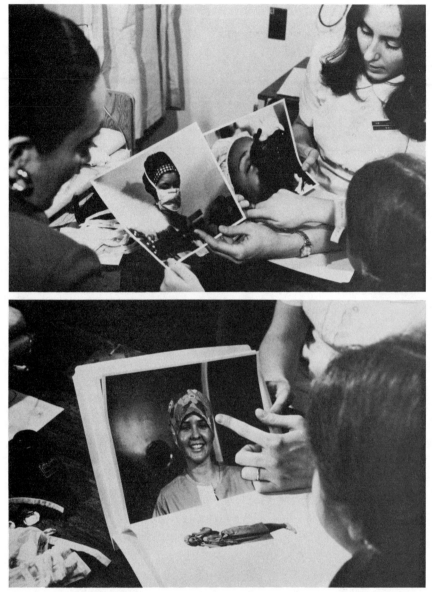

Fig. 6–7. Having a scrapbook showing doctors and nurses at work, children being cooperative with treatment (going to the operating room, waking up in the recovery room, using equipment, etc.) is helpful in explaining events.

PART 4. (Continued)
GENERAL INSTRUCTIONS FOR ALL PATIENTS ON THE DAY BEFORE TREATMENT

DIRECTIONS	COMMENTS AND EXAMPLES
6. Explain preparation for anesthesia, including blood pressure cuff, cardiac monitoring equipment and cap on head.	"Before giving you medicine by mask or by IV, the anesthesiologist (man or woman doctor or nurse who is in charge of giving you medicine throughout the operation) will place a blood pressure cuff on your arm and paste disks with wires on your body. (Show to child.) These will be hooked up to a monitor, a machine that shows a picture of your heartbeat on a TV screen. [Show patient a monitor or model of one.] And she will place a cap on your head to keep your hair off the face. All this will make it easier to take care of you during the operation."
	Variation of monitoring equipment: "You will lie on a back pad which contains disks (electrodes) attached to wires . . ."
	It is helpful to have a scrapbook with photos (from medical or nursing journal, or snapshots taken in the hospital) showing surgeons and nurses in working clothes, children on the anesthesia table, anesthesiologist at work, Recovery Room and ICU, etc.
7. Explain anesthesia—that he will not be awake because he will be given a sweet-smelling medicine by mask over the nose and mouth (modify for intravenous anesthesia); that he will not feel the operation or remember it. Show him a mask and allow him to try it and handle it.	Many children show preoccupation with waking during the operation, or disbelief that they will not feel pain. Reassure child that there is a special doctor whose entire job is to see to it that the mask is kept in place and that everything goes well.
	It is difficult to avoid the word "sleep" in describing anesthesia. Thus, it is important to differentiate between nighttime sleep and sleep induced by

PART 4. (Continued)
GENERAL INSTRUCTIONS FOR ALL PATIENTS ON THE DAY BEFORE TREATMENT

DIRECTIONS	COMMENTS AND EXAMPLES
	medication in order to avoid problems around bedtime later. Some children fear that procedures will be done while they are asleep.
8. Avoid giving any details of OR that child will not experience.	
9. Introduce Recovery Room.	Tell the child that he will not return to his room directly but will go to the RR until he is fully awake. Explain that the people working there are especially trained to take care of patients who have just had operations.
	Describe attire of staff and the number of other patients there.
	Explain that all children get a little oxygen through a mask, for a short while, to make breathing easier until they are wide awake.
	Tell him that the Recovery Room nurses will call his unit to let floor nurses know that he has returned and that his nurse will come to see him right away (if true).
OR 10. Introduce Intensive Care Unit.	Describe it as a place where the staff is trained to care care of his kind of surgery or illness. Explain the anticipated length of stay and the visiting policies.
	If the child is to go to an adult ICU, do not allow a visit preoperatively; it is much too threatening. If a child is to be sent to a pediatric ICU, arrange for him to visit in advance if you can determine ahead of time that it is not frightening. Otherwise, ask a member

PART 4. (Continued)
GENERAL INSTRUCTIONS FOR ALL PATIENTS ON THE DAY BEFORE TREATMENT

DIRECTIONS	COMMENTS AND EXAMPLES
	of the ICU staff to visit him in his own unit. Describe activities, noise and people of the ICU. Arrange for a member of the staff to accompany parents on their first visit to the ICU and to prepare them for child's appearance.
11. Discuss pain and its relief.	"After the operation, you may feel uncomfortable (feel some pain or hurt). The pain will mean that the operation is over and that the body is sore. We know how to take care of hurting with medicine. We usually know when you need it, or you can tell us when you need it."
12. Review information covered in Part 3. Ask simple questions to help child recall, in relation to body outline and doll. Evaluate how much has been retained. Repeat information as necessary. Encourage questions.	
13. Explain preoperative medications that he will be receiving—that one "shot" (or two) will make him drowsy and get him ready for the operation.	This aspect is covered at the end of the session because it is exciting for the child. We want to be assured of the child's attention to the preceding material. Demonstrate needle play again and encourage participation. See Needle Play, page 198.
14. Encourage parent or supportive adult to be present no matter how early surgery or procedure is scheduled.	The issue of whether or not the parents will be on hand should be settled out of the child's hearing, in order to protect the parent who is unable or unwilling to be present. However, every effort should be made to interpret the child's need for support at such a stressful time. Knowing that someone is

PART 4. (Continued)
GENERAL INSTRUCTIONS FOR ALL PATIENTS ON THE DAY BEFORE TREATMENT

DIRECTIONS	COMMENTS AND EXAMPLES
	waiting lessens the child's anxiety and makes the event more tolerable. This is true for any age group, from adolescents, who may appear indifferent or stoic, to babies, who cannot verbalize their distress, but may show it instead by excessive crying, restlessness or irritability.
	Dependency needs increase with illness. This is true for adults and is all the more so for children. When parents are absent, substitutes should be assigned from the staff.
15. Turn to Part 5.	

PART 5
INSTRUCTIONS FOR ALL PATIENTS ON THE DAY OF SURGERY

DIRECTIONS	COMMENTS
1. Allow parents to stay with child.	See Part 4.
	If parents are very anxious, just a brief visit to let the child know that they are there and will be waiting will suffice.
2. Review quickly the last-minute events that are to take place. Tell child or parents that you believe you have told them everything they need to know, but if there is anything that has not been explained, they should bring it up for discussion later.	Most children will demonstrate anxiety in some way. Helping them to verbalize feelings and letting them know you understand is immensely comforting.
	Despite the fact that young babies cannot comprehend what is happening, they are able to pick up anxiety

PART 5. (Continued)
INSTRUCTIONS FOR ALL PATIENTS ON THE DAY OF SURGERY

DIRECTIONS	COMMENTS
	in others. As a result, they may appear irritable or restless. Pacifiers and rocking help to calm them.
3. Prepare preoperative medications and place them out of sight in the child's room. When you are ready, tell him that it is time for his shots and proceed to administer medications immediately. Indicate that it will hurt a bit; that it is unpleasant but has to be done. Do not ask child if it is all right to go ahead; he has no choice. Permit him to object or cry but direct him to hold still so that it can go faster. Tell him you have brought a helper with you to make it easier for him to hold still. Do not imply punishment.	A lapse of a few minutes is enough for the child to develop extreme anxiety. Once you have informed the child that it is time for injections, follow through quickly, even though the child may find numerous ways to delay. There is no way to totally eliminate some discomfort—so the quicker the better.
Explain that the shots will make him sleepy, just as you told him they would. Allow quick needle play to help him master the situation. Young toddlers and babies respond well to cuddling.	A steady, calm voice communicates safety. Anything familiar is reassuring. Being friendly, scientific and chatty helps the older child during the procedure.
4. Allow child to wear clean underpants.	See Cory's story, page 171.
5. On call, accompany child (and parent or parents, if allowed) to operating room. If he is awake, discuss with him the events taking place (include him in any conversations) and point out different personnel encountered.	
6. Stay with child until he is anesthetized.	Most institutions will require the nurse or assigned staff member to change into appropriate clothing for this activity.
7. Turn to Part 6.	

PART 6
HELPING THE CHILD TO COPE WITH FEELINGS RELATED TO HOSPITALIZATION AND TREATMENT POSTPROCEDURAL PERIOD

DIRECTIONS	COMMENTS
1. Allow child to resume former activities as soon as possible, and to wear own clothing or hospital-supplied daytime clothing.	Dressing and getting out of bed are immensely reassuring to the child. Even young babies and toddlers with IVs can be picked up or positioned so that they may observe activities.
2. Allow opportunity for dramatic play. Have at child's disposal safe equipment that has been used in his treatment—stethoscope, tongue blades, blood pressure equipment; also doll, body outline and play materials representing equipment specific to his condition.	A hospital corner in the pediatric playroom provides an excellent opportunity for the expression of feelings and clarification of events.
3. For the verbal child, encourage talk about hospital experiences with staff, family, visitors and peers.	This can be done by merely asking the child what happened to him.
4. Encourage letter writing and telephoning as way of communicating with friends about experiences.	
5. Provide materials for child to draw or paint about hospital experience. Ask child to tell a story about his picture.	Covering walls in hallways and isolation rooms with brown wrapping paper and supplying crayons or chalk allows for additional recreation and diversion when playroom is closed and encourages expression of feelings. Graffiti are easily interpreted.
6. Some children prefer to make a scrapbook with pictures cut out of medical or nursing journals. Ask child to write or tell a story related to them.	
7. Organize patient discussion groups with focus on the expression of feelings and coping with treatment and disabilities.	

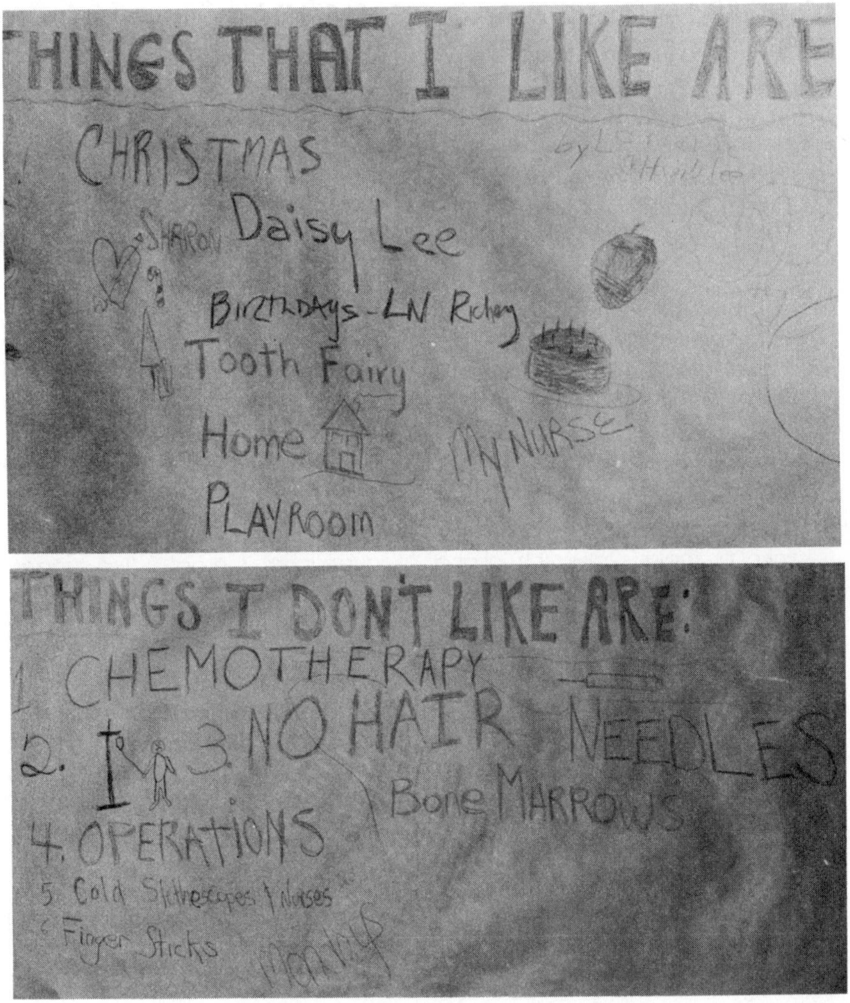

Fig. 6-8. Graffiti. (A) Things That I Like; (B) Things That I Don't Like.
Covering walls in hallways and isolation rooms with wrapping paper
and supplying crayons, chalk or paint allows for additional recreation
or diversion. In addition, graffiti alert the staff to areas that need
discussion of feelings. (Photos by Terry Hanna)

PART 6. (Continued)
HELPING THE CHILD TO COPE WITH FEELINGS RELATED TO HOSPITALIZATION AND TREATMENT POSTPROCEDURAL PERIOD

DIRECTIONS	COMMENTS
8. Encourage older children to keep diaries or to tape-record their experiences in a group or privately.	
9. Encourage parents to photograph hospital scenes related to their child, so that he may have a picture history of events and can be reminded of his bravery.	The preceding measures give the child the opportunity to gain ego mastery of difficult situations by giving conscious thought to them. They also provide the occasion for clarifying the difference between fantasy and reality, thus preventing the repression and retention of unrealistic fantasies.
10. Supply occupational and educational projects. Enroll in school and teen program if available.	Consult with schoolteacher, play and occupational therapists for suggestions.
11. Allow child to take home safe play materials.	
12. Interpret to parents the need to keep the subject of hospitalization and treatment open to discussion and clarification, in order that the experience can be integrated into the child's life.	This is especially true for the three- to six-year-olds, who need repeated assurance that they were in no way responsible for illness, as guilt is a major problem for this group (egocentric thinking).
13. Prepare parents for the kinds of behavior their child may demonstrate after discharge.	See Preparing Parents for Discharge of the Child, page 113.
14. Invite child to visit the unit after discharge, when he comes to clinic or the doctor's office. This provides the staff with an opportunity to evaluate the child's adjustment and helps the child maintain contacts with staff. For children requiring frequent hospitalization, this facilitates future adjustment.	This revisitation helps to correct the distorted memories and diminishes anxiety in the event of future hospitalization.

Before ending this chapter on diagnostic and surgical procedures, which has presented very specific suggestions, it is important to remember a few considerations. Coping reactions—which have both creative and defensive roles—develop best when the child can anticipate a stressful event. The effect of surgery on the child's life depends less on the type or seriousness of the operation than "on the type and depth of the fantasies aroused by it." This statement by Anna Freud goes on to say that "any intervention with the child's body may serve as a focal point for the activation, reactivation, grouping and rationalization of ideas of being attacked, overwhelmed and/or castrated."[21] We need to be cognizant at all times of how serious a measure hospitalization is, separating the child from his caretaker at the very moment when his body is threatened both internally and externally by danger.

Anesthesia is a mixed experience for a child in that it promises protection from pain and a form of magical "waking up and being all better." On the other hand, anesthesia also represents loss of control and defenselessness against mutilation and attack. Premedication is particularly threatening in that it causes loss of control without loss of consciousness. Children want to know exactly what will be done while they are helpless. Many children promise themselves that this loss of consciousness will not involve loss of control and, following surgery, may appear docile. This represents a feeling that they have been caught and punished, "put under," and must be careful so as to avoid further anesthesia in the future.

The foregoing considerations imply that elective surgery before the age of six is emotionally risky. The child has not integrated a strong sense of himself and is not possessed of effective, or mature, coping mechanisms. Furthermore, preop preparation of the under-six child may not be completely effective in allaying and constructively counteracting all the stress reaction. Further implications are that the time spent away from the family be as brief as possible and that rooming-in, bringing into the hospital familiar objects, delegation of a few professionals to be the main focus for carrying out treatment, all become dramatically important to the child, particularly to the younger ones. One of the usual postoperative situations —and one that is often neglected in the preparation of children for surgery—is that hazy, dizzy, dreamlike state after anesthesia, which may persist beyond the recovery room. Children having just clearly drawn the line for themselves between the real and the imaginary world will find this time particularly upsetting. Similarly, post-op complications ought to be carefully explained and worked through whenever they occur and the child's reactions given a chance to be expressed.

There is no substitute for knowing in depth an individual family and their child. For some families in various places the emergency room has been used as the general practitioner. This is particularly true in large urban medical centers. Children will have consequently already formed many impressions about the hospital structure and events and about medical personnel so that actual hospitalization may not be the discontinuous experience that it was for most children in the past. The hospital may be the one institution in the community that a family sees as relevant and useful to its needs, however imperfect that institution has been. For pediatric caretakers, to experience the family as supportive and effective, and to learn that they perceive the hospital as a useful resource, can be ego building.

For the pediatric staff to successfully help a child to work through an experience, for him to remember it, reexperience it with understanding and to go beyond coping with the memory to a mastery of that experience—the rewards are tremendous.

REFERENCES

1. Klaus, M. H., and Kennell, J. H.: Maternal–Infant Bonding, p. 85. St. Louis, C. V. Mosby, 1976.
2. Goren, C., Sarty, M., and Wu, P.: Visual following and pattern discrimination of facelike stimuli by newborn infants. Pediatrics 56:544–49, 1975.
3. Brazelton, T. B.: Psychophysiologic reaction in the neonate. II. Effects of maternal medication on the neonate and his behavior. J. Pediat. 58:513–18, 1961.
4. Condon, W. S., and Sander, L. W.: Neonate movement is synchronized with adult speech: interactional participation and language acquisition. Science 183:99–101, 1974.
5. Kagan, J.: Personality development. In Talbot, N., Kagan, J., and Eisenberg, L. (eds.): Behavioral Science in Pediatric Medicine, p. 288. Philadelphia, W. B. Saunders, 1971.
6. Klaus, M. H., and Kennell, J. H.: Maternal-Infant Bonding, pp. 10–14. St. Louis, C. V. Mosby, 1976.
7. Ibid., pp. 10–14.
8. Ibid., pp. 50–54.
9. Ibid., p. 2.
10. Chapman, J. S.: Effect of auditory stimulation on gross motor activity of short gestation infants. Unpublished Doctoral Dissertation, New York University, 1975.

11. Neal, M. V.: Vestibular stimulation and developmental behavior of the small premature infant. Nurs. Res. Report (Amer. Nurses' Foundation) 3(1):1, March 1968.
12. 2-Month-Old Can Distinguish a Stranger. Pediatric News, p. 32, January 1977.
13. Kagan, J.: Personality Development. *In* Talbot, N., Kagan, J., and Eisenberg, L. (eds.): Behavioral Science in Pediatric Medicine. pp. 288–91. Philadelphia, W. B. Saunders, 1971.
14. Stone, L. J., Smith, H. T., and Murphy, L. B.: The Competent Infant, p. 990. New York, Basic Books, 1973.
15. Robson, K. S.: The role of eye-to-eye contact in maternal–infant attachment. J. Child Psychol. Psychiat. 8:13–25, 1967.

16. Winnicott, D. W.: Mirror role of mother and family in child development. *In* Playing and Reality, pp. 111–18. New York, Basic Books, 1971.
17. Stone, L. J., Smith, H. T., and Murphy, L. B.: The Competent Infant, p. 997. New York, Basic Books, 1973.
18. Levy, D. M.: The Demonstration Clinic, p. 63. Springfield, Charles C Thomas, 1959.
19. Sarnoff, C.: Latency, p. 7. New York, Jason Aronson, 1976.
20. Fraiberg, S.: The Magic Years, p. 277. New York, Scribner, 1959.
21. Freud, A.: The role of bodily illness in the mental life of children. The Psychoanalytic Study of the Child 7:69–81, 1952.

BIBLIOGRAPHY

Adams, M.: A hospital play program: helping children with serious illness. Amer. J. Orthopsychiat. 46:416, 1976.

Barnett, C. R., Leiderman, P. H., and Grobstein, R.: Neonatal separation: the maternal side of interactional deprivation. Pediatrics 45:197, 1970.

Brazelton, T. B., and Robey, J. S.: Observations of neonatal behavior. The effect of perinatal variables, in particular that of maternal medication. J. Amer. Acad. Child Psychiat. 4:613, 1965.

Brazelton, T. B., School, M. L., and Robey, J. S.: Visual responses in the newborn. Pediatrics 37:284, 1966.

Brazelton, T. B.: Infants and Mothers. New York, Delacorte, 1969.

———: Toddlers and Parents. New York, Delacorte, 1974.

Bruner, J., Cole, M., and Lloyd, B. (eds.): The Developing Child. New York, Basic Books, 1977.

Cassell, S.: The effect of brief puppet therapy upon the emotional responses of children undergoing cardiac catheterization. J. Consult. Psychol. 29:1, 1965.

Cofer, D. H., and Nir, Y.: Theme-focused group therapy on a pediatric ward. Int'l. J. Psychiatry in Medicine 6(4):541, 1975.

Daniel, W. A. (ed.) Adolescent medicine. Pediatric Annals 2(6), 1973.

Danilowicz, D. A., and Gabriel, H. P.: Postoperative reactions in children: "normal" and abnormal responses after cardiac surgery. Amer. J. Psychiat. 128:185, 1971.

Davenport, H. T., and Werry, J. S.: The effect of general anesthesia, surgery and hospitalization upon the behavior of children. Amer. J. Orthopsychiat. 40(5):806, 1970.

Desmond, M. M., Rudolph, A. J., and Phitaksphraiwan, P.: The transitional care nursery: a mechanism of preventive medicine. Pediatr. Clin. N. Amer. 13:651, 1966.

Donovan, E., and Gold, M.: Modal patterns in American adolescents. *In* Hoffman, L. and M.: Review of Child Development Research, vol. 2. New York, Russell Sage Foundation, 1966.

Escalona, S. K.: The Roots of Individuality. Chicago, Aldine, 1968.

Hammar, S. L., and Eddy, J. A.: Nursing Care of the Adolescent. New York, Springer, 1966.

Hardgrove, C. B.: Emotional inoculation: the 3 r's of preparation. JACCH 5:17, Spring 1977.

Hofmann, A. D.: The hospitalized adolescent. Pediatric Annals 2:49, 1973.

Hofmann, A. D., Becker, R. D., and Gabriel, H. P.: The Hospitalized Adolescent: A Guide to Managing the Ill and Injured Youth. New York, Free Press, 1976.

Huntington, D. S.: Learning from infants and families. JACCH 4:5, Summer 1975.

Jessner, L.: Some observations on children hospitalized during latency. *In* Jessner, L., and Pavenstedt, E. (eds.): Dynamic Psychopathology in Childhood. New York, Grune & Stratton, 1959.

Josselyn, J. M.: Passivity. J. Amer. Acad. Child Psychiat. 7:569, 1968.

Kagan, J.: Change and Continuity in Infancy. New York, Wiley & Sons, 1971.

Kaufman, R.: Body image changes in physically ill teen-agers. J. Amer. Acad. Child Psychiat. 11:157, 1972.

Klaus, M. H., and Kennell, J. H.: Mothers separated from their newborn infants. Pediat. Clin. N. Amer. 17:1015, 1970.

Korner, A.: Individual differences at birth: implications for early experience and later development. Amer. J. Orthopsychiat. 41:608, 1971.

Korsch, B. M.: The child and the op-

erating room. Anesthesiology 43:251, 1975.

Leboyer, F.: Birth Without Violence. New York, Knopf, 1976.

Levy, D. M.: The Demonstration Clinic: For the Psychological Study and Treatment of Mother and Child in Medical Practice. Springfield, Ill., Charles C Thomas, 1959.

Mahler, M. S., Pine, F., and Bergman, A.: The Psychological Birth of the Infant: Symbiosis and Individuation. New York, Basic Books, 1975.

Meeks, J. E.: Dispelling fears of the hospitalized child. Hospital Medicine 6:77, 1970.

Moore, D., Hilton, C., and Marten, G.: Psychological problems in the management of adolescents with malignancy. Clin. Pediat. 8:464, 1969.

Murphy: L. B.: Individualization of child care and its relation to environment. *In* Chandler, C., *et al.*: Early Child Care: The New Perspectives. New York, Atherton, 1968.

Puppet Preparation for Surgery. The Children's Memorial Hospital, 2300 Children's Plaza, Chicago, Ill.

Richmond, J. B.: Child development: a basic science for pediatrics. Peditrics 39:649, 1967.

Sander, L. W., Stechler, G., Burns, P., and Julia, H.: Early mother–infant interaction and 24-hour patterns of activity and sleep. J. Amer. Acad. Child Psychiat. 9:103, 1970.

Senn, M. J. E., and Solnit, A. J.: Problems in Child Behavior and Development. Chap. 3. The newborn and young infant. Philadelphia, Lea & Febiger, 1968.

Silberstein, R. M., *et al.*: Autocrotic head banging, a reflection on the opportunism of infants. J. Amer. Acad. Child Psychiat. 5:235, 1966.

Smith, E. C., Liviskie, S. L., Nelson, K. A., and Mcnemar, A.: Reestablishing a child's body image. Amer. J. Nurs. 77:445, 1977.

Smith, M.: Ego support for the child

patient. Amer. J. Nurs. 63:90, 1963.

Stechler, G., and Latz, E.: Some observations on attention and arousal in the human infant. J. Amer. Acad. Child Psychiat. 5:517, 1966.

Visotsky, W.: Coping behavior under extreme stress. Arch. Gen. Psychiat. 5:423, 1961.

Vredevoe, D., Kim, A., Dambacher, B., and Call, J.: Aggressive postoperative play responses of hospitalized preschool children. Nurs. Res. 4:1, 1969.

Waechter, E. H.: The birth of an exceptional child. Nurs. Forum 10:202, 1970.

Wessle, M. A.: Training in neonatal pediatrics. *In* Solnit, A. J., and Provence, S. A. (eds.): Modern Perspectives in Child Development. New York, International Universities Press, 1963.

White, B., and Held, R.: Plasticity of sensorimotor development in the human infant. *In* Rosenblith, J., and Allinsmith, W.: The Causes of Behavior: Readings in Child Development and Educational Psychology, 2nd ed. Rockleigh, N.J., Allyn & Bacon, 1966.

Wolfer, J. A., and Visintainer, M. A.: Pediatric surgical patients' and parents' stress responses and adjustment. Nurs. Res. 24:244, 1975.

Wolff, P. H.: Observations on newborn infants. Psychosom. Med. 21:110, 1959.

Yarrow, L. J., and Goodwin, M. S.: The immediate impact of separation: Reactions of infants to change in mother figures. *In* Stone, L. J., Smith, H. T., and Murphy, L. B. (eds.): The Competent Infant. New York, Basic Books, 1973.

AUDIOVISUAL MATERIAL

Petrillo, M.: Staff Development Series: Preparing Children for Surgery or Teaching About Illness. Scarsdale, New York, Campus Films, 1975.

7

Emotional Care of the Dying Child

Chronic, terminal illness in children presents a notable challenge to professionals. Inundated with numerous books and articles on infant, child and adolescent development, on family and cultural forces, it is often easier to rely on the liaison psychiatrist,[1] nurse specialist or social worker than to integrate an effective emotional approach. But the satisfactions from skillful management of desperately sick children and their families can be profound. One child psychiatrist working with an oncology team, after several months of involvement, found that the nursing and house staff felt more free to bring up their concerns about a child and/or his family, more often stated the problem, related what they had done and requested information more frequently for continuing management.[2] The opportunities to lead a family in their anguish and bewilderment toward closeness, strength and maturity are abundant. This chapter aims to demonstrate how professionals working with dying children and their caretakers can counterbalance the depression and silence that often wear them down.

Just as the answer to the old saw "How do you get to Carnegie Hall?" is "Practice, practice, practice!" the acquisition of skills in the art of medicine and nursing requires preparation and deliberation, until such time that the material is well absorbed and its application automatic. For example:

Kathy's mother was called in from the waiting room. Dr. R told her that the diagnosis of acute leukemia was confirmed. After drying her eyes, she asked him what she should do, how she should present the illness to Kathy. Dr. R warmly and quietly told her to treat Kathy as normally as possible within the constraints of office and hospital visits. He outlined the probable course of leukemia and his availability to the family.

The doctor in the above case, except for his kind face and slightly moist eyes, could have been replaced by a computer printed form, mailed to this mother.

A basic skill is to listen and learn before giving reassurance and direction. Would Dr. R have said what he did had he known that Kathy had begun having nightmares and wetting her bed, and that the mother had already been crying uncontrollably, with the grandmother's tears adding to a regular scene just outside Kathy's bedroom door each night? Did he know that Kathy's parents had planned a separation prior to the onset of illness or that from remarks made to another patient overheard by the nurse in Dr. R's waiting room, Kathy was aware that her illness was terminal?

Think-before-you-speak has other dividends. In the thinking time, one can review a number of concepts: how children think, the many ways a family copes with stress, illness, death, and the nature of love and grief in young and old. With a mind more fully prepared, the professional becomes an intelligent, sensitive listener. The time added for this process is well spent.

The principle to "practice what you preach" finds important application here. That is, we urge families to pull together, to enjoy the present as much as possible and to talk about mutual concerns during an obviously stressful time. Are we, as professionals, doing likewise? Do we regularly turn toward individuals and groups to commiserate our own feelings, to share difficult decisions and intense stress? Can we, despite heavy responsibility, enjoy our present lives? When we become overly depressed, anxious, angry, are there regular and dignified channels for us to receive emotional help?

Another principle is that separation and loneliness are the enemies that invariably turn tragedy into horror.

When asked why he never told his mother that he was having painful breathing, but waited to ask for oxygen after she departed, Michael said that his mother kept her tears inside and he was doing everything he could to keep her from breaking down and crying. He was embarrassed for her

when she would leave the room with the story that something was in her eye.

Michael was suffering from the emotional separation that commonly follows alteration in patterns of family interaction once a
diagnosis of cancer is known. Even without so ominous a label, mere
hospitalization suffices to create awkwardness and estrangement
from their child for most parents (no matter how long they stay on
the floor or room-in).

It strains belief that life is ever the same once cancer is detected.
Adults uniformly report a year or more of arduous, uphill adjustment
when personally afflicted. The adjustment—to any impairment, but
particularly to a terminal one—in a child takes even longer and has a
rougher road than with adults. A sample of 18 children with malignancies, all between 5 and 14 years old, was studied, using psychological tests.[3] Compared to nonsick children, they showed a "pro-
pensity for distortion and unrealistic thinking processes . . . and more
negative phantasy. The child with cancer shows overt behavior
devoid of emotional response . . . inhibited and withdrawn." This
doesn't mean that the child is unresponsive to personal and impersonal stimuli. The tests showed that the children concealed their
feelings and displayed only subtle emotional responsiveness. The
necessary conclusion to be drawn from this study is that health
professionals must make the effort to elicit feelings and make an
equal effort to avoid vague ambiguous explanations that can readily
lend themselves to distortion.

Another careful study[4] comparing 25 children with leukemia
with 25 others suffering from a chronic nonfatal illness found that all
children with repeated hospitalization felt distance from parent
figures and that leukemics "not only perceive a growing psychological distance from those around . . . but for whatever reason, prefer it
that way." The depth of helpless rage against a condition that ends a
life before it has fully been lived is poignantly described in Gunther's
Death Be Not Proud.[5]

A pretense that the child knows nothing blocks the clinician
from helping the family to use their resources toward a creative,
honest and deeper way of coping. Of course, the family and child
may become distracted and temporarily forget the prognosis, to
allow entertainment and relief from the constant awareness of the

impending finality. Nevertheless, children from four years of age on will have pieced together a reasonably accurate portrait of their illness within a few months of the diagnosis. This occurs even if a most assiduous campaign of secrecy by the adults has been planned.[6, 7] Pretense wrecks the trust a child will have in his parents and other adults, moving him toward the eventual charade that he either doesn't know, has accepted the lies he has been told or is comfortable with the idea of dying. Would any professional, himself gravely ill, wish to be the last to know the nature of his illness!

The emotional care of children with cancer or other terminal illness both in the hospital and in the home has four facets:

preparation and support systems for professionals;

premorbid service to and support of families (including siblings);

approach to and study of the individual afflicted child, with the formation of a comprehensive strength and character-building program, and protection from pathology-inducing interactions;

postmorbid follow-up and continued caring for families

Complete patient care takes place when all four facets are effectuated.

PREPARATION AND SUPPORT SYSTEMS FOR PROFESSIONALS

The most important preparation for the clinician is based on self-exploration. How have personal separations and losses affected thinking and behavior? Were distinctive patterns such as disbelief, protest, disorientation, withdrawal, sadness, acceptance and reattachment to remaining persons discerned? What was the role of relatives and friends surrounding the bereavement? Were tears and crying an important part of the process? Were there changes in eating, sleeping, sexual and work patterns? How long did it take to fully recover from the acute phase of loss? Is the loved one from whom you are separated remembered and under what circumstances? As professionals the surest way we make it possible to care deeply for our patients in a comprehensive way is to empathize, to resonate ourselves to what they are experiencing with what we have experienced.

Another preparation is for the clinician to become familiar with the literature. There are well-written books and articles that can orient the reader for further exploration. Gunther,[5] Bowlby,[8, 9] Robertson,[10, 11] Lindemann,[12] Solnit[7] are classics. A reading and case conference, once made a regular part of the hospital schedule, can illustrate concepts by clinical examples.

More specific references regarding liaison teamwork in pediatric settings can be found in Mattson,[13] Schowalter,[14] Friedman,[15] Green,[16] and Sack.[17] Anthony and Koupernik,[18] with respect to family and culture, and Gaylin[19] on the relationship to depression. These are compendiums of many relevant issues needing consideration. Rochlin[20] writes convincingly about how grief and discontent are the "engines of change" that mature the individual. Parsons[21] eloquently describes the helplessness, anger, loneliness and sadness in very young patients. These emotions are often left untouched by adults, who themselves are reluctant to explore. She shows how the hospital, to children, is a symbol of a place where one suffers pain and separation and advocates that professionals intervene to help children adapt rather than to allow them to regress. Koocher[22] interviewed 75 children between the ages of 6 and 15, finding each one capable and wanting to talk about death. He notes that the child under eight needs simple direct explanation and that the child above eight years should be helped to correct misrepresentation. The subject of death must be discussed; the keeping of secrets and taboos prevents children from coping with feelings of loss. Much light can be shed from such literature to better understand patients and families.

The philosophy of reading and case conferences must be to present a balanced view of the role of terminal disease: the frustrations and triumphs of battling a destructive disease, the rendering of life more meaningful and precious during remissions. One needs to consider the humbling of professionals alongside the satisfaction of working at the frontier of life versus death when the healthy parts of a patient respond to the therapeutic efforts. There is also the condensed and intense view of families adjusting to the ultimate challenge. It is eerie, exciting, heartbreaking work. There is also the opportunity for the various disciplines of pediatrics, nursing, lab sciences, play, occupational therapy, psychiatry, social work, chaplaincy, etc., to unite in a common goal for mutual recognition and support.

PREMORBID SERVICE TO AND SUPPORT OF FAMILIES

The family unit, in the long run, has the total responsibility for the child and bears the emotional brunt of the disease. Professionals, therefore, need to equip themselves with general knowledge about family dynamics, communication patterns, cultural styles, economic factors and "nuclear" family tensions. To what extent will a given family behave predictably according to its socioeconomic category? To what extent is a family a small group of people needing a unique perspective? These questions can be discerned only with time and the cooperation of everyone who has had contact.

Delicate issues are common. The staff may see that a child is more upset when the family is visiting, or at the prospect of going home. In rare instances, medicolegal factors such as objections to transfusions and medications, quack treatments, abuse or neglect of therapeutic regimens frustrate treatment. At what point and on what basis is it justifiable to interfere with family wishes?

In knowing everyone of significance in a family, one is able to ascertain sources of power and influence. It is of no avail to obtain a mothers' promise to cooperate in a difficult therapeutic design when a powerful grandmother who lives in the home doesn't "believe in doctors." Fathers are seldom seen except during visiting hours, or may emotionally avoid closeness to wife or patient. Commonly, the mother becomes the medical surrogate and displaces the father and others in handling the sick child. If this exacerbates family dissension and isolates the child from his siblings, perhaps a series of family meetings with the professional who knows them best might remedy the family drift.

Conducting a family session either for diagnostic evaluation or brief therapeutic purpose is benefitted by familiarity with texts by Ackerman,[23] and Bell and Vogel.[24] Lansdown[25] describes families who grieve, mourn and get over the loss even before the child dies. These parents are then in an awkward position in trying to relate to the child who continues to live. Not surprisingly, the child is happier with the parents' state of coolness, as they no longer hover and become upset about every small detail. Others in the field report that weekly hour-long talks reduce parents' anxiety.[26, 27] Fears were transformed into more appropriate ways of adapting to the hospitalization. These studies found that the surgical and nursing staffs also noted reduced pressure on them and more cooperation from parents.

When such children are hospitalized, pediatric staff must be alert to signs that the child's support system—the parents—is becoming broken and dysfunctional. Marital counseling can prevent hidden family tensions from becoming so exacerbated by the fatal diagnosis that the family structure is in jeopardy.

The brothers and sisters of the patient also need attention.[28] They are usually forgotten and left to cope as best they can. What and how are they told about their sibling's illness? A meeting with the doctor and a visit to the office (later also to the hospital) offer them an opportunity to ask questions and find answers. They may build a truer picture of the efforts being made to treat the disease. They may want to be shown how to help, how to tolerate parental visits to the hospital, how to be supported when parents become discouraged, how to maintain their relationship to their sick sibling. In particular, siblings under five may think that the illness can strike them next, that they may have caused their sibling to fall ill, or that some bad action brought on the grave sickness. When they are jealous at the attention sickness attracts, siblings often hide their feelings out of shame for being meanspirited. Thus the illness itself and/or the absence of the mother can also lead to disturbance in a previously well-adapted sibling.

Parental tensions and upsets may block children's access to crucial emotional nurturance even when parents are at home. Siblings might be helped to find other adults for supplementary support, so long as disloyal thoughts toward parents are neutralized.

> Rachel had been in the hospital for almost a month and lived for the day she could return to her dolls, her dollhouse, and her stuffed animals who slept in a basket next to her bed. There hadn't been time to take the bikes out of her room, which had served as storage space during her absence. Even her basket and dolls had to be hastily retrieved

from other rooms. Rachel silently noted the signs of wear
and the idea that she had been forgotten took hold. Three
months later she fought vehemently not to go back to the
hospital. She demanded that her room be locked while she
was away and cried that her animals would forget the path to
the safety of their basket home. Her older sister, Jessie, cried
and tearfully said she'd never again touch Rachel's things.

Tensions may involve also the relatives and friends of the
family, resulting in isolation. Irrational fears of contagion, of enter-
ing an awkward situation, or of becoming attached to a child to
whom it would be hard to say good-bye make it easier to shun the
family.

APPROACH TO AND STUDY OF THE
INDIVIDUAL AFFLICTED CHILD

There is no substitute for knowing each child as deeply as
possible. Rather than creating a uniformity among children, terminal
illness heightens the preexistent individual differences. In other
chapters we have described getting to know children through play,
nondirective conversation and empathetic listening. Interview and
play techniques can be taught by means of a combination of one-way
screen observation and with the clinical supervision of the actual
interviews practiced by the learner. An experienced child therapist
can usually be called for a demonstration. However, the picture of a
child is complete only when personal, nursing, family, social, and
school histories are gathered; this should be augmented by observations of receptionists, caretakers, playroom persons, and social
work. The integrated picture of the formulation of the child's personality, capacity to relate to peers and adults, and current emotional state will emerge clearly.

Further study is indicated where there is uncertainty either in
making a diagnostic formulation or in predicting the effects of stress.
In-depth psychological testing, extended diagnostic play interviews
and more detailed personal history from the family can fill important
gaps.

A general focus for all professionals is on the future: how will
the stress of chronic and remitting illness affect this child's adjust-

ment? Will the child "merely" stop progressing? Will the child be pushed by stress toward greater maturity? Will this child trust adults who try to be helpful? Are adults seen as repositories of skill and knowledge?

Why this emphasis on an intimate knowledge of the individual child? The reason is important: this knowledge is the basis of all professional usefulness. Adherence to therapeutic programs, productive guidance to families, management of hospitalization to minimize separation effects and preparation of professionals to plan their time effectively—all depend on it.

> Seven-year-old Jeff saw the doctor's office and the hospital as places where he could break all the rules established at home—from dropping his coat on the floor to turning out the table lamps, ripping magazine pages to searching the nurse's desk for supplies to play with and stuff his pockets. The receptionist, nurse and physician rapidly became provoked, trying to contain the antisocial behavior as best they could. His misbehavior continued, to everyone's dismay. They dreaded his return visits. Mother was embarrassed and found that it took several hours of discipline after the return home for Jeff to control himself.
>
> After a few months a team conference ordered a systematic study. It was learned that Jeff had maintained a deep fear that his tumor would "grow back" and he would be tricked again with "We're just going for a checkup visit to the doctor's" and left without familiar people or objects to undergo a painful procedure on his insides. He also associated hospitalization and surgery with retaliation and punishment for his having damaged his father's camera, which he had taken without permission. It became evident that, until Jeff understood these distortions and the condensations of the past events were unraveled for him, he would continue to repeat provocative behavior.

An individual child's ideas about death stem not only from the parents' ability to deal with the facts of death and dying themselves but equally from the child's own experiences and level of ego development. Once a child has an awareness of his separateness from his parents and the language to know the words "death" and "dying," the concept begins to form itself. A child who will have had some immediate exposure to death, either with a pet or a relative, certainly has formulated early ideas about the finality of life. Other preconditions for the development of a concept of death are that the individual child has a stable concept of himself and inner representation of primary figures; a sufficient control of his behavior so that he is able to think rather than turn stressful ideas into action; the ability to know animate from inanimate; the ability to see time in past, present and future; and finally, to see the linkage between the inanimate state and the inability to function. Most children from age three on have the necessary components to develop the concept.

If, in taking a history of a child, the following have occurred, it is likely that the ability to grasp a concept of death has been interfered with: (1) the parents do not accept the reality of a loss; or (2) a death occurred when the child was very young in his character development (usually under three). In such children as these, when there is a death of someone vitally needed, the child usually pretends that death hasn't occurred. A child's concept of death may be distorted by a belief that higher powers caused the death; or that the child himself, in wishing death, had made it happen; or that death is reversible, resembling sleep. These distortions most frequently occur before the age of six or seven.

Just as in the adult world there is no such thing as a "little" heart attack in the emotional life of the cardiac, there are no medical/surgical procedures of minor impact on a child. The concept of death will vary throughout childhood as an individual becomes more sophisticated. Thus, there may be ideas that death resembles suffocation and entombment in a crypt, that some arrangement of the body or presence of objects will facilitate rebirth in the next world, that parts of a dead person may continue to live on after the major portion of that person has died, and that death will have achieved a kind of resolution whereby enemies are punished and friends rewarded. The anger that develops in the preadolescent is usually caused by adults who withdraw and convey thereby that death is too painful for discussion (a revulsion to be dealt with in silence). It is predominantly in adolescence that there is a sense of anger regarding projects, plans and hopes that have been thwarted. After a fatal diagnosis is established, adolescent children may rage toward and blame parents; they may feel they were neither protected from this invader nor made strong enough to resist the growth of the disease.

There may be also a spread of the rage to health professionals who have failed to cure this illness and who, instead, recommend irritating, painful, separating and repeating hospitalizations. The course of an illness in which there are exacerbations and remissions usually leads to depressive episodes in all children. This is not different from the response in adults to conditions that they think will not recur and that do.

Commonly, children avoid dwelling on the idea that life will be shortened. Their mental focus narrows, however, to the duration of the remission, time that is measured in weeks and months, or living to that next birthday or to Christmas. They also feel increasingly distant from family members and, during remission, from classmates. The latter often leads to transient "school phobia," exacerbated by fear of humiliation (their wig will be discovered, they'll be out of step in classwork, they won't be able to parry embarrassing questions) or fear that the mother will be out of reach if they suddenly have need of her.

The terror that adults feel regarding fatal diseases such as cancer is the one single factor that traumatizes their children. The panic of an invasive agent that causes progressive "liquefaction" or "hardening" of body organs and poses instant threat of unbearable pain and progressive loss of body parts cannot be overestimated. The helplessness of standing by and not being able to remove this cancer from their awareness leads parents to estrange themselves from their children. All prior bonds of affection and experience are stretched to their limits by this impotent terror; only the most strongly supportive families can survive without help. The individual child will show the effect of such an estrangement by turning away from his family and toward caretaking professionals. There is no point in hiding from a child the significance of the illness and the parental response. It is much more therapeutic to openly acknowledge and support the child's true estimate of what has happened and build a new relationship.

Leventhal and Hersh[29] emphasize the crucial need for candor and a trusting relationship. They give the patient and family as complete a share of the medical knowledge as possible, which they claim "provides a necessary illusion of control similar to that used by physicians and nurses." The creation of this illusion is a somewhat dubious undertaking, but the main thesis that what counts is a relationship is not to be disagreed with. This may occur with the physician, nurse, social worker, play specialist—anyone with whom the child has an individual recognition of friendship. After that friendship has ripened for a few days or weeks, it may be possible to talk about his disappointment in, and distance from, his family.

It is helpful to the opening up of this painful topic for the professional to have in mind the many positive acts the child has done to preserve what little relationship there is within the family— the efforts a child makes to talk about television, for instance, or ask about pets, or even his use of silence, which can often be seen as an effort to avoid words that may cause further distance. So many adults pretend and sham with a child who already knows his diagnosis and prognosis[30] that for the child to stop the adult from further misrepresentation is to control his own disappointment. Once the child is helped to explore and understand his position with respect to significant family and friends, he can now help others. It is axiomatic that one helps oneself and raises self-esteem through helping others. For a child to calm an anguished relative, to call in a nurse to show a friend around the hospital floor when the friend is about to cry, or to offer a tissue to crying grandparents is to diminish the potential for depression based on helplessness that fatally ill children feel. To cope with the somber mood they detect in their hospital visitors dilutes the paralysis of interaction and carries on life in the face of death.

At this point we recommend some cautionary words to all professionals regarding children with terminal illness. First, children will tolerate and maintain relationships with most helpful, kind people so long as they feel they will be dealt with truthfully. The telling of an untruth is so insulting and mystifying to most children that no subsequent efforts will be meaningful. This is not to recommend that everyone be blunt. Some children will be content if they know you are trying to explain or will in time further elaborate on something that may take a while to formulate. In very young children one avenue of approach is to talk of animals. Mahon and Simpson[31] suggest that "children (under 5) cannot mourn an object of such critical importance as mother or father . . . but that a pet can be mourned because of its lesser importance. The pet is a trial object, a transitional toy." So long as the child has a sense that the adults are sincere and not concealing, he will feel cared for.

Second, levels of maturity and experience in childhood are so variable that generalizations should be made lightly. Singher[32] states that for the younger child it is wise to express hope continually and with the older child professionals must keep the patient hopeful and let him know he will not be left alone. This author goes on to claim that the child rarely questions the finality of death. Singher generalizes that parents' hopes should be kept up even while telling them there is no certain cure; and that after the child's death the family should come back after an "appropriate" interval when the doctor can provide **"welcome support and constructive channeling of emotions"** (bold type is used here for emphasis). Well-meaning as it is, the above article offers advice that is simplistic and contradictory. False hope or social talk and cheer increase parental anguish when facing a child's imminent death.[33]

Clinical observations gathered from many children do serve as stimulants to thought and can create an atmosphere of receptivity for sensitive listening without preconceived bias.

Whether to tell a dying child he is dying is an issue created by adults in projecting their own ideas of childhood innocence and fragility. The children know! They reveal this knowledge indirectly on psychological testing[34] and directly in play. Their concerns are with fears of separation, abandonment, pain, mutilation—much the same as adults whose lives are in jeopardy. When children talk among themselves or note an empty bed, they convey fears based on the realities they see around them.

Even a humane and otherwise useful recent review[35] of the subject contains many of the old biases. The quotation "most children never ask directly if they are going to die" is a clinical artifact gathered from children who know they won't get a straight answer. "If a child wants to discuss death with doctor or parents, it can be done without indicating you are talking about him" is pure hypocrisy. The quotation ". . . If the child does ask if he is going to die, tell him, 'You have a very serious illness, but we will do everything possible for you,'" is true but sidesteps the question asked and effectively silences the questioner. The avoidance or sidestepping of a child's inquiry raises even greater anxieties than the simple, supportive statement of the truth.

If one listens to a child, one may also hear a reluctance to know too much too soon. Naturally, there is never a benefit from blunt confrontation or pure information giving. Anything told anyone, child or adult, must always be in context and clearly solicited.

Finally, there is the common advice to keep things as "normal" as possible . . . no special parties, such as "Christmas in July" parties, no favors, no special immunities. Well, why not! So long as the events give pleasure and are tasteful and appropriate, such projects offer group activity, assuage guilt, and allow for nonverbal expression of love and apprehension. This, we realize, does cause some differences of opinion among professionals. Instead of criticizing such families, professionals might try to help the child understand how his parents and friends are trying to cope. It is also easy to forget that to many children actions speak louder than words.

The story of Winnie's death illustrates many of the preceding points about how children cope with a fatal illness in themselves and in their friends.

Fran, Anita, Barbara and Winnie were a closely knit group. They shared the same room for many months and related to one another as belligerent siblings. The two things they had in common were chronic, debilitating illness and (with the exception of Anita) virtual abandonment by their families. Unfortunately for them, discharge from the hospital was not possible even during short periods of remission.

A major crisis developed for these children and for the pediatric staff when Winnie's condition unexpectedly deteriorated, necessitating the girl's transfer to the Intensive Care Unit. Frances was the first to react, by profound depression. She withdrew from adults and the group, covering her ears at any mention of Winnie. The staff tried to keep the situation open to discussion by giving the children progress reports, but Frances continued her silence and immobility. After consultation, it was decided to try another approach. Because Frances was the most competitive of Winnie's friends and was seen frequently in argument over possessions, it was assumed that she was feeling guilty over the events taking place.

Her nurse was directed to talk to her during morning care in terms of the staff's and other children's response to Winnie's serious condition: "We're quite worried about Winnie—more than we've ever been. We don't know if she can get better; we hope so, but it's too soon to tell. Some of the nurses and doctors remember now that they were so mad at her the other day. Quite often they scolded and punished her for taking things that didn't belong to her. You know how she behaves; it makes people very angry because eight-year-olds should know better. But as one of the nurses said, 'It's a good thing we can't make children sick by getting mad and wishing them harm, because it would make us feel terrible if we thought we had made Winnie sick.' Some children I have known thought they could make things happen by wishing it, but they learned better. Wishing is not the same as doing." Fran's response was, "Yeah?" and a big smile. Variations on the same theme were also carried out by other personnel. Fran became her old self again.

The next hurdle came soon after Winnie died. The children and parents were gathered together for discussion. Various fantasies were brought to light. Barbara thought that Winnie had been punished for being bad; Anita blamed the devil; Frances said the death had occurred because Winnie refused to eat; another child believed she had died because her mother did not love her. A great deal of time was spent in clarifying reality for these children. We placed emphasis on Winnie's congenital kidney disease. We explained that it had been a problem no one else on the unit had; that the doctors had tried hard to help but could not make her well; and that fortunately we knew how to help all the other children. In addition, we talked about missing Winnie, stating that she was a friend even though we were sometimes angry with her and that we felt sad about not seeing her any more.

Additional opportunities for clarifying reality developed in the following days. When Winnie's bed was returned to the unit, Anita was the first to speak, "Well, the devil got her and you're next, Frannie." A great deal of work needed to be done before Anita could understand that the staff neither believed in devils nor were in league with him. Anita traded one fantasy for another. In the ensuing days she began to eat large amounts of food; this was a complete turnabout in her normal habit. It was discovered that Anita's mother was concerned about her lack of appetite and had told her that Winnie's death was caused by starvation.

Fran worked out most of her feelings in puppet play and painting. In puppet play she looked for missing dolls, and she painted pictures that asked questions about lost people. These occasions provided additional opportunities for reassurance.

Barbara's reaction was to cry a great deal, especially at night. Once she had to be moved into the hallway so that she would not disturb the other children. To Frances it meant that Barbara was also being sent to the Intensive Care Unit. Fortunately, the night staff was alerted to the treatment plan, understood the problem and was able to continue the day-time regimen.

It was a difficult period for the nurses and resident pediatricians as well. In addition to coping with the reactions of children, they were finding their own feelings un-manageable. Winnie's death created much tension among the staff. There was an undertone of blame and anger that was subtle at first; however, as the days passed, the nurses made openly hostile remarks that indicated they believed that Winnie had been incompetently treated. Defensively, the physicians accused the nurses of overinvolvement and subjectivity. The stress felt by many became the subject of a nursing–medical conference. As a result, the doubts and antagonisms regarding the medical management were dis-pelled because they were not based on facts. Review of the records indicated that heroic measures had been taken on Winnie's behalf. Once the staff were able to view the distortions in their thinking as reactions to grief and loss, they were able to be friendly toward each other.

The children rallied too. Within a few days, they wel-comed another child into their group. Play continued, and they were able to talk about Winnie warmly and vividly.

POSTMORBID FOLLOW-UP AND CONTINUED CARING FOR FAMILIES

Any program that has fulfilled the aforementioned criteria for comprehensive care has continued responsibility to families after the child has died.

It is too easy, unfortunately, for busy professionals to let their work absorb and neutralize the grief they themselves feel and to separate from a family they may have been working with for many years. Efforts need to be made earlier, before the child's death, to discuss how the survivors will relate to each other. There isn't anyone who does not imagine what the world would be like without the significant people with whom they are in contact. Thus, it will not come as a surprise when professionals explore with parents or siblings what they think it will be like before the impending death occurs.

Will the family allow a place for an ongoing relationship? When professionals limit their role to talking only about the illness and procedures, families cannot picture any other role. Although there may not be the kind of leisure to imitate the country doctor who would take coffee with the family and even join in family celebrations, rapport must be established on a broad front. If the professionals are to have a continuing relationship, this must be started not at the moment of death, but earlier, over the course of many months. Again, as in getting to know the individual child, if the health care team can create a larger role for themselves, the way is open for its continuation as a support system for the grieving family.

Conversations can take place on a number of subjects: general health, the pleasures the family have been able to enjoy, the nature of their vocations, attitudes about medicine and even the exploration of families' beliefs in religion and philosophy of life. Professionals who are pressed for time and who fear overextension often worry that they will gather upon themselves the unwanted burden of the friendship of these families.

Actually, no such thing happens. Most people want merely to know that if needed, the professional would not be aloof from contact. The number of actual instances when families have misused and overly pressed themselves on a professional are quite few. However, the opposite is unfortunately only too common—that is, families at the time of acute pain get the impression (soon after the loss of their children) that professionals are too busy and removed. It is unfortunate because this isn't true of the professionals we have known. Mostly, the nursing, medical and ancillary staff personnel experience very deeply the loss of each and every child they have treated. It remains for the professionals to develop techniques to maintain and express what is already there between them and their patients' families. In order to effect a post-patient-death relationship, professionals need to institutionalize meetings, conferences and projects that involve families.

Surprisingly, though all too frequently, siblings at home are expected to manage on their own when their sick brother or sister dies. Professionals need to introduce the subject of how the children at home are affected by the illness, what questions they ask and what answers they get during the parents' long absences before the child's death. This would reveal that even with the milder experiences of long separations, explanations to siblings are inadequate, since these children are not totally ignorant of what is happening around them. Children are seldom completely in the dark. Even a very young child senses a change in mood or picks up anxiety. Silence itself can have a foreboding, ominous quality. In these circumstances, children who are not informed about the seriousness of the sibling's condition will be left to bear the complete burden of dealing with these complex feelings. Families who deal poorly with the fatal illness also mismanage the eventual final loss—death.

Children deserve an explanation, but many parents fear that a discussion of illness and impending or actual death would break down their own controls and lead to their own disintegration. Hence these parents assume that their children would be likewise beset, and so they keep silent. Parents need reassurance that exposure of their feelings would reveal that they have cared and have the strength to feel deep compassion. They need to be told that children also have the strength to withstand grief reactions. This may come as a surprise to many adults who have a Pollyanna view of childhood.

When children are allowed to hear their parents openly discussing their hopes and concerns about the sick child, they too should be given permission to participate. They may take the opportunity to ask questions about the nature of the illness and treatment. In the absence of questions, information can be interjected by the parents. After initial talks, parents are then ready to comment on the possibility that the patient may not get well despite all that is being done, and later on that he is not expected to live. When there is adequate time, this explanation can be carried out gradually.

Children of all ages can and do tolerate the witnessing of a very sick sibling. The total impact obviously depends on the child's understanding, the reactions of the adults and the constancy of the parents' support of the sibling.

After the child has died, the parents should not tell the remaining children to remember the deceased as he was in the fullest bloom of life. This statement would cause the children to believe that life is tenuous and can easily end despite good health. On the other hand, the sudden viewing of a dead body without foreknowing that the grown-ups may be upset can cause the children to have a lasting painful memory of seeing an immobile, dead figure.

Statistics from the family courts in California show that 100 percent of children under five experience personality disintegration for as long as a year after the parents' divorce.[36] The same is very likely to be true when a brother or sister dies. Even up to the age of eight or nine, 50 percent of children are deeply upset.[37] This finding is supported by another study showing that in half the families who lost a child with leukemia one or more siblings developed psychosomatic symptoms. Uniformly, siblings would benefit from a series of interviews both before and after experiencing a loss.

Discussions before death occurs allow siblings to make amends for their hostilities toward the sick child. Ambivalence in families is usual. Children need to come to grips with both positive and negative feelings about the sick child and need to know that each is acceptable. A sick child in any family is quite an irritant, usually causing short- or long-term neglect of the siblings by parents and requiring much sacrifice in finances and mobility. It is only natural for siblings to wish that the sick child either be well or dead. They may also welcome the idea of performing small acts of kindness before death—visiting, sending gifts and writing letters.

Ms. H accompanied her eight-year-old to the hospital in the terminal stages of his illness. During ten weeks of rooming-in she won the respect of the staff, who were constantly impressed by her stoicism. However, her courage failed her temporarily after Matthew was placed in protective isolation. The isolation made it difficult for her to take frequent small breaks from his bedside because of the inconvenience of washing, masking and gowning. Consequently, she remained with Matthew for long, uninterrupted periods and found the tension unbearable.

On one occasion Ms. H ran out into the hallway in tears, asking to talk with someone. She explained that she feared losing control in Matt's presence and that her feelings of grief were so intense she could not hide them from him. The mental health nurse took the opportunity to discuss with her what she believed Matt knew about his illness. She sincerely thought that he had no knowledge of the seriousness of his condition and that she had succeeded in protecting him. However, the fact that she and Matt had become more and more withdrawn from one another indicated otherwise. Her reactions were observed. Because she could not discuss her preoccupations with Matt, she did not commmunicate with him at all. It was suggested that if she broke down again, she should tell him that it was because she was sad about his sickness and that sometimes she became discouraged and upset. Ms. H's pretense that she was not sad only denied the child's perceptions and made it impossible for him to confide in her and assuage his own anxieties.

On the same occasion Ms. H discussed with the nurse the reactions of other members of the family. Her husband was her main support, but he was not available because they lived a distance from the hospital. He was caring for their two sons with the assistance of several neighbors who took turns inviting them for meals. Ms. H confided that she and her husband were unable to be truthful with the older children, fearing that if they were aware of impending death for a long period of time, they might become insecure. The possibility was mentioned of her visiting the boys over the weekend in order to prepare them for Matt's death, and in order to find a housekeeper so that the family could maintain a semblance of normal living. It made sense to her.

A few surprises awaited Ms. H on her arrival home. Both boys were quite aware of their brother's condition. The older boy disclosed that he had embarked on a project of scientific inquiry. His science teacher directed the class to investigate a problem by collecting data, discarding the irrelevant material and coming to a conclusion on the basis of facts. Twelve-year-old Steven decided to research his brother's illness. His conclusion—leukemia.

The response of 10-year-old Luke to his brother's hospitalization was massive regression—demonstrated by clinging behavior, soiling, enuresis and learning difficulty.

Mr. H was coping poorly. He found the questions the two boys asked about Matthew harassing because he was trying to divulge as little information as possible. Disorganization in the household led to his quick consent to acquiring a housekeeper.

On her return to the hospital Ms. H was eager to recount her experiences. In particular she wanted to find psychiatric help for Luke, whose regression in this crisis gave impetus to her wish to have him see a professional. She was able to disregard what the antipsychiatry neighbors would think. She said that something constructive had to come of this ordeal—and helping Luke would be it.

Ms. H tried a different approach with Matt. Instead of leaving his room the next time she was tearful, she stayed, and a big teardrop fell on Matt's hand. He kidded her, saying, "You're pretty sloppy in your old age, Mom." Before long, Matthew was telling his mother that he was worried about himself too.

Similarly, grandparents and others need to be looked after by the concerned professional. Shaw[38] advises one-to-one staff for parents in general, as there is a tendency to seek quack cures, obtain bad advice and blame doctors for poor medical care. Parents question God as well for bringing the fatal illness on. At times, parents blame themselves for not having recognized the illness before it became hopeless. Shaw presents in detail how he tells parents bad news with dignity in a quiet room and avoids giving them tranquilizers.

All too often one family person is a focus of professional support and others become neglected. Both parents, all siblings, relatives who live in the home, close support people of the child no matter where they live—all may need strengthening for themselves and consequently for the afflicted child concerned.

VARIATIONS OF TERMINAL ILLNESS

As the cure rate for childhood malignancy is 20 percent five years postdiagnosis, there is realistic support for the hopes of children and their families that they will be the one in five who "makes it." Where the recovery is complete,[39, 40] as in acute meningitis, poisoning, trauma, seizures, and nephrotic syndrome, parents and children (recalling the sudden fearful onset, loss of consciousness, elaborate intensive care procedures) may resist accepting the good prognosis. In that group of children who almost died but have made some form of recovery, there can develop the fiction that they died and were reborn. Parents may join this fiction, with the added twist that now their child has knowledge of a spiritual or forbidden realm. Minor personality changes in the child become magnified, with parents idealizing the child's preillness personality. To have a child who is near death recover is a fright requiring a series of exploratory individual and group conversations. With the conquest of most infectious diseases, hovering near death, then recovering, is no longer an experience common to our culture; many people, therefore, lack the necessary coping mechanisms for it that they may have had in former times.

Where the recovery from fatal illness is incomplete, as in remission from acute leukemia, concerns about relapse and the child's fragility may influence parents to overprotect while, at the same time, doubting their own competency to follow a medical regimen.[41] Concurrently, the child may be denying that he is ill at all. Discussions with both parents and child need to focus on a realistic appraisal of the indefinite status and to expose apprehension, lingering grief, guilt and anxiety reactions.

A life-threatening episode or the diagnosis of a fatal disease, such as cancer, affects a family permanently. That the unthinkable has now occurred makes it more likely that it will recur. Observable changes in the body, such as weight loss, amputations or hair loss, or in the personality, such as regressive behavior, makes it more difficult to hide the painful thoughts. Continuing medication, clinic visits and arranging financing for catastrophic costs force the family toward depression. Dealing with home care, siblings, school and the child himself consumes a great deal of energy. A crisis in the home should be expected whenever a patient returns, whether for a visit or a long-term stay. The parents need support in their marital relationship. The special medical and emotional needs of the patient must be reconciled with those of siblings. With assistance, fathers can be guided to involvement equal to that of mothers.

Everyone in the family can use the opportunity of the remission to integrate their continuing fears of death with their abilities to live fully and constructively. Most children want to die at home. Yet parents may hesitate in the face of heroic physical and mental efforts to accommodate this wish. Larianne Stanciu, 13, dying of leukemia, says, "Don't hide yourself or your illness; you are still a person. If others can't deal with you honestly, it's their problem. I've been able to get close to my Mom and Dad, and we've even had a good cry together. I've talked about what I want and what I don't want at my funeral. I've asked a chaplain to give the service and I don't want a sob story."[42]

With the British system of hospices and hospice care now spreading to this country, there will eventually be a more available support structure for those families who wish to have their dying child cared for in their own home. For the child to be in his familiar surroundings, surrounded by his possessions, his family and his pets, the security offered is invaluable. He doesn't have to cope with the physcial day-to-day separation at the same time as he has to cope with his impending permanent separation. For the family to have their very ill loved one close at hand away from the impersonal machinery of a forbidding institution is reassuring when they are still able to have continuance of the necessary medical–nursing care unit (and after) the end.

Wherever preventive services have been offered families, more effective utilization of health care professionals has been the result. Wherever professionals, including students in the health professions,[43] are fully prepared, they can meet the demands. Whether this requires a greater effort or results in greater efficiency is less important than that the management of the dying child is comprehensive and of the highest quality.

REFERENCES

1. Bernstein, N. R., Sanger, S., and Fras, I.: The functions of the child psychiatrist in the management of severely burned children. J. Amer. Acad. Child Psychiatr. 8:620–37, Oct. 1969.
2. Lansky, S. B.: Childhood leukemia: the child psychiatrist as a member of the oncology team. J. Amer. Acad. Child Psychiat. 13:3, Summer 1974.
3. Goggin, E. L., Lansky, S. B., and Hassanein, K.: Personality characteristics of children with malignancies. 21st Annual Meeting of the American Academy of Child Psychiatry, San Francisco, October 1974. *In* Sandoz Psychiatric Spectator 9:12, 1975.
4. Spinetta, J., Karon, M., and Rigler, D.: Study of death anxiety among fatally ill six to ten year olds. J. Consult. and Clin. Psychol. 42:6, 1975.
5. Gunther, J.: Death Be Not Proud. New York, Harper & Row, 1949.
6. Oremland, E. K. J. D.: The Effects of Hospitalization on Children, p. 200. Springfield, Ill., Charles C Thomas, 1973.
7. Solnit, A. J., and Green, M.: The child's reaction to the fear of dying. *In* Solnit, A. J., and Provence, S. A. (eds.): Modern Perspectives in Child Development. New York, Harper & Row, 1963.
8. Bowlby, J.: Attachment and Loss. Vol. I: Attachment. New York, Basic Books, 1969.
9. Bowlby, J.: Attachment and Loss. Vol. II: Separation. New York, Basic Books, 1973.
10. Robertson, J.: A mother's observations on the tonsillectomy of her four-year-old daughter. *In* Psychoanalytic Study of the

Child. pp. 410–27. New York, International Universities Press, 1956.

11. Robertson, J.: Young Children in Hospitals, 2nd ed. London, Tavistock, 1970.

12. Lindemann, E.: Symptomatology and management of acute grief. Amer. J. Psychiat. 101:141–48, 1944.

13. Mattson, A.: Child psychiatric ward rounds on pediatrics. J. Amer. Acad. Child Psychiat. 15:2, Spring 1976.

14. Schowalter, J. E.: Death and the pediatric house officer. J. Pediat. 76:706–10, 1970.

15. Friedman, S. G.: Management of fatal illness in children. *In* Green, M., and Haggerty, R. J. (eds.): Ambulatory Pediatrics, pp. 753–59. Philadelphia, W. B. Saunders, 1974.

16. Green, M.: Care of the child with a long-term life-threatening illness. Pediatrics 39:441–45, 1967.

17. Sack, W., Cohen, S., and Grout, C.: One year's survey of child psychiatry consultations in a pediatric hospital. J. Amer. Acad. Child Psychiat. 16:4, Autumn 1977.

18. Anthony, E. J., and Koupernik, C. (eds.): The Child in His Family—The Impact of Disease and Death. New York, Wiley & Sons, 1973.

19. Gaylin, W. (ed.): The Meaning of Despair. New York, Science House, 1968.

20. Rochlin, G.: Griefs and Discontents—The Forces of Change. Boston, Little, Brown, 1965.

21. Parsons, E.: Effects of experiences with loss and death among preschool children. Child. Today 4 (6):3–7 (Nov.–Dec.) 1975.

22. Koocher, G. P.: Talking with children about death. Amer. J. Orthopsychiat. 44 (3):404–11 April 1944.

23. Ackerman, N. W.: The Psychodynamics of Family Life. New York, Basic Books, 1958.

24. Bell, N. W., and Vogel, E. F. (eds.): A Modern Introduction to the Family. Glencoe, Free Press, 1962.

25. Lansdown, R.: The dying child's view. Psychol. Today, April 1975.

26. Irwin, S., and Lloyd-Still, D.: The use of groups to mobilize parental strengths during hospitalization of children. Child Welfare 5:305, May 1974.

27. Cherry, R. L.: When cancer strikes at children. New York Times Magazine 80: April 7, 1974.

28. Binger, C.: Childhood leukemia: emotional impact on patient and family. New Eng. J. Med. 280 (8), 1969.

29. Leventhal, B. G., and Hersh, S.: Modern treatment of childhood leukemia: the patient and his family. Child. Today 3:3, May–June 1974.

30. Vernick, J.: Childhood cancer emotional consideration. Symposium sponsored by the American Cancer Society of Los Angeles County and the Children's Hospital of Los Angeles, Los Angeles, January 8–9, 1971. *In* Zeligs, R.: Children's Experience with Death, p. 88. Springfield, Ill., Charles C Thomas, 1974.

31. Mahon, E., and Simpson, D.: The painter guinea pig. 22nd Annual Meeting of the American Academy of Child Psychiatry, St. Louis, October 1975. *In* Sandoz Psychiatric Spectator 10:6, 1976.

32. Singher, L. J.: The slowly dying child. Clin. Pediat. 13:10, 1974.

33. Guimond, J.: We knew our child was dying. Amer. J. Nurs. 7:248, Feb. 1974.
34. Waechter, E. H.: Death Anxiety in Children with Fatal Illness, p. 86. Unpublished Doctoral Dissertation, Stanford University, 1968.
35. Zeligs, R.: Children's Experience with Death, p. 84–86, 87. Springfield, Ill., Charles C Thomas, 1974.
36. Wallerstein, J., and Kelly, J.: The effects of parental divorce; experiences of the pre-school child. J. Amer. Acad. Child Psychiat. 14:600–617, Autumn 1975.
37. Wallerstein, J., and Kelly, J.: Parental divorce: later latency. Amer. J. Orthopsychiat. 46:256–69, April 1976.
38. Shaw, A.: Dealing with the parents of a dying child. Med. Econ., Jan. 24, 1977.
39. Benjamin, P. Y.: Psychological problems following recovery from acute life-threatening illness. Amer. J. Orthopsychiat. 48:284–90, April 1978.
40. Green, M., and Solnit, A.: Reactions to the threatened loss of a child: a vulnerable child syndrome. Pediatrics 34:58–66, 1964.
41. Kagen-Goodheart, L.: Reentry: living with childhood cancer. Amer. J. Orthopsychiat 47:651–58, Oct. 1977.
42. Woodward, K. L., et al.: Living with dying. Newsweek, May 1, 1978.
43. Griffith, J. A., Fabri, P. J., Kies, M. S., and Sinibaldi, M. R.: Three medical students confront death on a pediatric ward. J. Amer. Acad. Child Psychiat. 13:72–77, Winter 1974.

BIBLIOGRAPHY

Benoliel, J. Q.: The concept of care for a child with leukemia. Nurs. Forum 11:194, 1972.

Easson, W. M.: The Dying Child. Springfield, Ill. Charles C Thomas, 1970.

Green, M.: Care of the dying child. Pediatrics 40:492, 1967.

Heffron, W. A., Bommelaere, K., and Masters, R.: Group discussion with parents of leukemic children. Pediatrics 52:831, 1973.

Karon, M., and Vernick, J.: An approach to the emotional support of fatally ill children. Clin. Pediat. 7:274, 1968.

Kübler-Ross, E.: On Death and Dying.

Martinson, I.: Home Care for the Dying Child. New York, Appleton-Century, 1976.

Mills, G. C.: Books to help children understand death. 79. Amer. J. Nurs., Feb. 1979.

Miya, T.: The child's perception of death. Nurs. Forum 11:214, 1972.

Natterson, J. M., and Knudson, A. G.: Observations concerning fear of death in fatally ill children and their mothers. Psychosom. Med. 22:456, 1960.

Rothenberg, M. B.: Reactions of those who treat children with cancer. Pediatrics 40:507, 1967.

Schowalter, J. E., Ferholt, J. B., and Mann, N. M.: The adolescent patient's decision to die. Pediatrics 51:97, 1973.

Stoddard, S.: The Hospice Movement: A Better Way of Caring for the Dying. New York, Stein & Day, 1978.

Waechter, E. H.: Children's awareness of fatal illness. Amer. J. Nurs. 71:1168, 1971.

Literature

1. The Hospice of Marin, P.O. Box 72, Kentfield, CA 94904.

2. Hospice, Inc., 765 Prospect Street, New Haven, CT 96511.

8

The Mental Health Team in Action

This chapter is a sampling of typical adaptational difficulties that come to the attention of pediatric mental health personnel. Each case illustrates the environmental approaches and background skills described in the other chapters. The dramatic, immediate results in many children are usual and a major factor in gathering support for this type of program from uninitiated staff. The lack of complication in the case descriptions is partly in the interest of clear exposition. In fact, as often as not a treatment plan is arrived at through negotiation and compromise. This then has to be implemented against the resistance of those who are outwardly compromising to the plan but still have degrees of subtle emotional opposition. Open disagreement is always more productive, because it allows clarification and healthy debate. This often leads to an arrangement in which a trial change of environment teaches everyone the most effective approach.

ANTHONY—EIGHT MONTHS

Failed to Thrive

Ms. C was concerned because Anthony was not growing as well as her three older children. He was not hearty, did not eat as well, vomited easily and did not respond happily to his environment. In effect, his mother derived little pleasure from caring for him.

One look confirmed Ms. C's description. Anthony appeared to be suffering from a nutritional or malabsorption problem. Thorough diagnostic work was performed, but the results were negative.

The possibility of inadequate sensory and tactile stimulation was considered. Thereafter, Anthony was bombarded with stimuli—music, singing, rocking, cuddling and much activity—but nothing about him changed. This circus atmosphere came to an abrupt stop one afternoon after several members of the staff witnessed Anthony and his mother together. They discovered that his mother also believed in highly stimulating interactions; she petted, stroked, shook and jostled him without mercy until he vomited. On this occasion his vomitus was bright red. Panicked, Ms. C rushed him into the hallway, screaming for help. Anthony screamed too.

The chaos diminished when one of the nurses casually reported that he had eaten beets for lunch. It took a while to calm Ms. C, who kept expressing concern that the staff would blame her for doing something wrong.

It was a valuable experience. This convinced the staff that it was not a case of understimulation—just the wrong stimulation. A detailed account of Anthony's daily home routine confirmed this. He was fed in front of a television set, in the company of three young children who were all competing for the attention of their harassed mother.

We succeeded in gaining Ms. C's cooperation in trying a different approach in the hospital environment. Anthony was:

1. Placed in a quiet room.
2. Assigned to the care of one nurse and his mother, who gave him one feeding daily with the support and supervision of the nurse assigned. Ms. C was assured that her mothering techniques were very good but that some babies were more sensitive and needed more subtle management.
3. Received quiet stimulation such as rocking, soft music, gentle handling, subdued lighting and bright mobiles. His nurse was directed to repeat his vocalizations as a method of rewarding and encouraging him.

   The results were dramatic. Anthony quickly settled down to a routine. He stopped vomiting, gained weight and smiled readily. Without any persuasion, his mother decided that she could find a quiet place to feed the baby at home as well as providing activities for the others at the same time. She was grateful to be assured that she was a good mother.

After his discharge, Anthony was followed in the outpatient department. He continued to thrive and developed into a robust boy from whom his mother derived much satisfaction.

CALTON—EIGHT MONTHS

Ruminated

Calton was admitted because of low body weight and rumination (chewing and gargling of partly digested food and a dribbling form of vomiting). The usual vigorous hospital diagnostic workup proved negative.

A conference was held to pool the knowledge everyone had about this baby. The nurses had learned that throughout this child's first months of life, he had been sleeping in a succession of temporary locations and had been handled and fed according to the mother's schedule as an amateur entertainer. A chance remark that his mother made to a staff member indicated that she resented this child, who was interfering with her career. Also, the staff reported that Calton was unable to maintain eye contact, arched his back and became stiff when held, moved his fingers in front of his face and rolled his head from side to side. A tentative conclusion was that this child was suffering from maternal deprivation. One nurse on each shift was assigned to care for him, and interfering contacts were kept to a minimum. His nurses were directed to respond to his crying immediately and to ignore the rumination. In this way, crying was reinforced as a more satisfactory way of getting attention and showing distress. Within 12 days the rumination diminished and Calton was able to maintain eye contact for several seconds.

Because the vomiting did not stop completely and because weight gain was minimal, the medical staff decided to reinstitute further vigorous diagnostic testing to account for calories that were being swallowed but not reflected on the scale. The rumination returned in full force, and eye contact stopped with a change in the nursing assignments. The staff became anxious as the child slowly continued to lose weight despite the introduction of nasogastric tube feedings.

Another conference was held, at which time the staff disagreed about the validity of the small improvement made initially and about the feeding techniques to ensure adequate nutrition. With reluctance and amid the rumor that the psychiatrist's recommendation of low stimulation actually meant an isolation room, a maternal regimen was finally reinstituted. Calton was placed in a quiet room, assigned one nurse per shift and protected against sudden changes of light and noise.

It took several days for the infant to begin to thrive. Before long, however, he gained significant weight, became more sociable and rarely ruminated. Over a period of several weeks he began to sit, crawl and progress developmentally. Eventually, he was ready for foster family placement. The follow-up was uneventful.

At a later staff conference, the management of Calton and others with similar symptoms was reviewed in the light of growing literature on the failure-to-thrive syndrome. As a result, the doctors were willing to accept a less rigid approach to the treatment of these children. A meeting was planned at the departmental level to establish policy in these cases because bias prevented an individualized approach.

TINA—AGE 2 YEARS, 4 MONTHS

Was Helped to Accept Radiation Therapy

Because she failed to cooperate with radiation treatment following brain surgery, Tina was referred to mental health nursing. As is consistent and normal for toddlers, she had only a limited understanding of what was happening and refused to have anything to do with it. She was required to remain perfectly still and alone while being radiated for two periods of three and six minutes.

The pediatricians were disturbed by the fact that sedation was unsuccessful. Her reactions were too unpredictable: she became either hyperactive or slept for hours after the procedure. The radiologists concluded that general anesthesia was required for 30 consecutive procedures. Actually, it was tried once, but even under light anesthesia Tina managed to move slightly. Anyhow, the nursing staff objected to this method and asked how this child could be managed without such drastic measures. This was the plan.

In the playroom, Tina, her mother and Ms. S, one of the mental health nurses, made a mold for a little doll, like the plaster mold used to immobilize Tina during radiation. Ms. S placed the doll on the x-ray table of the play hospital and explained that this was a treatment that didn't hurt at all; that sometimes dollies wondered if it would. She directed the doll to hold very still while she read a story to make the time go very quickly—a three-minute story. She praised her for being cooperative, learning so quickly and doing a good job.

Next Ms. S helped Tina to make a bigger mold for her own teddy bear and to practice giving needles because of the many tests she underwent that required parenteral sedation. Before long, Tina was ready to wheel the doll and teddy to the radiology department, accompanied by her mother and the nurse. By appointment, a practice session was arranged with the radiology staff.

Tina placed the doll to one side of the treatment table and the teddy face down in the plaster mold previously used for her. She immobilized his head with three velco straps that came together at the back of the head, making a great deal of noise. His arms were positioned to his back. Then Tina had fun raising and lowering the table to suit her. When satisfied, everyone went out to observe the bear and doll on the TV screen. Tina pressed buttons to get different views of the room as Ms. S talked to the doll and bear reassuringly over the intercom. Periodically, all went to see how the patients were doing.

Soon Tina consented to wear the same headgear and to assume the difficult position in order to show the doll and animal how to do it better. Ms. S held her hand, and her mother spoke to her over the intercom. She tolerated this for more than two minutes.

To complicate this process, the radiology staff congregated to make derogatory remarks about what was being done. They said that all this had been tried before without success. Before long, there was a large defensive audience.

When they observed that Tina was cooperative during rehearsal, the radiologist and the technician decided to proceed immediately with the actual treatment, although Ms. S objected. It was much too premature, in her judgment. Having no influence over this decision, however, she talked reassuringly to Tina. Everyone was amazed. It worked! Tina understood, trusted and cooperated.

During the afternoon, Tina resumed play in the miniature hospital, this time by herself as her mother and the nurse watched nearby. She stuffed a baby doll into the mold and said it was her sister. Next a nurse doll received equally bad treatment. Finally she picked up the doctor figure and smacked it across the face, looking very pleased with herself. Play is self-healing.

On the following day, Tina was scheduled for two full treatments of three and six minutes and, remarkably, she proved equal to the task, behaving like a six-year-old. On the third day, her mother took over as the supportive person who talked and read stories, as the nurse supported her. The whole project was so successful that her pediatrician decided Tina could be treated on an outpatient basis. Initially, this occurred with both the nurse and the mother in attendance until both agreed that her mother could manage independently.

It was encouraging to see Tina's mother develop confidence and pride in her ability to cope with her child. Formerly, she was impatient to the point of threatening to hit or leave Tina unless she cooperated. Although it was obvious that Ms. P loved her child, she was under great stress—pregnant and worried about the possibility that the same illness might develop in the unborn child. Tina's problem was believed to be hereditary.

This mental health intervention was particularly constructive because it produced change not only in the behavior of both mother and child, as was anticipated, but in the radiology staff as well. Once resistance to the interference of outsiders was overcome, they decided to modify the management of other young patients as the result of their experience with this toddler.

PHILIP—AGE TWO-AND-A-HALF

Resumed Growth—Physical, Emotional and Intellectual—During Hospitalization

Despite his hearty eating, Philip's mother noted that he had ceased to grow after the age of one-and-a-half years. He was admitted for diagnostic testing and observation that required long-term hospitalization. Separation from his family appeared to pose no problem for this toddler; he was immediately at home and courted relationshps with all members of the staff indiscriminately.

A charmer, he had everyone vying for his attention before long. He was able to manipulate people into giving him extra treats and privileges forbidden to the other children. Whenever he was refused a request, he found personnel from other floors to do his bidding. He had a following from every department connected with his unit. His maneuvers were so successful that it became obvious that he was completely undisciplined. His tantrums were catered to, and no limits were placed on his behavior.

At first Philip seemed excessively concerned with cleanliness. He became upset if his clothes and hands were soiled; he was rigid in his eating habits and became anxious whenever he dropped or touched food. He wanted everything cleaned up at once.

Philip became the subject of a nursing conference because of the premature versatility of his relationships and his overconcern with cleanliness, and also because his parents were not visiting regularly. The following plan was put into operation:

1. Assign one nurse as chief mother substitute and another staff member to relieve her. Others are to resist involvement with Philip and to direct him to his mother substitutes for gratification.
2. Disregard tantrums and do not reinforce this behavior by giving in to it.
3. Send Philip to the playroom regularly and introduce him to finger painting, play dough, soap and water play.
4. Mother substitutes are to (a) encourage autonomy by

preserving the skills already mastered—toilet training, dressing, feeding himself without help; (b) play games, sing and read to him, teach him rhymes and new words; (c) allow dramatic play related to procedures experienced, especially needle play.

5. Encourage parents to visit regularly, to leave family photos and to allow Philip to telephone home daily.

6. Ask for a social service intervention to determine the home situation and to counsel the mother.

7. Observe Philip's relationship to his parents during visiting periods.

At first, both Philip and the staff balked at the curtailment in his relationships; it was gratifying for some personnel to be Philip's rescuers. The restriction for Philip meant the curbing of his manipulative power. It took constant vigilance initially to ensure adherence to the plan. Before long, Philip learned that his needs were supplied by two people. As his relationships were strengthened with them, he naturally preferred them to others. After these relationships developed, it was easy to set limits on his behavior, because disapproval from his special nurses was now meaningful to him.

Philip's first experience with play dough and water caused him some difficulty. He frequently looked to those around him for their reactions. Once convinced that the staff would not be punitive, he derived great pleasure from these activities. He showed less concern about soiling, often eating with his hands, and once he was seen playing with feces.

With encouragement and praise, Philip maintained his former skills. In addition, he showed much curiosity, learned games and songs and increased his vocabulary rapidly. He enjoyed playing doctor on his patient doll and displayed understanding of the procedures. Thus, his tantrums subsided when avenues for expression were provided.

It was difficult to persuade Philip's mother to visit because she had no one to care for her other children. Furthermore, she did not enjoy visiting because Philip refused to go to her voluntarily. Every time she visited, she disapproved of his disheveled appearance and would wash his hands and rearrange his clothes. She believed that the staff had spoiled him and it took some effort to convince her that we did not intend to usurp her maternal role. We explained that Philip's reaction to her was his way of expressing his anger at not having seen her for a long time. She agreed to call daily and to accept social service help.

During the latter part of his hospitalization, Philip began to gain weight. In order to ensure his progress, the staff arranged close social service follow-up with tentative plans for foster home placement if counseling of parents was not influential in his being more welcome at home.

NICOLAS—AGE THREE

Refused to Sleep in His Room

The night staff reported that Nicky had not slept for six nights. He cried to be let out of his room: sometimes he called for his mother. Medication was not effective in promoting sleep. On a few occasions he was taken into the dayroom, where he promptly fell asleep on a chair or a sofa. During the day Nicky was groggy and liked to curl up for catnaps in any area other than his own unit. It was difficult to keep him in his room except when his family was present. Most of the time he closed the door and remained outside, directing everyone else to do the same.

This behavior began the night following surgery for hypospadias repair. His mother believed that it resulted from separation anxiety; Nicky was obviously calmer and more cooperative in her presence. This possibility was considered, but it did not account for his sleeping at night when the location was changed. This led to the supposition that Nicky's difficulty probably was related to an association between sleeping in bed and going to the operating room. He had received preoperative medications in his room and was transported to surgery in bed.

We decided to observe Nicky's play in the miniature hospital. The plan was to use the miniature hospital as a diagnostic tool to externalize the child's problem; to use dramatic play as a therapeutic tool as a way of relieving tensions and setting the boundaries between reality and fantasy.

In the first session he vacated all patient dolls and furniture from the bedroom areas; he then placed the patient dolls in the nurses' station, the toy chest, and outside of the hospital area. When asked what the dolls were doing in these places, he said that they were asleep. When he was asked, "Why there?" he said it was better that way. We asked him what happened to the boys and girls when they remained in their own rooms. He said that fires happened there, and then he labeled the anesthesia and treatment rooms as fire areas too.

This episode made it possible for us to point out to him, over and over again, where the fire rooms were (anesthesia and treatment rooms). We explained that fires did not happen in the bedrooms and that it was safe to sleep there. Also, we made the distinction between nighttime sleep and drug-induced sleep. Nicky ended his play abruptly, stating that he did not like to play because it made fires. When asked where the fires were, he clutched his penis.

The staff and his mother, who was an eager participant, were directed to reinforce the explanations made during the day. There was no change in Nicky's behavior after the first session. However, he was keen on playing in the model hospital again. During the second session, essentially the same themes prevailed—that is, removing beds and dolls from the "boo-boo" rooms. On this occasion he was asked what brought little boys to the hospital. He had a quick answer, "because they make do do in their pants and touch their pee pees." Therefore, as previously, the staff took the opportunity to clarify reality for him. This time the session ended differently. Before he left the playroom Nicky returned the dolls and beds to the bedroom areas. Thereafter, his sleep problem disappeared, and we knew that he understood our explanations.

However, we did have reason for concern later. Just before discharge it was decided that Nicky needed to have deep sutures removed under anesthesia. Precautions were taken in order to prevent a recurrence of the old problem. This time he was given medication in the treatment room, and he was transported to the operating room on a stretcher. This procedure proved to be a good move because there was no more difficulty.

Because of egocentric thinking at this age, the relief Nicky experienced would only be temporary. His parents were encouraged to reinforce reality by keeping the subject of hospitalization and treatment open for discussion and by assuring him that he was not responsible for his condition.

JACK—AGE FOUR

Suffered Acute Depression

Jack was originally admitted for repair of a chest deformity. He acquired a staphylococcus infection postoperatively. As a result, he was placed in isolation for two weeks and received medication intramuscularly every six hours.

Following the period of isolation, severe depression brought him to the attention of the mental health consultant. It was reported that Jack had not been prepared for hospitalization. His parents appeared overwhelmed by the experience and attempted to keep information from their child for his protection. Jack's response was to withdraw from all activity, shun the company of his parents and staff and vomit repeatedly when forcibly fed by his parents.

On the basis of the information brought out in a staff conference, the following plan was initiated:

1. Assign nursing personnel to him consistently.
2. Ascertain Jack's understanding of his hospitalization and treatment and clarify misconceptions; communicate with him by the use of drawings and encourage the expression of feelings by playacting treatments on his teddy bear.
3. Deal with separation anxiety by (a) encouraging his parents to visit consistently; (b) allowing Jack to telephone his family daily; (c) asking parents to bring in family photos and (d) talking to him in terms of when he is home again.
4. Interpret to parents the necessity for giving explanations to children and of visiting regularly in order to maintain the child's trust.
5. Gain parents' cooperation in managing the eating problem by deemphasizing it.

Initially Jack talked to no one; thus, it was not possible to elicit his understanding of what had happened to him. Instead, his nurse explained to the teddy bear, who had the role of the patient, the nature of the surgery and the kinds of routines and procedures that Jack had personally experienced. She gave teddy his first injection and had the bear object loudly and demand a proper explanation for the painful needle. Following this, Jack gave injections too but remained silent until he received his next intramuscular injection. His first expression to the nurse was, "Now you're really getting me mad."

Safe equipment such as syringes without needles, bandages, and adhesives were left at his bedside for leisurely play. On one occasion he taped the bear to the bedside and explained that teddy was being punished for not eating. When he was asked what kept him from eating, Jack replied, "Teddy won't eat because he feels choked."

Before long, Jack was telling us how much he missed his mother, although he continued to ignore her presence when she visited. His mother believed that he did not need her and decided to stop visiting altogether. When she explained this feeling to Jack's nurse, the latter took the opportunity to interpret his behavior. She explained that Jack's behavior was his way of retaliating for what he perceived to be his mother's abandonment of him (in fact, it is not unusual for young children to react in this manner). It was made clear to her that he asked for her frequently and that no one could adequately substitute for her.

As a result of the discussion, a regular visiting pattern was established and other measures to lessen the mother's separation anxiety were carried out. The parents were included in Jack's teaching and were encouraged to reinforce it. Also they agreed to avoid being present at mealtime, because they believed that they could not refrain from force-feeding.

Within two days, Jack's vomiting stopped, even during times when his parents coaxed him to eat (other than mealtime). He began to relate to other children and was able to object verbally to what he considered "choking" treatment.

The staff was delighted with his behavior and did not anticipate that Jack's parents would be less so. Apparently, his parents did not consider an outgoing, expressive child to be an asset. At a staff conference, we discussed the reasons for the parents' hostile attitude to what we termed Jack's improvement. We had assumed that Jack's former behavior was a problem to his parents, when in actuality it was not. In retrospect, no one could recall the parents' voicing any concern. We agreed that there had not been enough work done with the parents to explore their ideas and feelings regarding the events taking place. We had not adequately considered the mother's belief that Jack did not need her any more. To her it probably meant that she had no more function and that the staff could do better.

The best recommendation for this kind of problem is psychiatric evaluation of the mother. Had our relationship with this family been better, this might have been possible. Under the circumstances, however, we could not expect Jack's behavior at discharge to be long lived.

ROBINSON—AGE FIVE

Acted Out His Castration Fantasy

Uncircumcised in infancy, Robbie, age five, was admitted for elective surgery to correct the situation at his father's request.

Robbie was told that the procedure involved the removal of foreskin, that his penis would be sore afterward but that it would all be there. Nevertheless, he was not a willing candidate; preoperatively, he was uncooperative and hyperactive.

Postoperatively, Robbie was agitated and cried a great deal. He was observed on several occasions sitting on the edge of a chair in the hallway, pulling up his gown to expose his genitalia as different staff members passed. Each time he was told that his penis looked sore but that it was all there and that before long he would notice that it looked better too. At first he was encouraged to repair broken toys (restitutive play) and then to use syringes and water pistols to play out the pleasure in the function of the penis. He appeared to progress well on this regimen and the staff was greatly relieved. By chance, however, just prior to his discharge, Robbie was examining his penis at his bedside as a woman visitor approached him. She reacted hysterically— screaming for a nurse to come see what had happened to the poor child. Robbie's reaction was even more intense. He began to howl like a wounded animal and was inconsolable. Not long afterward, he was found wearing a girl's dress. He was assured over and over again that his penis was intact and that he was still a boy. The staff was unanimous in recommending further treatment. He was referred to Child Psychiatry on an outpatient basis.

Although this child's reaction was more prolonged and intense than usual, it is not atypical for children between the ages of three to six, since preoccupation with mutilation and castration is prominent. Ideally, the stage of emotional development is one of the criteria considered in the selection of patients for elective surgery. The staff can assume that regardless of age, however, a child will have castration fears from procedures involving the genitals.

In Robbie's case, he was predisposed to difficulty. At a vulnerable period, he was to have surgery on a highly symbolized area of his body and for no apparent flaw. The parents' motivation for having Robbie circumcised at this particular time and other factors that predisposed him to a major disturbance were unclear.

The plan for managing this child involved (a) a thorough explanation of the surgery and related events, (b) repeated clarification of reality; that his penis was intact; (c) use of restitutive play and (d) psychiatric follow-up.

ALEX—AGE FIVE

Showed Bereavement and Feelings of Guilt

Alex was a five-year-old boy whose mother died three months before he was admitted for the correction of a congenitally deformed penis (hypospadias). He clung to all the nurses who came by his bed, cried and whimpered continuously. Despite this, the entire staff found him likable and was sympathetic to him. He spoke about his mother and to one intern in particular of how he missed her. However, this talk was illogical, and he often stopped in the middle of a sentence or changed the subject.

At a staff conference, it was decided that a boy of this age, who had already had two stressful experiences (loss of mother and surgery), would tend to view these experiences as being related. They believed that he needed to talk about his ideas of how his mother died, whether her death was caused by anything he had done, and whether the hospitalization and surgery were evidence of his badness and were punishment for his mother's death and his other wrongdoings. One person was assigned to Alex to talk with him and play out his ideas on his own mortality and his feeling that his mother might not have left him if he had been a more lovable person.

Unfortunately, Alex was discharged before the plan could be carried out. On a return visit to the surgical follow-up clinic, it was noted that Alex was depressed, more taciturn and unwilling to attend school. At this time, the mental health nurse went over most of the issues that had been discussed at the conference. Alex became almost instantly loquacious and happier in his mood. His aunt was informed of the conference and was told to reinforce Alex's confidence by telling him whenever the opportunity arose how much his mother loved him. She was also to tell him that doing wrong does not result in horrible consequences, that it is unlikely for him to die, and that his mother would be proud of his ability to talk about his worries. He was given a photo of his mother to carry with him and a hospital card with the names of staff he could visit in the coming months.

RUTH—AGE FIVE

Developed Nightmares After Cardiac Surgery

Ruth was a cooperative, docile child. She participated in the elaborate preparations indicated for major cardiac surgery and appeared to tolerate the stress remarkably well.

Postoperatively, Ruth's difficulties did not become apparent until she was returned to her own room after 48 hours in the Intensive Care Unit. Her mother, who stayed with her continuously, reported that Ruth was having such frightful nightmares that she was trying to avoid sleep altogether. The usual reassurances of telling her that the dreams were not real, of leaving a light on, and of having her mother close by did not help. Medication for sleep was tried without success.

During the day, Ruth was irritable, clinging and uncooperative. Her mother was alarmed and asked for direction.

There was no doubt that Ruth was reacting to the ordeal

that she had undergone and was attempting to work out her experiences during sleep. The objective was to help her master the problem in her waking hours. Our routine practice of helping children to cope with hospitalization by allowing them to reenact experiences in dramatic play was completely rejected by Ruth. She refused contact with her preoperative doll on which she had practiced so compliantly those procedures she herself would undergo. It was too direct an approach for her. Instead, the staff used a method that Ruth found tolerable and that also employed her mother's artistic talents.

We avoided talk and play that concerned Ruth directly. Instead, we focused attention on a fictious character named Evelyn, who was to be admitted to the pediatric department for chest surgery. Ruth and her mother occupied themselves with preparing a booklet on the kinds of things Evelyn needed to know—the people she would meet, the procedures she would undergo, and the fun activities in which she would participate. In addition, other patients on the unit were singled out as having experiences similar to or different from those of Evelyn and their reactions were discussed openly. Eventually it was possible for Ruth to identify with Evelyn and to talk about herself and Evelyn interchangeably. When this occurred, she had no difficulty in playing with her own doll—inserting and removing chest tubes, IVs, bandages and giving countless injections—with appropriate effect, sometimes in the role of doctor or nurse and at other times as the victim. Within two days, the nightmares disappeared. Convalescence proceeded satisfactorily. Her mother was encouraged to continue the play activities after discharge.

The plan for this child focused on helping her to cope with traumatic experiences by bringing them into conscious awareness. This involved (a) recalling the events and lessening her anxiety by using indirect methods (that is, substituting a fictitious character and other children as the subjects); (b) turning passive experiences into active ones in order to master them and giving alternative meanings to real events; (c) using her mother, the most trusted person in her life, as the therapist; and (d) encouraging the expression of feelings and the enacting of events through play after hospitalization.

VALERIE—AGE FIVE

Was a Champion Manipulator

Although Val came to us with a variety of behavior problems in addition to chronic kidney disease, nothing about her provoked so much response from hospital personnel as did her refusal to eat at mealtime. In short order, she managed to win the attention of people from many different departments—physicians, nurses, dietitians, cleaning and laundry personnel and ever-changing visitors. She was so appealing—cute, little, sick and abandoned by her mother. Everyone wanted to make it up to her by feeding her whatever she wanted. It appeared that there were as many ideas on how to solve her problem as there were people involved. She was bribed, coaxed, petted and punished to no avail. Val had never had so much attention, and she was not willing to give it up.

After a few weeks of struggling, it became apparent that Val was eating no better and was obviously emaciated. The head nurse decided to call a halt to all personal remedies and asked for the intervention of the mental health nurse.

Although some staff members disagreed, the mental health consultant decided to remove altogether the gratification Val received and to substitute other pleasures. The plan adopted was to:

1. Serve her minute portions of food without comment; refrain from praising her for eating as well as to refrain from scolding for not eating; remove the tray at the usual time.
2. Offer her the usual between-meal snacks given to all the children, and nothing more.
3. Assign one person as a consistent mother figure.
4. Arrange for pleasurable activities within and outside of the hospital environment.

Our purpose was to get Val to eat because of hunger, and not for the purpose of pleasing anyone. We also wanted her to stop using mealtime as a way of retaliating and expressing her anger. We needed to show her that her eating habits did not matter to us one way or another.

It was not easy going. Some of the staff thought that the plan was a sadistic one: a form of starvation. A number of people were slipping her goodies just before meals. It took a few days before everyone, including visitors, understood what was required of them.

Gallantly, Val held out for ten days. It was difficult for her to believe what was happening. She was stunned by the small quantities of food and the seeming lack of interest in her antics. On several occasions she demanded different kinds of food and was ignored; she tipped over her tray and was sent out of the dining room; she announced that she would eat if she were fed, but no one agreed to feed her.

When all Val's maneuvers were thwarted and every illicit source of food cut off, she surrendered. She ate voraciously. It was difficult to keep the staff from praising her.

Soon after, Val was deriving much pleasure from her outings and from the concentrated attention of one nurse. The eating problem dissolved except when new personnel were assigned to the floor. On these occasions she did attempt to manipulate them by refusing to eat, but it did not work. The staff was finally united on this issue.

WHITNEY—AGE SEVEN

Had Violent Postoperative Episodes

Whitney accepted admission for a skin graft on his leg with equanimity, yet he expressed some concern about the gas mask that had frightened him in the past. He had been hospitalized previously for multiple surgical procedures for correction of ptosis of the eyelid. All the procedures had proved to be failures.

In preparing Whitney for his operation, both the physical and psychological factors were considered. A great deal of dramatic play was performed, with the emphasis on anesthesia. He seemed to understand what was to take place.

On the morning following surgery, an emergency situation concerning Whitney occurred. He accused the nurses and doctors of having lied to him—of pretending to graft his leg when they really had done something else. He attempted to remove the pressure dressings, splint, and IV; he threw his bedpan and urinal at the aides and actually succeeded in moving pieces of equipment to different parts of the room while remaining in bed. He terrorized the children and staff without too much difficulty. Intervention of the mental health nurse was requested.

In this immediate upheaval, Whitney was told that his anger was obvious from how he had reacted and what he had done. Since he would not have been destructive without a reason, everyone wanted to find out why he was so angry. Clearly Whitney was confused about what had happened to him because he had bandaged both eyes of the patient doll that was used in preoperative teaching. In addition, the staff reported that his leg's appearance postoperatively was considerably different than that which was anticipated: a splint and pressure bandage had been applied to his leg unexpectedly as a measure to prevent damage to the graft site.

He was reminded of what he had been told preoperatively and that his expectations were different; also, that sometimes boys and girls were confused after surgery when things were not familiar to them. He was assured that the staff had not lied to him but rather had not anticipated his appearance correctly and that they were sorry about it. He was then invited to ask anything he wanted to know. He responded by exposing his genitals and waited for a reaction. He was told that he looked all right and that the only place he had been operated on was his leg. With this, Whitney jumped out of bed into a wheelchair, unassisted, and announced that he was going to the playroom.

Later in conference, the staff discussed the clues Whitney had given preoperatively that were forewarnings of difficulties. A plan for future management ways:

1. Assign one nurse consistently to care for him.
2. Repeat all preoperative teaching, including the changes; use dramatic play as necessary to communicate with him; make clear the operative site, since children around the ages of three to six are fearful of injury to the genital area.
3. Show him that the staff is not afraid of him; let him know that we are able to stop him if he gets out of control.
4. Request psychiatric evaluation and medication.
   On medication, Whitney was cooperative for two days. However, there was a second violent episode that was precipitated by a disagreement he had with

a visitor; this time he threw furniture. The staff and patients fled, and several mothers barricaded themselves in a room. The atmosphere was chaotic.

This time, the staff approached Whitney by telling him that "the law" (the "boss") (the mental health consultant) was there to see to it that he did not get hurt and that he did not hurt anyone. Fortunately, it was not necessary to use physical restraint: verbal limits were sufficient. He immediately stopped his activities and meekly went along to a side office. Once there he related his persecution fantasies to the mental health consultant—how people were trying to hurt him, especially with the operation. The opportunity was used to explore the reasons for his beliefs and to clarify reality for him.

It was important to show this child that people were not afraid of him and that others were in control. By confronting him with "the law," there were now external controls to bolster his shaky inner controls. By asking him for evidence to justify his persecution fantasies, those fantasies could be dispelled and the events of hospitalization could be explained to him.

All these measures were palliative, however. Whitney required long-term treatment. Psychotherapy on an outpatient basis and social service counseling for his mother were arranged.

ELLIOTT—AGE EIGHT

Reacted with Anxiety to a Change in Relationships with His Parents

On admission, the medical staff thought that Elliott had pneumonia. However, further investigation led them to believe that his condition was more serious. The findings strongly suggested a malignant growth in the chest.

His parents were informed of this possibility and were presented with a tentative plan for more diagnostic testing and eventual surgery and radiation. They were completely stunned by the knowledge and lost their self-control. In their son's presence they were unable to keep up appearances. The parents were in anticipatory mourning and did not attempt to hide it, nor did they offer Elliott an explanation for their behavior, which was extreme considering the child's understanding of his illness. Instead, they summoned their large family to come from distant places. Relatives congregated and visited with expensive gifts. Elliott panicked and appealed to his nurse to tell everyone he was not sick enough for all the fuss.

The staff attempted to intervene without success. A conference was called to determine how we could be helpful to this family. The following plan was initiated:

1. Assign one nurse to support the parents and to encourage them to express to her their feelings regarding Elliott's hospitalization and diagnosis.
2. Interpret to the family how their behavior was affecting Elliott and how their denials of his perceptions served to confuse and alarm him.
3. Curtail visitors and gifts and reestablish former disciplinary measures.

In a series of conferences held with their nurse, the parents were able to explore how they were reacting to the events taking place. They blamed themselves for the child's condition—for not insisting on a more complete diagnostic workup when Elliott was previously hospitalized with a diagnosis of pneumonia. They believed that had they been more astute, their child could have been treated earlier. It was pointed out to them that the responsibility for medical diagnosis could not be placed on them, and that most likely the possibility of malignancy would not have been considered at an earlier date by any physician. The medical staff was particularly influential in conveying this information.

By dealing with their feelings outside of Elliott's room, his parents were able to assume a more normal attitude in his presence. They told him that they found it difficult to see him suffer and had probably overreacted to what was happening. The main point was that they were able to communicate with him again. Subsequently they were able to assist in preparing him for more studies and surgery and to give him the support he deserved. Elliott's confusion and anxiety lessened appreciably, and he was able to tolerate his experiences with remarkable courage once he realized that his parents would not withdraw and that his immediate and greater family relationships would be maintained in the usual way.

CHARLIE—AGE EIGHT

Wanted to Know What Happened to Him

Soon after trying out his new bicycle, Charlie was struck by a truck and knocked unconscious. Examination in the Emergency Room revealed that his left leg was almost completely amputated. Although immediate surgery was scheduled, it had to be delayed until agreement could be reached on his management. The pediatricians argued that every effort should be made to save the limb, but the surgeons believed that this was an impossibility. They recommended hip disarticulation. The specialists could not come to a decision, so they considered the parents' wishes. The leg was reattached, but there were grave doubts about the final results.

Charlie returned from the operating room in traction. He was in constant pain and required large doses of medication. After several days, the staff began to wonder why his pain could not be alleviated even with increasingly large amounts of analgesics. He began screaming uncontrollably until he "tuned out"—that is, he withdrew and was unresponsive for long periods. Neurological examination ruled out the possibility of brain injury. Therefore, Charlie was evaluated by a psychologist and a psychiatrist, who agreed that he was emotionally disturbed. They recommended treatment after convalescence.

But the nurses objected. They could not accept this recommendation, since the screaming persisted. The night staff complained that Charlie could not sleep and that other patients were distraught by his behavior. They demanded that something be done for Charlie and everyone else on the unit. The mental health consultant was elected to do it.

In preparation for the assignment, she collected several photos from magazines that represented important aspects of Charlie's experiences. They were to be the basis for a story about an injured boy. The object of this technique was to promote full integration of the dissociated or repressed experience by helping him recall the accident and deal constructively with related feelings. His disturbed behavior indicated that he was reacting to events that were out of his conscious awareness.

Charlie was asked to paste pictures in a scrapbook and

encouraged to dictate a story about each one. He was quickly involved. "That's a picture of a boy who got a bike for his birthday. He took it out to the street to try it out and it felt good. And then this big truck came and knocked *me* down." "Who is this boy?" she asked. "His name is Douglas," he said, without noting the slip.

On page two, Charlie reacted to a photo of a nurse standing by a door marked EMERGENCY ROOM. "That's where the boy went," he said. "That's where they had all the fights. Some said take it off; some said try to save the leg. And a mother was crying. He was scared. Hurry up with the writing, nurse. Turn the page." She asked him what he expected to find, and he cried out, "I want to see if he's alive. I want to find out what happened to him."

On the following page, they examined a photo of a child on a stretcher with several persons in attendance. They agreed that Douglas looked allright; that he was being helped. Charlie fell asleep.

The screaming stopped completely, and he slept through the entire night. On the following day, there was a new development. Charlie began exposing himself and masturbating openly. The nurses ignored him, but his mother slapped his hand. No one dealt with his unspoken question. Under stress he had regressed to an earlier phase of development (phallic) and was showing concern about injury to or loss of his genitals.

Clearly, it was time for Part 2 of the story. "I wonder," said the mental health nurse, "what Douglas will tell his friends when they ask about his injuries? I brought this body outline of a boy about his age. Let's paste it in the scrapbook and write what he needs to know on it. For instance, was his head hurt? [Charlie nodded no.] Okay, let me write that down. What about his face, neck, arms and chest?" [Charlie nodded no again as she continued to write, then he volunteered, "This leg is hurt bad."] "Yes," she said, "and the right leg is fine. His penis and scrotum are swollen because of the swelling in the leg, but of course, they weren't hurt. [This material was depersonalized and delivered casually so that he could hear it.] And his back is allright too." Charlie had the reassurance he needed. The masturbation stopped.

The conclusion of the story concerned Charlie's guilt about riding in the street against orders. He said that Douglas had been bad and so was punished. The mental health nurse said that she had known other boys like Douglas before. And because she knew how they felt, she wanted to tell a part of the story. Her version: "Douglas was so happy with the red bicycle and curious about how it would feel to ride in the street like the older boys. He was so excited that he forgot what his mother said. And before he knew it, the accident happened.

"Douglas was there because he wanted to find out what it was like, not because he wanted to disobey. He wasn't bad, just curious. And usually being curious and wanting to be grown-up are good things. His parents wanted him to wait until he was older and understood the rules of bicycling. They weren't angry with him, but happy that he would be well again."

Once events and feelings related to the accident were discussed, all signs of disturbed behavior vanished. Scientific–technical aspects of his treatment became his focus, as was consistent for his age. To help him understand how traction worked, the mental health nurse and he built a replica from scraps of wood donated by the carpentry shop, a cardboard box, miniature pulleys, string and tea bags for weights. The model and attached dummy shuffled back and forth from hospital to home or school. It served not only as an educational tool but as a conversation piece as well, to promote further integration of traumatic experiences.

A close relationship with his parents and staff and improvement in his emotional health strengthened Charlie's ability to withstand, without the recurrence of regression, the numerous complications that followed. Within a week, and frequently thereafter, there was evidence of impaired circulation to the reattached leg, which threatened to undo the initial good results. Heroic surgical measures were taken to correct these developments. And slowly over a period of months, with the help of physical therapists, he regained function of the leg.

Five months after the accident Charlie walked out of the hospital limping slightly and with his psyche intact.

KATE—AGE EIGHT

Was Rewarded for Positive Behavior

No one could doubt that Kate was acutely ill on admission for the treatment of rheumatoid arthritis and complica-

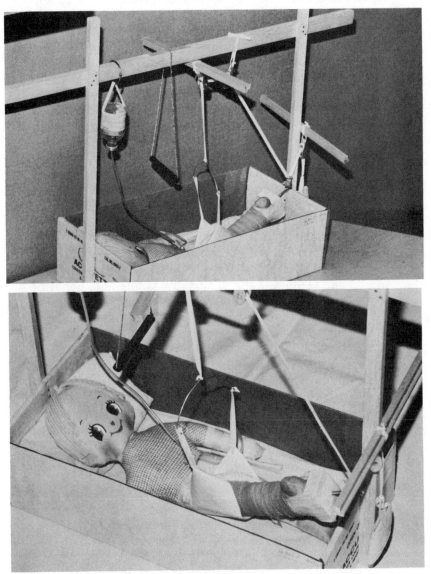

Fig. 8–1. A model of a dummy in traction served as an educational tool and as a device to promote integration of traumatic experiences for a severely injured child. (Photo by Steve Campus)

tions caused by medications. She was unable to walk and vomited repeatedly. Intravenous therapy was necessary to restore electrolyte balance and adequate hydration. Despite the seriousness of her condition, little compassion was felt among the staff for this miserable child. It was difficult to disregard her appearance and behavior: she shrieked for attention from her mother and nurses, refused to eat and to cooperate with treatments, vomited medications at will and accused the staff of deliberately causing her pain. And unfortunately, the side effects of prolonged medical therapy had distorted her face and body grotesquely.

Although her physical treatment was a challenge to everyone, the emotional component of her illness proved to be the more taxing aspect of her management. A many-faceted approach was required. At conference the following plan was outlined:

1. Reward positive behavior (when she communicates in a normal speaking voice, when she is not vomiting and whenever she demonstrates tolerable behavior attitudes) by (a) showing more attention; (b) reading her stories, playing games and records; (c) and giving her the prestige of a special relationship with one person.
2. Reduce the secondary gains derived from sickness by (a) ignoring the eating problem by withholding praise or reprimand; (b) carrying out physical care in minimal time as casually as possible; (c) anticipating her requests and meeting them before she has a chance to demand.
3. Administer tranquilizers to reduce anxiety and to make her more responsive to the positive aspects of the environment.
4. Refer her to the Physical Therapy Department for a daily program of movement and walking.
5. Support and counsel the parents regarding the child's illness and its effect on their family life.

The effects of the tranquilizers were immediately apparent. Screaming stopped and it was possible to gain Kate's attention for short periods. When she was calm and approachable, she received the concentrated attention of one person, who provided companionship and pleasant activities so long as she remained sociable. As soon as Kate began vomiting or complaining, her special friend left, explaining that she would call someone to attend to her. Then one or two staff members appeared to clean her or turn her as quickly as possible and with little concern. This procedure was followed approximately four times daily.

Initially it was possible for Kate to enjoy her special attention for about two minutes before reverting to the sick role. However, by the end of the first week, the pleasant periods grew to 15 minutes, and it became apparent that the amount of attention she derived from positive behavior exceeded that which she gained from short episodes of self-induced sickness, albeit without her conscious awareness.

Kate's parents were eager to cooperate and found some relief in this approach. By this time, they had become exhausted by their daughter's demands, however legitimate. They expressed anger toward Kate for the financial burden and the disruption of family life that her illness imposed. Subsequently, they felt guilty for this anger and tried to atone by indulging her. This action, in turn, led Kate to derive further gratification from the sick role. The vicious cycle was one they could not break until the environmental approach took effect.

Within three weeks, Kate's communication improved dramatically. She was able to ask for what she needed in a reasonable manner; she expressed anger toward treatment, hospitalization and having to share her mother with her two younger siblings. In addition, she was cooperating with her physical therapist to the point of walking satisfactorily and tolerating her program graciously.

As her improvement became obvious, it was then possible for the staff to socialize with her. She smiled spontaneously, stopped vomiting and demonstrated a sense of humor. Regrettably, her progress brought forth an unexpected reaction from a few of the staff. There was the unfortunate connotation that the approach used in this case denied the child's illness, when no such meaning was intended. It was a difficult notion to dispel and one that influenced future management.

Kate fared well at home for approximately one week. In ten days' time, however, she was readmitted because of vomiting and lethargy. At home, without support, it was difficult for her parents to continue the regimen followed in the hospital because of the stress of other children and household routines. On this second admission, Kate's treatment was considerably different; she was treated in a physical sense only; behavioral care aspects were avoided because of opposition to them. Instead, Kate was transferred to a hospital for the chronically ill, essentially unchanged.

MICHAEL—AGE NINE

Was the Terror of the Pediatric Department

Michael, along with his twin sister, was the youngest of eight children. The staff was mystified by his violence at night toward other patients and nurses. During the day he threatened the doctors that his father would avenge any needles he received for the treatment of a massive cellulitis of the leg. It usually took four adults to hold him down for his injections. His language was pungent. He had a deadly spitting aim and was far stronger than his size indicated. Often pilfering from other children's night tables, he was once found with a ten-dollar bill belonging to one of the visiting parents.

A small staff conference was held with the liaison psychiatrist, at which time it was discovered that there was much known about this family from the social service department and from a city court social worker. It was learned that the father, a construction worker, was violent and abusive; that his mother was equal to him in her pugnacity; and that the older siblings, as each reached approximately 15, got into trouble with the law. On interview, this child told the liaison psychiatrist that he was very jealous of his docile, favored twin sister and that he often misbehaved in order to get attention. He said that his father and oldest brother praised him for his toughness and would often punch him to show how much tougher he would have to be before he could face the world. Michael said he missed the fights he got into at home.

A treatment plan was made to establish strong external controls on his behavior. The staff was to use force, if necessary, to show the child that they were not frightened of him. They were to resist being provoked into aggressive action by him but were to be quick in apprehending him with the first sign of misbehavior and in arranging appropriate punishment (with the assistance of his family). It was hoped that after a semblance of self-control was achieved, some tenderness and reciprocity of relationship could be attempted in order to help him learn to be more sociable. A diagnosis of dissocial personality was made—that is, he made an excellent adaptation and identification with an antisocial family pattern, within which he did have a conscience (albeit it was different from that of the prevailing American culture).

An opportunity to implement the treatment plan came soon after conference. Michael attempted to bar the medical staff from his room by threatening to spear, with his IV pole, anyone who approached him. His screaming and swearing attracted a large audience. He taunted the onlookers, daring them to come in.

The mental health consultant, who was standing by, asked people to leave the area in order to lessen the gratification Michael was receiving. She remained in the vicinity. By chance, a passing psychiatrist looked in the room, and Michael told him not to come closer or else he would be hit. The doctor took him off guard by saying that there were too many trees in the way. This unexpected response so disorganized Michael that he dropped the pole and allowed the mental health consultant to enter his room. When he objected to her presence, she commanded him to get out of the way, stating that she was there to make an empty bed and that he was interfering with her schedule. The boy withdrew to his bed, shouting obscenities and trying to provoke a reaction, but she ignored him. When he was quiet, she told him a story incorporating much of the information she had about his home life. She said:

"You know, you remind me of a boy who was here recently. His name was Giovanni. He went around carrying a shovel. Every time someone told him to do something he didn't like, he tried to hit out with it. Of course, he was smaller than you and he wasn't very bright, so we thought he didn't know any better. People kept asking one another what made Giovanni behave that way. Some said that it was because his mother didn't like him, that his father beat him, and that his brothers and sisters were cruel to him. Some people even said that because his family treated him that way, he believed that everyone else was going to do the same. That's why he carried the shovel to protect himself. Can you imagine, he thought the whole world was like his mother, father, sisters and brothers! Of course, he was little, and he wasn't very bright; in fact, he was really stupid. He didn't know everyone wasn't like the people at his home."

As she made the bed, she offered him variations of the story. Within a few minutes, he dropped his weapon and announced that he was joining the other children for lunch.

Regrettably, this approach was not well accepted by some of the medical staff, who regarded it as negative and excessively punitive. They sought further consultation from the psychology department for an alternate plan. The psychologist made the alternative recommendation that a kid-gloved approach would lessen Michael's anxiety and thereby enhance his security. It was explained that Michael's behavior was a response to the threat he felt from staff anxiety and anger. Consequently, Michael was taken off all injections; he was allowed to play, eat, swear and wander as he pleased; also, he was given many toys.

The staff divided into two factions—one maintaining that the staff's threats and anxieties were being communicated to the child, the other maintaining that the problem lay within the child and his family.

Indeed, with the kid-gloved approach, Michael did not experience frustration. He became angelic and was chosen by the department to be presented during grand rounds as an example of deconditioning behavior therapy. Just as he was to be ushered onto the podium from the backstage room, the large audience heard several loud crashes and a stream of four-letter words. Michael never appeared. His favorite syringe, which he carried everywhere with him, was missing just prior to the conference, causing Michael to become enraged and completely out of control.

This incident taught the staff that in this case permissiveness had accomplished nothing. The first treatment plan was reinstituted. Thereafter, Michael was subjected to the pressure of a total environment. Once he realized who was in authority on the unit, he became remarkably well behaved and was able to form constructive relationships with a number of people.

Social Service tried to keep in touch with the family to maintain the discipline and direction that had begun in the hospital. After a month of weekly visits, neither parent kept further appointments.

BETTY—AGE NINE

Developed Personality Changes
After She Was Hit by a Car

Betty was struck by a car while crossing the street with her five-year-old sister. Her leg was fractured but otherwise she was unharmed, whereas her sister sustained multiple internal damage and was on the critical list. The mother, an intelligent and volatile woman, let the staff know that she was in the process of a divorce and that there had been many illnesses in the family during the past year. The factor that brought Betty to the attention of the staff was her complete personality change from a sweet, cooperative, almost prissy little girl to a screaming, ill-mannered brat whenever her family visited. In addition, despite the minor abrasions to her body, she kept the night nurses frantic by requesting assistance while writhing in pain. Because she caused such an uproar, the psychiatrist interviewed her at the bedside, with the staff and her mother standing by. Betty revealed that she fervently wanted to be more damaged than she really was. If she were hurt as much as her sister, this would expiate her sin of carelessness in crossing the street and regain her mother's love. She could not believe that her mother could continue to love her after the accident. She also revealed that for a long time she had suspected that her mother preferred the younger sister, and she believed that everyone thought she had arranged the accident. Finally, she showed a thinking disorder in which she felt magically empowered to cause all sorts of tragedies and distant events by the sheer power of her mind.

The staff devised the following plan for Betty's management:

1. Show the child the difference between thinking and doing.
2. Question and doubt the fact that Betty had enormous magical powers and inform her that the way to be powerful was to develop skills.
3. Insist that the things that had happened in the family and to her directly could be talked about with feeling and put in perspective without placing blame.
4. Indicate that others had similar feelings and that she could get angry at her sister and mother without losing her mother's affection.

After three days of following this regimen, the staff noted that Betty became more helpful, calm, pleasant, less rude to her family, and happy to be rapidly recovering. She did not revert to the saccharine, prissy girl she had been prior to the accident. In a follow-up conference, her mother reported that her emotional change was maintained. The staff felt they had in the short space of a few weeks averted the need for long-term psychotherapy that at first appeared indicated for this child, on the basis of current trauma and long-standing emotional difficulties.

BOBBY—AGE TEN

Resisted Taking Medication

Bobby was admitted for treatment of kidney disease. A rather unattractive, overweight child who had difficulty making friends, he was frequently made a scapegoat. Although bright, he was immature and lacked ambition. One of the chief problems in his hospital management was his inability or unwillingness to swallow pills. Many of the children teased him because of this. Although at first tolerant and patient, the staff became exasperated and ordered Bobby to cooperate, explaining to him that he was old enough and big enough and was expected to do so.

Bobby responded by vomiting, explaining that he was too sick to take medication. The staff realized that forcing him was dangerous and futile because he was too large to restrain. When it was possible to get medication into him by coercion, he vomited it quickly.

He became the subject of a staff conference, and the following plan was agreed on:

1. Assign one nurse to promote a special relationship and to support his mature behavior. (He was singled out by Ms. K, who played games with him, visited and won his confidence.)
2. Encourage him to express his feelings regarding his hospitalization and treatment and to talk about the attitudes toward illness in his family and the kinds of responses his sickness elicits from each family member.
3. Ask Bobby for ideas on how his medication problem

could be solved. Then incorporate his suggestions, thus making hospitalization more palatable for him.

Bobby quickly responded to the attention given him. He demonstrated the confidence he had in his nurse by revealing difficulties he had in establishing friendships and the loneliness he felt. He discussed the family pattern of sickness—that he was like his mother in the frequency of illness; that his family paid him much attention because of his chronic ailment; and that his brother was not of special concern to the parents because he was healthy like his father. It was clear that this family rewarded sickness, which was also seen as a feminine characteristic.

Bobby's solution to the medication problem was to ask for intramuscular injections. Luckily, it was the alternative measure the medical staff had considered taking. This course was agreed on and Bobby was directed to tell his nurse when he was well enough to change treatment. He was placed in charge. We were careful to avoid a punitive connotation to this plan.

Throughout, his nurse maintained the one-to-one relationship, with the idea of building up Bobby's self-esteem by praising him for jobs reasonably well done and for mastering new activities. Also, he received a great deal of admiration from the children and staff for tolerating the injections so well. Emphasis was placed on his manly behavior.

All teasing stopped and he began making friends with his roommates. On the fourth day after the intramuscular therapy was initiated, Bobby announced that he was ready to take pills because he was considerably better. He was successful immediately: there was no hesitancy, no vomiting.

Once Bobby found gratification through new relationships and achievement, he no longer needed to gain attention by means of the sick role he played in the family. There was more pleasure in mastery and in his newly found status.

ABBY—AGE TEN

Competed for Attention in a Sick Role

Abby was hospitalized to have a complete and rigorous workup for the possibility of blood dyscrasias or arthritis. All tests proved negative; yet Abby persistently complained of pain in her arms. The staff observed that analgesics and placebos were equally effective in alleviating her discomfort, except in her mother's presence. On those occasions no medication helped. A number of staff members suspected malingering. Although Abby was not confronted openly, the staff conveyed their skepticism to her through a lack of concern and inattention. This attitude, unfortunately, only intensified the child's symptoms and increased her mother's anxiety. Abby's pediatrician asked the mental health consultant for an evaluation of the situation.

It was not difficult to converse with Abby once we assured her that we (the staff) appreciated how difficult it must be for her to be hospitalized and to experience such pain. She was told that we would continue to pursue the cause of her problem so that we could help her. This approach removed the need for her to prove her illness. Once convinced that she had a sympathetic listener, she was able to talk freely about school, friendships and hobbies, none of which were especially satisfying for her. At first she hesitated to discuss family relationships, but with help she was able to discuss her problem. After the birth of her five-month-old sister, she believed that her mother no longer had time for her and did not love her any more. The discussion focused on both the positive and negative feelings that family members have for one another and how difficult it is to express some of those feelings overtly.

On the basis of this interview with Abby, the following suggestions were offered to the staff and to Abby's pediatrician:

1. Accept her symptoms as real because they indicate that a problem exists. (Once a problem is solved, symptoms may disappear. Attacking symptoms directly may result in their intensification or in a substitution of symptoms.)

2. Focus on the problem. (a) Advise parents to discuss sibling rivalry openly—how hard it is for Abby to share her parents with a young baby; how she must think they no longer have time for her; the negative feelings she must harbor toward her little sister for displacing her as well as her positive feelings; how she cannot hurt anyone through her thoughts but

only by her actions. In short, communicate with Abby that she is allowed to say what she is thinking without fear of criticism. (b) Ask the parents to spend time with Abby at home, when she does not have to share them or compete for attention. (c) Encourage Abby to develop peer relationships and new skills (social, scholastic, physical). As Abby acquires more abilities, she will rely less on her parents for emotional support and feelings of worth, using instead her own achievements as a basis for self-esteem.

Fortunately, Abby's parents were open to suggestions and were able to adopt the plan. This made additional intervention unnecessary. A few weeks after her discharge from the hospital, Abby's pediatrician reported that she had "straightened out."

ALLISON—AGE TEN

Regressed on Learning That She Required Cardiac Surgery

Soon after she learned that she had a cardiac problem, Allison developed the fear of vomiting, which became her preoccupation. Because her behavior became unmanageable—she was abusive and had hysterical episodes—her parents arranged for psychiatric treatment.

Several weeks later she entered the hospital, protesting and armed with a carton of eggs to defend herself against the staff. The fear of vomiting intensified. Her parents were equally distraught. They pleaded for her to be reasonable and bribed her with gifts, including a horse, to buy her cooperation for a few minutes at a time. Mother said she couldn't take it all, talked inappropriately in Allison's presence, and demonstrated her own anxiety constantly. Father was the stronger parent; he tried to be supportive but was overwhelmed by the behavior of his wife and daughter.

This family needed help, and they got it. The staff managed the parents and child separately. It was clear that the parents themselves required so much support that they could not offer it to Allison. Actually, their presence aggravated the child's behavior. Further, they interfered with her forming relationships with staff and peers. So, as one nurse counseled the parents, another provided the type of preparation best suited for Allison. As on the toddler level, all the teaching was depersonalized and toys more appropriate for a young child were used. Sessions were short and more numerous because it was difficult to hold her attention for more than a few minutes.

The nurse talked in terms of the doll's problems, and of other children who had had cardiac surgery, and verbalized fears and concerns about future events. Immediately, Allison began talking about how scary it was, and the fear of vomiting subsided. On the day of surgery, she was still frightened but could be comforted by her nurse, to whom she had developed a strong attachment. She said Ms. M was the only person who could help her.

In the ICU Allison reexperienced the fear of vomiting, which was intensified by the sensation of the endotracheal tube. Once extubated, however, she resumed talking about feelings, and the fear of vomiting disappeared once again.

When Allison returned to her own pediatric unit, she was angry and offensive to everyone. To help her deal with her feelings, her nurse helped her make a scrapbook record of her hospital experiences. They cut out photos of ICU scenes, monitors, oxygen tents, IVs, syringes, needles, hospital personnel and mood pictures (of people expressing feelings of fear or distress) from medical and nursing journals. With encouragement, Allison wrote about events and feelings (actually replayed her experiences). At one point, as planned, Ms. M said to her, "You were acting like someone who didn't expect to make it." This precipitated discussion of her basic fear. She blurted out that soon after she learned about her heart problem, a well-known entertainer undergoing cardiac surgery died in the operating room. And following this, her friend's uncle died of complications as a result of cardiac surgery. The fear of vomiting began during this period. Once this was revealed, Allison was able to link the sensation of nausea to these terrifying thoughts.

It was the turning point. Allison became more verbal, relaxed and, in addition, volunteered to assist in the preparation of hew new roommate, who was scheduled for similar surgery. She said, "Of course, I won't tell how bad it really is." Thereafter, she developed an interest in the welfare of other patients and identified with caretakers of children. She convalesced quickly and was discharged in record time.

Soon after, the family returned to visit. There was further evidence of integration of the hospital experience. Allison confided that she was in the process of making a play hospital and had put to use old dolls that had been rejected long ago because she was too old. She collected more equipment to make her production as authentic as the playroom's. Authenticity was important because she and her teacher were preparing a program and scientific exhibit on cardiac surgery for her classmates. At this stage, her experiences could be utilized to her advantage and prestige.

Her parents said that she had matured several years in three weeks' time. As evidence of maturity, they told of Allison's writing letters of gratitude on her own initiative to her nurses, cardiologist and surgeon. They explained that she continued to discuss feelings because they had learned to allow and tolerate it. They added shyly that it meant they had grown up too.

JILL—AGE TEN

Demonstrated Postsurgical Confusion

Jill was a pensive, well-mannered girl who became a puzzle to the house staff and a trial to the nurses because of her constant crying, screaming, incoherent speech and angry outbursts for several days postoperatively. The neurologist's findings were unremarkable, and a review of her anesthesia showed nothing unusual. Psychological testing showed nonspecific organicity.

A psychiatric consultation was requested. When the liaison psychiatrist saw Jill at her bedside, he noted that she was immobile, had a terrified look in her eyes and kept her head turned toward the wall. A medical student noticed that from the blinking of her eyes, Jill was following closely the conversation between the nurses and the doctors. On interview, she talked coherently about the happy times of her life:

her grandmother's visits, trips to an aunt's, birthdays, parties, and school activities. With any mention of her parents, illness, and events related to hospitalization and surgery, she reverted immediately to gibberish and screaming. Repeatedly, a return to conversations on subjects that Jill did not associate with anxiety resulted in a complete change in mood and greater relatedness.

In the staff conference, it was learned that Jill's illness had brought her parents together for the first time since their divorce, and that her father, whom Jill rarely saw, was keeping a constant vigil at the bedside. The nurses described their futile attempts at gaining her mother's cooperation in preoperative teaching and discussion of illness with the child. They wondered if adequate preparation could have averted the extreme behavior.

A tentative diagnosis of psychotic reaction was made, and the following plan was outlined for the staff:

1. Talk to Jill simply and as if she were responding appropriately; be matter-of-fact with her, chatty and friendly, but when she reverts to gibberish, tell her that she must be having painful thoughts—that sharing thoughts helps children begin to feel better.
2. Structure the environment by explaining every noise, activity and roles of staff.
3. Administer Stelazine, an antipsychotic medication.
4. Set up a regular visiting pattern for the parents and explain to them (a) that their constant attendance implies serious illness to the child; (b) that it is necessary to discuss Jill's illness and treatment with her.

It was hoped that this approach would direct Jill back to the more usual modes of communication and at the same time gratify her as little as possible in her aberrant behavior.

Within two days, her communication changed to the point where she could express anger at her mother. Her mother had withheld information about surgery and had implied that only tests would be performed to find out how to get rid of her pain, dizziness, and lethargy. In subsequent conferences with the liaison psychiatrist, Jill's desperate unhappiness and depression emerged and long-term psychiatric treatment was recommended.

SYLVESTER—AGE TWELVE

A Manipulative Hemophiliac

Sylvester arranged for his family to indulge him in every way. This was not difficult, because his parents were in constant marital strife which this youngster exploited to his own advantage. He rarely did homework, never controlled his temper and felt entitled to watch TV continuously. Whenever his machinations failed, he used his ultimate weapon of complaining of joint pain.

This behavior on the part of the parents and child, which was also continued in the hospital setting, so distressed the emergency room staff that several nurses and doctors dreaded being on duty. It was on one of Sylvester's regular 3 A.M. visits to the emergency room, while he was issuing orders to everyone, that his mother divulged the information that the child swallowed any pain-killing pills he could find, even when he was not complaining of joint pain. The home medicine cabinet contained tranquilizers prescribed for the mother, sleeping pills and antispasmodics used by the father, and analgesics for Sylvester.

Curiously, in spite of the obvious maladaptation of this boy and his family, and the knowledge that he was a virtual recluse at home and rapidly becoming an addict, no one in the hospital could muster sympathy for him. Many conferences were held regarding his management, both in the outpatient department and on the pediatric units. For a while, different members of the team such as the teacher, play or physical therapist would be able to work with him, but eventually he would alienate them. The staff recognized that he was a patient who was manipulative in such subtle ways that he angered them in spite of their intentions to resist provocation.

The staff discussed Sylvester at a large conference. They believed that over the years he had become a psychopath—that is, he was without a conscience. Unless everyone in his environment could unite in carrying out a single policy, he would exploit them and obtain sufficient gratification to resist changing. The staff devised a plan for his management. They were to tell him that his behavior was obnoxious, thwart his successful manipulation, use social isolation as punishment for his gross antisocial acts, praise him only for genuine achievements and challenge his know-it-all attitudes. The social worker explained this approach to the parents. While Sylvester was in the hospital, he became a more pleasant person. However, Sylvester's change in behavior was only a superficial compliance in the face of having been overwhelmed by the floor treatment plan. He continued to be sly, to cheat at games and to test out new doctors and visitors.

He was discharged in early summer, and for the remainder of the season he was scarcely seen in the emergency ward. The staff were congratulating themselves on their beneficent influence until the usual 3 A.M. visits began in September. It was apparent that no fundamental changes in Sylvester's behavior had taken place.

At this time the parents were seeing a psychiatrist for marital counseling. Cultural disharmony added to their individual incompatibilty. The father was from an expressive, emotional family of foreign origin; the mother was from a rigid, puritanical family. Each was afraid to leave the other, yet they were too bitter to try to make a workable relationship. So far as is known, there has been no change in the family or in Sylvester.

TONY—AGE THIRTEEN

Mastered Fears and Matured During Hospitalization

Following open-heart surgery, Tony was uncommunicative and passively uncooperative. In the hope of avoiding procedures and contact with the staff, he frequently feigned sleep or ignorance of what was expected of him. In this he had the support of his parents, who gave him permission in their native language to resist what they viewed as barbaric treatments. They believed that they alone understood him and insisted on carrying out his every need (feeding, bathing, and toileting), although Tony was physically able to manage these activities. The staff felt helpless in the face of the family's infantilizing behavior and Tony's progressive withdrawal.

At a mental health conference, a clear picture of the boy's character emerged. He was described by a pediatric resident as a child who initially made feeble attempts to deal with difficult situations, but would give up as soon as he encountered opposition. For example, he had shown interest in preoperative teaching until the realities of the Intensive Care Unit were mentioned; thereafter, he literally refused to listen. He was obviously irritated by his family's hovering and at first attempted to push them away or rolled his eyes upward in exasperation; then he resigned himself to their suffocating attentiveness. Eventually he just grunted or pointed in the direction of what he wanted and it was granted.

A report from the ICU staff (Tony had spent 48 hours in the unit postoperatively) indicated that Tony may have witnessed several emergency situations, including the cardiac arrest of a patient nearby; however, he would not mention them.

The staff developed the following plan in order to encourage and support more effective communication and independence:

1. Let Tony know that the staff appreciates the difficulty of his having to accept hospitalization, surgery and constant procedures. Recognize his bravery and talk with him about the ICU, including other patients' reactions, in nondirect terms.
2. Encourage him to express anger verbally rather than by negativism and refusal to cooperate with medical procedures; let him know in a bantering manner that when he pretends sleep, the staff realizes that he's trying to escape interaction; tell him that nothing changes when he behaves in this manner and, to bring about change, he has to participate actively in the process.
3. Explain that the staff cannot know what he is thinking unless he expresses himself verbally and that no one can read his mind. Act obtuse when he expects his needs to be met without asking. This ignores his unacceptable passivity and forces him to take a more mature role.

4. Allow him choices in deciding when and where treatments are to be done. Make clear that all treatments have a purpose and that they are not punitive. Ask parents to leave during procedures.
5. Draw him into discussion about his parents' attitude regarding the treatment plan. Offer Tony practical suggestions on how he can deal with his family when they overpower him. For example, the staff person could say, "Tony, your parents mean well but maybe they try too hard, not letting you do for yourself. If you tune out, how will it ever change?" Tony could be encouraged to try saying to them, "That's enough now," or "I want to do it myself," or "If you do it for me, how will I ever learn?"
6. Refer parents for social work counseling as a way of altering their relationship to Tony.

The staff was quite unprepared for the immediate and unexpected response to their approach. When they expressed sympathy with his plight and discussed the Intensive Care Unit (couched in terms of the experiences of others), Tony let forth a stream of four-letter words. There was little doubt that Tony interpreted events there as diabolical—crazy people doing crazy things. He talked about the constant strange noises, his inability to sleep and his impression of several people beating a man in the next bed and how he kept thinking it would never be over. Once he was able to recount the frightening incidents, the staff was able to put them in perspective, with the connotation of the staff helping instead of hurting patients. The effect of expressing his feelings was seen in his greater tolerance for treatments, although he continued his protests verbally.

The nurses' pretended insensitivity to his obvious demands and moods—their refusal to understand his pointing to objects or responses to treatment—had a humorous side. Tony accused them of stupidity—"What's the matter with you? It's water I want, not my shoes." Their only defense was that they were not mind readers. This point was reinforced by his older sister, who was a willing accomplice in this ruse. She suddenly developed an obtuseness that was difficult for him to comprehend. When she asked him if he needed help in getting out of bed, he gave his usual grunt. "What's that supposed to mean? I can't read your mind," she asked. In great annoyance he responded, "Why don't you know? You're a teacher, aren't you?" All these occasions provided opportunities to negate the divining power of adults, which his parents fostered, and forced him to express openly his feelings and requests.

Tony's parents were bewildered by his newly found expressivity and wondered if it was a late surgical complication. His bluntness was remarkable. It took him some time to refine his statements so that his assertiveness came through without the obscenities which completely shocked this incredulous couple. He needed the assistance of the staff, who supported his independence although suggesting more acceptable ways of communicating. Social work counseling of the parents was instrumental in helping them accept a change in relationship after many years of justified overprotectiveness.

The staff wondered what they had unleashed as Tony's sexual preoccupations became apparent. He read "girlie" magazines, pinched and attempted to fondle the nurses, and demanded kisses. Frequent consultation with the mental health team relieved the nurses' perplexity. Discussions revealed that he was merely testing out different forms of expression. The nurses told Tony that although his feelings and curiosity were positive, his actions were turning people against him. They told him that he was allowed to ask any questions he liked; that it was obvious that he was thinking a great deal about what was and was not a permissible way to be curious; that although his interest in women was natural, his behavior could easily be interpreted as a rude attack because he did not have permission to touch. The staff pointed out that he had the same right to the privacy of his body.

Within two weeks, the beneficial results of the original plan were obvious to everyone. The staff believed that the maintenance and development of Tony's new skills—independence, responsibility and communication—were dependent on the parents' willingness to follow the same regimen after his discharge. They discussed with the parents the possibility of convalescent hospital care (for the purpose of consolidating his achievement). The parents refused this possibility; however, they agreed to continue with social work in the interest of Tony's continued growth.

HILARY—AGE FOURTEEN

Was Quietly Suicidal

Hilary was 14 when she came to our pediatric department for the first time, but she had been admitted to other hospitals on many occasions because of nephrosis over a six-year period. She suffered relapses of her kidney disease each time she had a cold, so she was admitted for intensive evaluation and treatment.

This pretty, redheaded girl seemed unusually apprehensive about the least discomfort; and when an intravenous infusion caused her mild phlebitis, she became clinically depressed and began to stroke her hair repeatedly. At first, although her change in mood was noted by the house officer in his daily notes, there was little concern. However, by the third day, her mother reported to the nurse on duty that Hilary was depressed and had quietly mentioned suicide. Such a strong idea from so mild an adolescent alerted the resident and the head nurse to the possibility that this youngster was asking for help.

At the liaison conference it emerged that Hilary had had several bouts of depression in the past; each one lasted a few weeks and then left spontaneously. She was the youngest child after her mother had many miscarriages. Her parents adored her, as did her much older siblings. The family all lived in the same neighborhood and socialized only with each other. She had never exerted herself in the least to make friends or to excel at school, though she had the modest ambition to be an assistant teacher. This picture of her was put together from information gathered by different members of the staff and offered by the patient while being interviewed at the conference. Her bland, dull answers showed her to be a self-contained girl who felt entitled to having a painless existence and to being unresponsive to the needs of others. Obviously overindulged and egocentric, Hilary was passive emotionally because everything had been done for her. Now being forced to undergo procedures that were uncomfortable and beyond her control, she became furious and saw no reason for continuing to live unless she could live completely on her own terms.

The conference decision was to make an intensive impact on Hilary by undercutting her passivity and egocentricity. This was done on a 24-hour basis by being pleasant to her but talking with her only when she initiated the conversation; having nurses compliment her only when she did something actively; and limiting severely the doctors' generously given assurances. The plan also included urging Hilary to help herself as much as possible and to assisit with the younger children, and emphasizing the prerogatives and pleasures of being older and more responsible.

Within a week, Hilary's mood began to change. She was talking of a career in nursing and volunterring her services on the unit. Six weeks after discharge, however, even though the parents were informed of the milieu treatment, Hilary was noted, on a clinic visit, to be returning to her little-girl role. Unfortunately, the parents were not able to see prospects beyond her egocentric behavior, her limited ambitions and her dependence on them.

ANGELA—AGE FIFTEEN

Was in Search of an Identity

Angela had a marvelous reputation as a patient. We had anticipated some rebelliousness because her condition (subacute bacterial endocarditis) required prolonged intravenous therapy and bed rest. Her recovery was slow and complicated by setbacks. In spite of it all, she remained cooperative and understanding.

In retrospect, it was clear that all was not as ideal as we had supposed. The problem became apparent just prior to her discharge. Instead of displaying joy at the prospect of returning home, she was impassive. Soon after, we learned that Angie was seeking out visitors and staff indiscriminately to recount tales of her complex social life—the numerous substitute mothers she had had since her own mother's death two years previously, and her father's in-fidelities and stories indicating that she was unloved.

Two days before discharge, an incident involving three-year-old Jimmy alerted the staff further. Jimmy's permanent ileostomy appliance was lost. At first, there was little concern. We searched his personal possessions, bed linens and wastebaskets to no avail. We knew that there was a duplicate, so it was not a problem until it became obvious that the second appliance could not be located either. Another thorough search was made, and Angie, who was in the area, was asked if she had any idea what Jimmy could have done with it. She wanted to know if it really was important. When assured that it was, she admitted to having taken it and reluctantly retrieved it from the suitcase in her closet. The staff tried not to shame Angie but merely asked her to disclose the contents of the suitcase. She refused, stating that it was her "secret sack."

The head nurse directed the night staff to investigate the suitcase as a safety measure. Examination of the suitcase revealed an assorted collection of equipment used in genitourinary treatments—scalpels, needles and catheters—most of which had been denied Angie when she had asked for them previously.

A conference was held and as a result, a number of other incidents were brought to light. Each staff member was unaware that others had previously had similar experiences. Angie had demonstrated repeated bursts of anger when admonished for her behavior with Jimmy, whom she had adopted as her own patient. For example, Angie was observed feeding him juice with a contaminated irrigating syringe. When she was stopped, she was indignant, stating that the syringe was his own and that his infection was in his kidneys, not his mouth. She added that she could care for the child better than anyone else. Other difficulties showed in her involvements with several mothers on the unit and her requests to live with them.

Angela's behavior was discussed with the liaison psychiatrist. His impression was that this young girl had a low frustration tolerance and had not yet worked out feelings regarding the death of her mother—also, that she was in search of her identity. During her two-month hospitalization she had some stability in her life and had patterned herself in the image of doctors and nurses. Consequently, any criticism of her in these roles incurred her anger. The impending discharge also threatened her security.

The plan outlined for her future management was: (a) to praise her efforts in the roles of medical personnel, (b) to arrange for long-term psychotherapy through her pediatrician and (c) to continue contact with one of the nurses after discharge.

Following discharge, there appeared little urgency in carrying out this plan until Jimmy's mother received a letter from Angie threatening suicide. At this time, the liaison psychiatrist contacted Angela's father directly and he consented to treatment without delay.

Further information from Angie's father corroborated the impression that the "secret sack" (a play on her surname) referred to secrets within the family. We learned, too, that within her home she was encouraged to have her own way and entitled to do as she wished. She was self-centered, narcissistic and was a party to destructive family gossip about her father and his fiancée. Her father soon arranged for Angie to have intensive psychotherapy. Within a few months, she attained a modest social success at school and was planning a career as a veterinarian.

WALTER—AGE SIXTEEN

Was Surrounded by Chaos

Wally, an overweight, torpid adolescent, was admitted to the hospital frequently for the treatment of ulcerative colitis. He was generally disliked because he related to no one, refused to attend school, watched television for hours and ignored customary daily hygienic routines. In addition, he took pleasure in thwarting the work of the staff with crude practical jokes such as flushing his stools before they could be examined.

Each admission revealed to the staff the chaos that totally surrounded Wally. His parents' marriage was a series of smoldering disagreements. Undeterred by the hospital setting and the presence of strangers, they continued their daily combats without interruption. No domestic issue was too sacred or too picayune to go unaired. The mother, with her outwardly calm and sweet facade, usually initiated the drama. On one occasion she berated the father for having forgotten their wedding anniversary. He retorted that in 20 years of marriage he had had only six good months; therefore, she was undeserving of a gift.

Wally responded to these episodes with increased bleeding. Staff intervention was required to halt the most violent scenes. The mental health team attempted to decide the best way to approach this family. A plan to protect Wally from the continual parental battles was made, with the strong suggestion that his mother and father visit separately for short periods. Wally was referred to child psychiatry, and the parents were referred to social work. Unfortunately, they were unwilling to fully participate in casework. Wally's bleeding continued and was no longer responsive to steroid therapy. Consequently, an ileostomy was performed.

Open hostility reemerged when the father discovered that his wife had consented to the surgery without his knowledge. The father's chronic peptic ulcer was exacerbated, forcing his admission to a nearby hospital. Paradoxically, the mother appeared calm in the face of all this difficulty. She compared Wally to her husband and considered them both the products of genetic weakness.

Wally went into a depression after surgery and required daily visits from his psychiatrist. After several weeks, Wally became more talkative and alert. About this time his father, having been discharged from the hospital, happened to visit when his wife was at Wally's bedside. This caused renewed difficulties. Wally became careless in caring for his ileostomy and petulant with his roommates. He displayed a new behavior that was to demand exclusive attention from the nurses and to seek opportunities to detain them.

Because at this time the psychiatrist could see him only twice a week, a plan was made in which the day nurse and the pediatric resident were to use every opportunity to talk about how he felt when his parents fought. From the information he supplied, it was easy to piece together a picture of a boy who had become so preoccupied with the marital strife that early developmental tasks—the resolution of the oedipal struggle with its outcome of appropriate gender identification—never were mastered. All the accomplishments that should have taken place in the subsequent years did not take place; he was like a child of five. Because he had missed the experiences of learning to get along with peers and developing pleasure in skills and achievements, Wally needed a long posthospital program in which inpatient, outpatient, pediatric, psychiatric, school and summer camp personnel were involved.

By the time Wally left the hospital, he was helping at the nurses' station, making amateur diagnoses of new patients and socializing comfortably with his roommates.

The staff's reaction to Wally was mixed. They were pleased that the hospital milieu could be so effective but dismayed to learn that his improvement was not long-lasting because he was not able to hold out against the toxic emotional climate at home.

It became increasingly important to treat the family problem. However, the parents could not be persuaded to seek further help for their unhappiness. Wally suffered a series of complications that necessitated frequent rehospitalization. Eventually, he consented to placement in a convalescent hospital from which he attended school.

BIBLIOGRAPHY

Abram, H. S.: Psychological aspects of the intensive care unit. Hospital Medicine 5:94, 1969.

Binger, C. M., et al.: Childhood leukemia. Emotional impact on patient and family. New Eng. J. Med. 280:414, 1969.

Caelho, G. V., Hamburg, D. A., and Adams, J. E. (eds.): Coping and Adaptation. New York, Basic Books, 1974.

Chapman, A. H.: Management of Emotional Problems of Children and Adolescents. Philadelphia, J. B. Lippincott, 1974.

Caplan, G.: The Theory and Practice of Mental Health Consultation. New York, Basic Books, 1970.

Cofer, D. H., and Nir, Y.: Theme-focused group therapy on a pediatric ward. Int'l. J. Psychiatry in Medicine 6(4):541, 1975.

Gardner, R. A.: The guilt reaction of parents of children with severe physical disease. Amer. J. Psychiat. 126:636, 1969.

Guerin, P. J. (ed.): Family Therapy: Theory and Practice. New York, Gardner Press, 1976.

Hannaway, P. J.: Failure to thrive: a study of 100 infants and children. Clin. Pediat. 9:96, 1970.

Korsch, B. M., et al.: Experiences with children and their families during extended hemodialysis and kidney transplantation. Pediat. Clin. N. Amer. 18:625, 1971.

Lewis, M.: Clinical Aspects of Child

Development. Philadelphia, Lea & Febiger, 1968.

Mack, J. E.: Nightmares and Human Conflict. Boston, Little, Brown, 1970.

MacKennon, R. A., and Michels, R.: The Psychiatric Interview in Clinical Practice. Philadelphia, W. B. Saunders, 1971.

Murphy, L. B., and Moriarty, A. E.: Vulnerability, Coping and Growth from Infancy to Adolescence. New Haven, Yale University Press, 1976.

Noland, R. L.: Counseling Parents of the Ill and Handicapped. Springfield, Ill., Charles C Thomas, 1971.

Oremland, E. K. and J. D. (eds.): The Effect of Hospitalization on Children: Models for Their Care. Springfield, Ill., Charles C Thomas, 1973.

Pearson, G. (ed.): A Handbook of Child Psychoanalysis. New York, Basic Books, 1968.

Rutter, M.: Helping Troubled Children. New York, Plenum Press, 1975.

Schowalter, J. E.: The utilization of child psychiatry on a pediatric adolescent ward. J. Amer. Acad. Child Psychiat. 10:684, 1971.

Schulterbrandt, J. G., and Raskin, A. (eds.): Depression in Childhood: Diagnosis, Treatment and Conceptual Models. New York, Raven Press, 1977.

Talbot, N. B., Kagan, J., and Eisenberg, L.: Behavioral Science in Pediatric Medicine. Philadelphia, W. B. Saunders, 1971.

Winnicott, D. W.: Therapeutic Consultations in Child Psychiatry, New York, Basic Books, 1971.

Appendix

I

Basic Supplies for Teaching/Preparation Program

1. Teaching protocol manual:
   (a) Select protocols from Chapter 6; (b) develop others that are frequently needed for your pediatric unit.
2. Visual aids manual
3. Work sheet—see Appendix II
4. Stuffed dolls:
   Ideally the supply allows every child to take home a doll and appliances, which are easily made.
5. Body outlines—see Appendix III
6. Beds and IV poles sized to dolls
7. Miniature IV sets:
   Miniature IV sets can be made from empty 30 cc. water vials or discarded antibiotic bottles and approximately 14 inches of washed, discarded IV tubing. Puncture rubber top of vial with sharp point of scissors. Push in tubing with Kelly clamp. Attach string or twill tape to top of vial with paper tape so that it hangs freely from IV pole on miniature bed.
8. Miniature collecting system—to be used as Foley catheter drainage, chest tube drainage or hemovac:
   Miniature collecting system for Foley catheter, hemovac or chest tube drainage can be made from discarded butterfly needle packages. Remove butterfly needle from one end of package so that paper back is not detached from plastic case. Insert approximately 12 inches of clean, discarded IV tubing into open corner of package. Secure with paper tape.
9. Models of familiar equipment, such as monitor and suction machines.

10. Needle play equipment:
    tongue blades for armboards, small tourniquets, clean used syringes, sterile needles and butterflies, medicine cups, sterile water vials (labeled PLAY), alcohol wipes, tape and Band-Aids
11. Gauze sponges (2×2)
12. Paper tape
13. Puppets
14. Preparation booklets
15. Books to help children adjust to hospital
16. Scrapbooks:
    Scrapbooks for stories about the hospital can be made inexpensively with about 12 sheets of plain paper stapled into a manila folder. Choose appropriate photos from medical/nursing journals and allow child to write or dictate stories about each.
17. Supply of photos (from medical/nursing journals) to use in scrapbooks
18. Paste

II

Work Sheet for Preparing Children and Parents for Treatment or Teaching About Illness Summarized from Chapter 6

PRELIMINARIES

1. See guidelines for working with specific age group in Chapter 6 or in manual for unit.
2. Consult pediatrician or surgeon on treatment plan.
3. Review with parents their understanding and how they have prepared child.
4. Determine whether parents and child will be taught together.
5. Decide on suitable explanation, language and teaching tools.
6. Plan two to three teaching sessions.
7. Outline the teaching plan. Use as guide during preparation sessions.
8. Gather necessary teaching aids: body outlines, doll (dummy), model equipment, visual aids, equipment for demonstration and practice, etc.

SESSION 1

1. Determine patient's understanding of problem or fantasy before teaching. Ask about symptoms, for example, "What do you know about being in the hospital?"
2. Ask what may have caused problem.
3. Reassure re: blame, punishment.
4. Clarify or reinforce understanding. Give simple explanation of anatomy and physiology. Make notes of key points:

5. Explain treatment and expectations. Use body outline for patients over three and a half years. Repeat exact area of treatment/surgery. Use playful repetition for children under seven years. Make notes here:

6. Play up positive aspects: new things and people to talk about to family and friends. Encourage discussion about hospitalization.
7. Ask simple questions to help patient recall teaching. Use body outline or allow young child to attach appliances to doll or dummy, in answering questions.
8. Allow needle play if appropriate for age.   End of Session 1.

SESSION 2   (if indicated)

1. Plan demonstration of equipment to be used postoperatively and allow practice time.

SESSION 2 or 3:   Preparation before treatment and routine. Delete areas that do not apply.

Explain:
1. Fasting; NPO sign.
2. Bath with special soap
3. Transportation to O.R. or treatment room.
4. O.R. personnel, how dressed.
5. Monitor, electrodes and leads, or pack pad with electrodes inserted.
6. Anesthesia: explain "sleep"
7. Recovery Room.
8. Pain and relief.
9. Ask simple questions to help patient recall teaching. Help young children prepare doll.
10. Explain premeds last.
11. Allow needle play if age-appropriate.
12. Discuss with parent(s), out of child's hearing, the need for their presence on day of treatment or surgery.
13. Explain who will accompany to O.R. or treatment room.

DAY OF TREATMENT OR SURGERY

1. Review quickly events of day.
2. Prepare meds before telling child. Have assistance to hold child. Give immediately. Allow quick needle play for young children.
3. Allow child to wear clean underpants to O.R.
4. On call, accompany child.
5. Follow-up: Coping with hospitalization and treatment. Methods?

III

Body Outlines—Infants to Adolescents
Figures 1–13

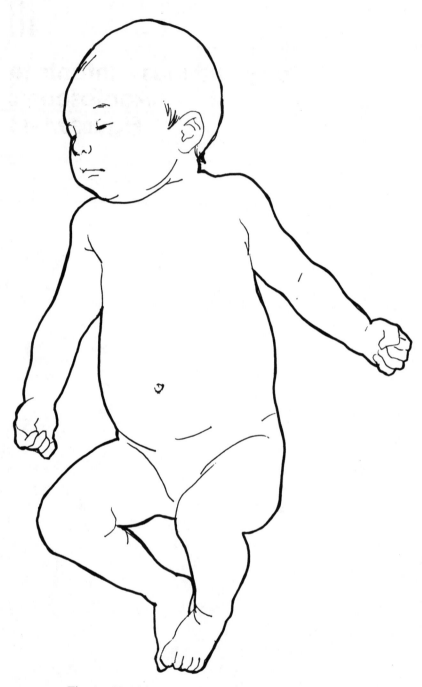

Fig. 1.   Newborn. Drawing by Nancy Cole.

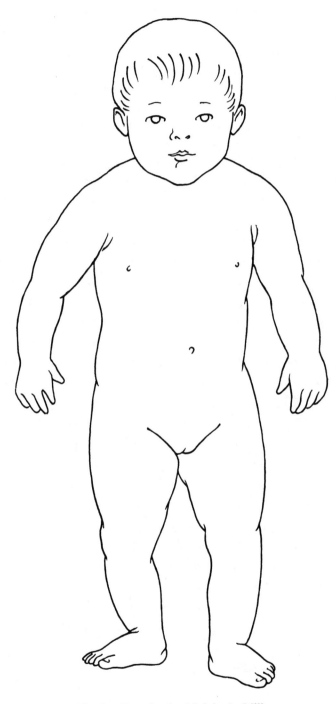

Fig. 2. Drawing by Melvin A. Miller.

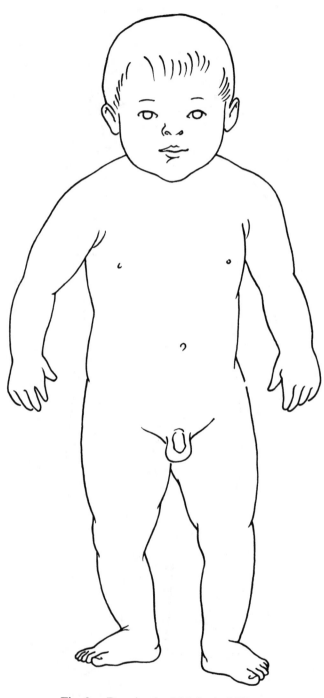

Fig. 3.   Drawing by Melvin A. Miller.

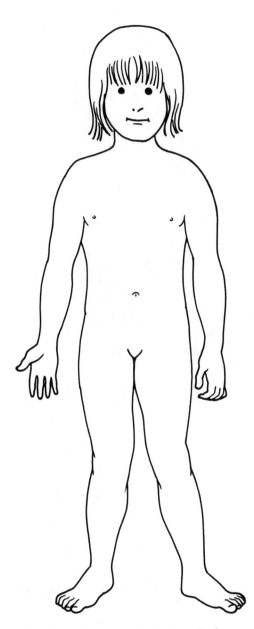

Fig. 4.   Drawings 4–11 by Lou Barlow.

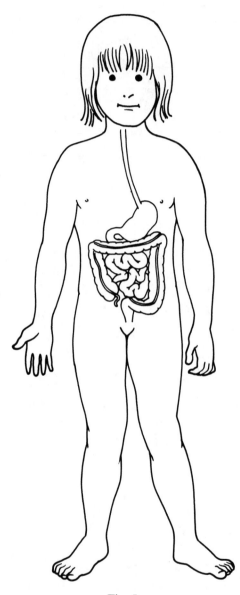

Fig. 5.

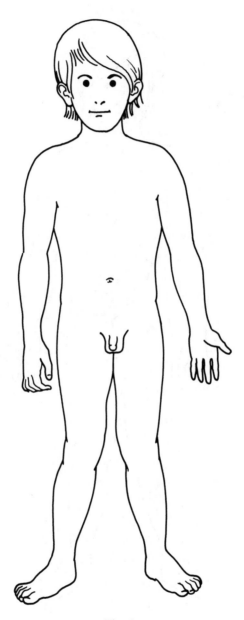

Fig. 6.

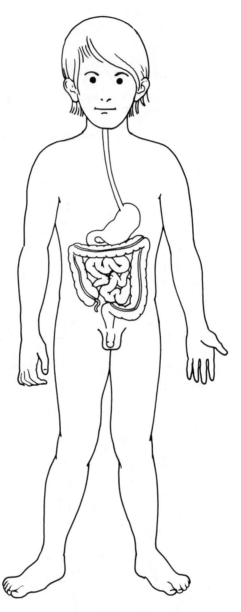

Fig. 7.

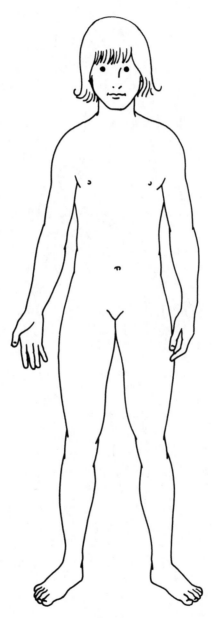

Fig. 8.

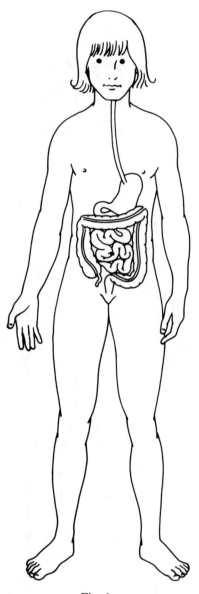

Fig. 9.

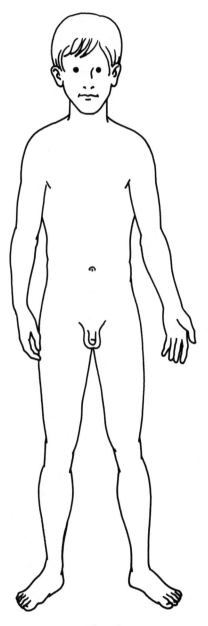

Fig. 10.

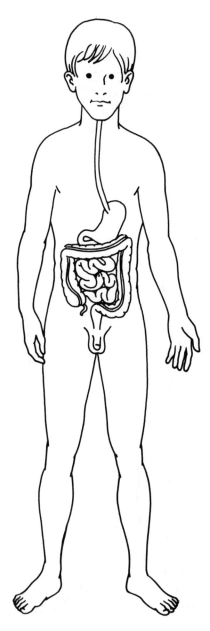

Fig. 11.

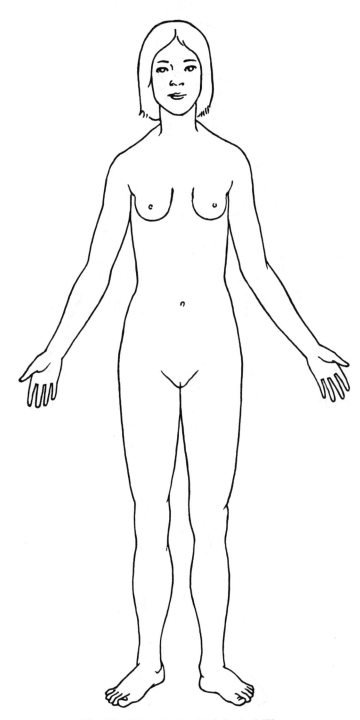

Fig. 12.   Drawing by Melvin A. Miller.

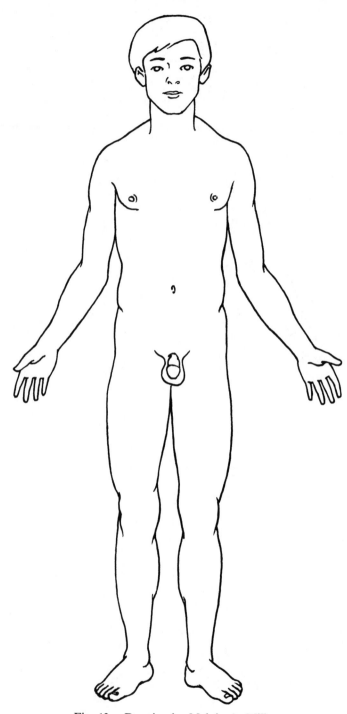

Fig. 13.   Drawing by Melvin A. Miller.

IV

Specialized Materials for Working with Hospitalized Children

ITEM	SOURCE
Body outlines	Appendix III
Stuffed dolls (wholesale)	*Mel Posin Associates 200 Fifth Avenue (Lower Lobby #4) New York, NY 10010 (212) OR 5-5010
Hospital play equipment: beds, cribs, IV poles, wheelchairs, examining tables, x-ray units, etc.	*V. C. Dye Hospital Play Equipment 1122 Judson Avenue Evanston, IL 60202 (312) 869-1269

All the following are available at all places to the right:
 Open-top dollhouse (can be used as play hospital as well)
 Modular dollhouse furniture
 Pliable family dolls
 Pliable hospital personnel dolls
 Brother and sister dolls (anatomically correct)
 Large body puzzle
 Water play trough
 Water play kit
 Animal puppets
 Family hand puppets

*Childcraft Education Corporation
20 Kilmer Road
Edison, NJ 08817
(201) 572-6100

*Community Playthings
Rifton, NY 12471
(914) 653-6561

*Constructive Playthings
1040 East 85 Street
Kansas City, MO 64131
(816) 444-4711

*J. A. Preston Corporation
71 Fifth Avenue
New York, NY 10003
(212) 255-8484

*Playskool Manufacturing Co.
200 Fifth Avenue
New York, NY 10003
(212) 675-3255

*Brochure available

PREADMISSION PREPARATION BOOKLETS

SOURCE

Available at nominal cost:

Azarnoff, P. (ed.): The Hospital (English and Spanish editions)	Wright Institute of Los Angeles 1100 S. Robertson Boulevard Los Angeles, CA 90035
Roberts, J. B., and Mano, J. S.: What It's Like to Be in the Hospital.	U.S. Military Bookstores
Sesame Street Hospital Preparation Kit: Booklet, Crayons, Finger Puppets and Poster.	Children's Television Workshop One Lincoln Plaza New York, NY 10023
Suhr, C.: What to do in the Emergency Room.	Child Study Program Prince George's County Public Schools Upper Marlboro, MD 20870
Mr. Rogers's *Let's Talk About the Hospital* Series: Going to the Hospital Having an Operation Wearing a Cast When Your Child Goes to the Hospital (for parents) A Guide for Hospital Staff Mr. Rogers' Wall Posters (based on each program)	Let's Talk About It Family Communications 4802 Fifth Avenue Pittsburgh, PA 15213

V

Gifts for Hospitalized Children

AGE LEVEL

Neonate to 3 months	Nursery mobiles, bright balloons, music box with moving figures, see-through crib bumpers
3 to 7 months	Rattles, cradle gym, soft hand toys, steel mirror, mobiles, toys that attach to crib
7 to 12 months	Teething toys, soft animals, activity box, bath toys (plastic or foam rubber), drinking cup, stacking rings or squares
Toddler	Pull toys, dolls, teddy bears (all without sharp edges or loose parts), play dough, Fun Factory for producing play dough in a variety of patterns and shapes, crayons, finger paints, doctor/nurse kits, books, dolls with clothes that button and lace to help a child learn to dress, simple puzzles, records, flowers, family photo album.
3- to 5-year-olds	Dolls, crayons, paints and paper, simple puzzles, doctor/nurse kits, balloons, records, books, erector sets, simple games, puppets, flashlight, family photos, dimes for telephone calls, flowers, goldfish in a bowl and fish food.
6- to 8-year-olds	Playing cards, checkers or dominoes, games with rules to play with other children, erector sets, felt tip pens, magic markers, scrapbooks or autograph books, plants, records, tape recorder and tapes, models, dimes for telephone calls, flowers.

8- to 11-year-olds	Playing cards, books, magic games, riddle book, scrapbook, diary, tape recorder and tapes, instamatic camera and film, autograph book, model plane or boat, stationery, stamps, dimes for telephone calls, T-shirt with inscription, flowers.
12 through adolescent	Books, records, stationery and stamps, instamatic camera and film, record player (if permitted by hospital), age-appropriate games, transistor radio, T-shirts, seeds, potting soil and small gardening equipment (for long-term hospitalization)

Gifts to provide tactile-sensory stimulation, for use as recreational/occupational projects, for diversion and as tools for coping with hospitalization, are always appropriate. They should not be given as rewards for illness. Parents and visitors may need direction in exercising restraint so that the pattern of gift giving within the family is maintained and relationships continue as usual. These measures serve to decrease anxiety and enhance socialization of the child.

VI

Suggestions to Parents Before Discharge from the Hospital (For Distribution to Parents)

Hospitalization and the period immediately following are frequently as difficult for parents as they are for children. The pediatric staff is interested in helping to make the adjustment from hospital to home as smooth as possible.

It is not unusual after hospitalization for children to demonstrate behavior that is not typical of them. Most likely, the change is related to the experiences of illness and separation from the home. It may be seen, for example, in a change in eating, sleeping or play habits or in the development of fears.

In the event that any of these problems arises while your child is still hospitalized, the staff is available to give you assistance. For helping your child at home, the following suggestions may be beneficial in preventing or dealing with the aftereffects of hospitalization. We encourage you to:

1. Return your child to his/her former routines quickly and give responsibilities equal to his/her abilities.
2. Avoid making your child the center of attention because of illness.
3. Be kind, firm and consistent in handling your child, especially in disciplinary measures. In this way, your child will know he/she is back in his/her normal situation.
4. Be truthful with your child in order to preserve his/her trust in you.
5. Provide play materials such as clay, paints, doctor/nurse kits and equipment given to him in the hospital. Allow him to play on his own.
6. Permit your child to talk about feelings regarding illness and hospitalization. Correct any misunderstandings. It is common for children to be concerned about hospitals for some time afterward.
7. Avoid leaving a young child for long periods or overnight until he is well adjusted and trusting of your return.
8. Allow your child to visit pediatric staff between admissions when he is in the hospital vicinity or after clinic appointments.

VII

Films About Children and Hospitalization for Staff Development

A HOSPITAL VISIT WITH CLIPPER
15 min., color, 16mm. Media Center, Children's Hospital Medical Center, 111 Michigan Avenue, N.W., Washington, DC 20010.

A film adaptation of the puppet program at Children's Hospital. Children and their families are given an entertaining introduction to hospital routine, procedures, equipment and personnel. It is appropriate to show to three- to 10-year-old children in doctors' offices, hospitals, clinics, and schools—wherever the children can be gathered together with adults who can answer questions and reinforce the film's message.

TO PREPARE A CHILD
32 min., color, 16mm. Media Center, Children's Hospital Medical Center, 111 Michigan Avenue, N.W., Washington, DC 20010.

A documentary film that follows the stresses of three young children in real hospital situations—a cardiac patient, an emergency case with a febrile seizure, and a child admitted for ear surgery. The film portrays the sensitive handling of the general apprehensions and fears of children and their families by a hospital staff acutely attuned to verbal and nonverbal distress signals.

WHEN A CHILD ENTERS THE HOSPITAL
19 min., color, 16mm. Polymorph Films, 331 Newbury Street, Boston, MA 02115.

A film that follows a child, accompanied by his mother, through the hospital experience, with emphasis on the role of the parent.

THE HOSPITAL
13 min., b/w or color, 16mm. Encyclopedia Britannica Educational Corp., 425 North Michigan Avenue, Chicago, IL 60611.

A survey of hospital services as experienced by two children.

A NEW WORLD FOR PETER
22 min., color, 16mm. A New World for Peter, P.O. Box 23, Ithaca, NY 14851.

Helpful to parents and staff for preadmission preparation to the hospital. Narrated in the first person by an experienced young patient.

A PLACE TO GET WELL
17 min., color, 16mm. Merck, Sharp and Dohme Film Library, 1617 Pennsylvania Blvd., Philadelphia, PA 19103.

A general preadmission orientation to the hospital.

MR. ROGERS'S NEIGHBORHOOD SERIES: LET'S TALK ABOUT THE HOSPITAL VIDEOCASSETTES OR FILM.
Family Communications, 4802 Fifth Avenue, Pittsburgh, PA 15213.

a. GOING TO THE HOSPITAL. An overview of the hospital experience, with emphasis on the sights, sounds and feelings children may experience. Suitable for a preadmission tour, for inpatient viewing, individually or in groups. (Three- to eight-year-old level)

b. HAVING AN OPERATION. Designed for patients scheduled for minor surgery, preparing them for typical events and encouraging the expression of feelings in words and play. Also suggested for postoperative viewing to encourage further discussion and play.

c. WEARING A CAST. A physician explains about casts and demonstrates on Mr. Rogers's arm. Activities permitted while wearing the cast are emphasized. Also discussed are the use of slings and the removal of the cast with a cast-cutter, stressing safety measures.

GOING TO THE HOSPITAL WITH MOTHER (James Robertson)
45 min., b/w, 16mm. New York University Film Library, 26 Washington Place, New York, NY 10003.

The benefits of parent participation and rooming-in facilities for a 20-month-old child.

A TWO-YEAR-OLD GOES TO THE HOSPITAL (James Robertson)
50 min., (abridged version 30 min.), b/w, 16mm. New York University Film Library, 26 Washington Place, New York, NY 10003.

Camera record of an eight-day hospitalization of a 29-month-old child and the events to which she is subjected. Although appearing to withstand the experience with unusual self-control, follow-up data suggest much greater psychological disturbance than was immediately apparent.

SEPARATIONS AND REUNIONS (Dermod MacCarthy, M.D. and Harold Lowenstein)

Film Studies I and II (25 min., b/w, 16mm) deal with the emotional convalescence of Susan, 17 months, after cleft palate repair; and of Robert, 20 months, after 18 days in isolation for salmonella.

Film Studies III and IV (10 min., b/w, 16mm) deal respectively with the short-term hospitalization of Vanessa, 14 months, for gastroenteritis, and of Alicia, 15 months, for celiac disease. Both films show the intensity of reactions to separation from the mother—what is sacrificed when the mother is absent and what is gained when she is present.

ROBIN, PETER AND DARRYL: THREE TO THE HOSPITAL

50 min., b/w, 16 mm. New York University Film Library, 26 Washington Place, New York, NY 10003.

Cameras record unrehearsed interactions of various hospital personnel with three toddlers hospitalized for minor surgery. Their reactions to separation from parents and effects of hospitalization are dramatically presented. Useful for prompting discussion on appropriate intervention.

SUDDEN DEPARTURE

28 min., b/w, 16mm. McGraw-Hill Film Division, 330 West 42 Street, New York, NY 10036.

Children's responses to maternal departure at various ages of development, dramatically recorded.

POINT OF VIEW

28 min., color, 16mm. J. Schulman, M.D., Children's Memorial Hospital, 707 Fullerton Avenue, Chicago, IL 60614.

Strong portrayal of the psychological impact of seemingly routine hospital events through the eyes of children.

THE WORLD OF CHILDREN'S HOSPITAL

20 min., b/w, 16mm. Public Relations, Children's Hospital, 4614 Sunset Blvd., Los Angeles, CA 90027.

A realistic account of a 13-year-old's experience with hospitals and procedures. Gives insightful portraits of staff and fellow patients.

STAFF DEVELOPMENT FILMSTRIP SERIES (Madeline Petrillo)
Approximately 15 min. each, color, Campus Films, 2 Overhill Road, Scarsdale, NY 10583.

Preparing a Child for Herniorrhaphy; Preparing a Child for Renal Transplant; Preparing a Child for Appendectomy; Preparing a Child for OR, RR and ICU; Teaching a Child About Leukemia; Teaching a Child About Nephrosis; Needle Play.

Focus is on techniques of psychological preparation for treatment or teaching about illness, types of problems encountered and their management, as well as specific content.

PUPPET PREPARATION FOR SURGERY
12 min., color, 16mm. Children's Memorial Hospital, 2300 Children's Plaza, Chicago, IL.

A preparation for surgery program through puppet play by a specially trained volunteer corps.

LINDA: ENCOUNTERS IN THE HOSPITAL
32 min., color, 16 mm. University of California, Los Angeles, UCLA Instructional Media Library, 405 Hilgard Avenue/Royce Hall, No. 8, Los Angeles, CA 90024.

A candid, unstaged film that documents the successful preparation of a four-year-old for major cardiac surgery by a play therapist.

PLAY IN THE HOSPITAL
50 min., color, 16mm. Campus Film Distributors, 2 Overhill Road, Scarsdale, NY 10583, or American Hospital Association Film Library, 840 North Lake Shore Drive, Chicago, IL 60611.

The use of therapeutic play for hospitalized children. Basic to advanced practical information for play therapists and pediatric staff of all disciplines.

LET'S PLAY HOSPITAL
50 min., color, 16 mm. Children's Hospital at Stanford, 520 Willow Road, Palo Alto CA 94301.

Demonstrates the use of supervised hospital play for helping children master traumatic hospital experiences.

PLAY THERAPY AND THE HOSPITALIZED CHILD
26 min., b/w, 16mm. The American Journal of Nursing Co. Film Library, 600 Grand Avenue, Ridgefield, NJ 07657.

Play therapy techniques for helping children cope with the hospital experience. Produced by the University of Missouri School of Nursing.

CARE THROUGH PARENTS: CREATING SPACE IN PEDIATRICS
(Carol Hardgrove)
15 min., color, 16mm. University of California Extension Media Center, Berkeley, CA 94720.
The creation of a rooming-in program where space is limited but staff motivation is high.

PARENTS AND STAFF IN A CHILDREN'S WARD (Dermod MacCarthy, M.D., and Harold Lowenstein) 45 min. for 4 parts, b/w, 16mm. Abridged version 1: Parts 2, 3 and 4, 29 min. Abridged version 2: Part 1, 16mm. Concord Films Council, Nacton, Ipswich, England; or The Psychological Cinema Register, Audio-Visual Services, Pennsylvania State University, State College, PA 16802.
Part 1: Parents' experiences during the hospitalization of their children.
Part 2: Every day on the ward—seen in part from nurses' point of view.
Part 3: Fantasies of anxious young mothers.
Part 4: Characteristic emotional situations based on actual incidents, staged and analyzed.

MEDICAL CARE FOR ADOLESCENTS
30 min., color, 16mm. Merck, Sharp, and Dohme Film Library, 1617 Pennsylvania Blvd., Philadelphia, PA 19103.
Focuses on the needs of adolescents and patient/staff collaboration required for successful treatment.

SECOND CHANCE
10 min., color, 16mm. Jerome L. Schulman, M.D., Children's Memorial Hospital, 707 Fullerton Avenue, Chicago, IL 60614.
Well-documented and photographed account of a failure-to-thrive child's response to surrogate mothering. Features "The Mother Bank."

GROWTH FAILURE AND MATERNAL DEPRIVATION
28 min., b/w, 16mm. The American Journal of Nursing Co. Film Library, C/O Association-Sterling Films, 600 Grand Avenue, Ridgefield, NJ 07657.
Demonstrates the clinical characteristics of infantile marasmus and the degree of recovery as the result of extensive human stimulation.

MOTHERS OUT OF TOUCH
15 min., b/w, 16mm. Clifford R. Barnet, Stanford University School of Medicine, Stanford Medical Center, 300 Pasteur Drive, Palo Alto, CA 94304.
The effects of maternal–infant separation in the neonatal period and modifi-

cations in patient management as proposed by the Departments of Pediatrics, Anthropology and Psychiatry.

DEATH OF A NEWBORN

32 min., b/w, film or 3/4″ videocassette. Health Sciences Communications Center, 2119 Abington Road, School of Medicine, Cleveland, OH 44106.

Dr. Marshall H. Klaus interviews the parents of a newborn who died 28 days after birth. The film portrays each parent's grieving process—reactions of guilt, depression, difficulties with friends and relatives. Support from the medical staff is emphasized, along with the parents' need for guidance and encouragement. In addition to the film, a brochure and a 30-minute audiocassette are provided to assist in planning group presentations at other institutions. The audiocassette discusses the interview technique used at Case Western Reserve, the kinds of questions asked during the interview sessions, the grieving of the pediatric staff and its effect on parents, and the selection of personnel who are able to support bereaved parents.

TO DIE TODAY

50 min., 16mm. Film Makers Library, Inc., 290 West End Avenue, New York, NY 10023.

The management of dying patients by Kübler-Ross.

VIII

Books to Help Children Cope with Feelings and Hospitalization

For a comprehensive listing see:

Bernstein, J. E.: BOOKS TO HELP CHILDREN COPE WITH SEPARATION AND LOSS. New York and London, R. R. Bowker Co., 1977.

Flandorf, V.: BOOKS TO HELP CHILDREN ADJUST TO A HOSPITAL SITUATION. Chicago, Association of Hospital and Institution Libraries (division of The American Library Association), 1967.

Mills, G. C., et al.: DISCUSSING DEATH: A GUIDE TO DEATH EDUCATION. Palm Springs, California, Etc. Publications, 1976.

AGE LEVEL

2–5   Corey, D.: YOU GO AWAY. Chicago, Albert Whitman, 1976.

The pattern of maternal separation and return in simple to challenging experiences from infancy to school-age children is the theme of this book.

2½–4   Cameron, P.: I CAN'T, SAID THE ANT. New York, Coward-McCann, 1961.

A broken teapot and spout get mended with great effort and rhyme.

2½–4   Eastman, P.: ARE YOU MY MOTHER? New York, Random House, 1960.

A bird hatches while his mother has gone to find him a worm; he misses the mother and goes on a long walk to find her. A happy reunion ensues.

2½–4   De Regniers, B. S.: HOW JOE THE BEAR AND SAM THE MOUSE GOT TOGETHER. New York, Parents' Magazine Press, 1965.

Very dissimilar animals find, after much negotiation, that they both like ice cream.

2½–4   Mayer, M.: THERE'S A NIGHTMARE IN MY CLOSET. New York, Dial Press, 1968.

A boy's premonition of a monster in his closet comes true. However, the monster is more afraid than the boy. The child manages very well in the end.

2½–4   Piper, W.: THE LITTLE ENGINE THAT COULD. New York, Platt and Munk, 1954.

An engine almost gives up but finally climbs over a mountain to deliver its toys.

2½–4   Sendak, M.: WHERE THE WILD THINGS ARE. New York, Harper & Row, 1963.

A boy who is punished by his mother revels in his badness and returns to a warm supper.

2½–4   Watson, J. W., Switzer, R. E., and Hirschberg, J. C.: MEN-NINGER SERIES. New York, Golden Press.
LOOK AT ME NOW (1971)
SOMETIMES I'M JEALOUS (1971)
SOMETIMES I GET ANGRY (1971)
SOMETIMES I'M AFRAID (1971)
MY FRIEND THE DOCTOR (1972)
MY FRIEND THE DENTIST (1972)
MY BODY—HOW IT WORKS (1972)

Parent and child read-together books focusing on fears and feelings common to all young children.

2½–4   Wezel, P.: THE GOOD BIRD. New York, Harper & Row, 1964.

A fish, all alone, is befriended by a bird, and they stay together all night. Told without words.

3–6   Bemelmans, L.: MADELINE. New York, Simon and Schuster, 1939.

A girl has an operation, and her friends envy her scar. At first the teacher is hysterical, but then she calms down.

3–6   Brown, M. W.: THE RUNAWAY BUNNY. New York, Harper, 1972.

A devoted, patient mother rabbit reassures her bunny that she will find him despite his intentions to leave home.

3–6   Lapsley, S.: I AM ADOPTED. Scarsdale, New York, Bradbury Press, 1975.

A simple, happy account of day-to-day family activities of Charles and Sophie. Charles mentions casually that they are adopted.

3–6   Lippman, P.: ARCHIBALD or I WAS VERY SHY. New York, Windmill Books and E. P. Dutton, 1975.

Archibald thought he would never be lonely or shy if he looked like other animals. But he learns that it's good to be himself.

3–6   Stein, S. B.: THAT NEW BABY. An Open Family Book for Parents and Children Together. New York, Walker, 1974.

Deals with feelings of jealousy, hostility, helplessness and anger in two older siblings before and after the arrival of the baby. A parallel parent section explains the psychodynamics of loss of a position in a family and gives constructive advice on management of behavior.

3–6   Welber, R.: GOODBYE, HELLO. New York, Pantheon, 1974.

The theme of separation from mother as a part of growing up is described first through young animals and leads to a child's first day at school. Told in rhyme.

3–6   Wells, R.: NOISY NORA. New York, Dial, 1973.

On the theme of jealousy and sibling rivalry, Nora's story is told in rhyme, charmingly.

3-6+   White, E. B.: CHARLOTTE'S WEB. New York, Harper & Row, 1952.

Life, death, love and hard work as illustrated by the relationship between the spider and a pig.

3-6+   White, E. B.: THE TRUMPET OF THE SWAN. New York, Harper & Row, 1970.

How a very human swan overcomes a terrible defect to lead a normal, even exemplary life.

3-6   Williams, B.: ALBERT'S TOOTHACHE. New York, E. P. Dutton, 1974.

No one would believe that Albert Turtle had a toothache. He had trouble making himself understood until his grandmother asked the right question.

3-6   Whitney, A. M.: JUST AWFUL. Reading, Mass., Addison-Wesley Publishing Co., 1971.

James hurt his finger in the school yard and felt awful until he met a jolly nurse who knew just what to do.

3-7   Alexander, M.: WE NEVER GET TO DO ANYTHING. New York, Dial Press, 1970.

A boy finds a way to enjoy himself despite the rules.

3-7   Blaine, M.: THE TERRIBLE THING THAT HAPPENED AT OUR HOUSE. New York, Parents Magazine Press, 1975.

Deals with changed relationships and stresses within the family when mother returns to a career. Humorously told.

3-7   Brown, J.: FLAT STANLEY. New York, Harper & Row, 1964.

A boy makes the best of an accident.

3-7   De Regniers, B. S.: A LITTLE HOUSE OF YOUR OWN. New York, Harcourt, Brace and World Inc., 1954.

The delights of a secret place from which to observe the world.

3-7   Hoban, R.: BEDTIME FOR FRANCES. New York, Harper & Row, 1960.

A bear has night fears but eventually gets to sleep.

3–7   Greenfield, E.: SHE COME BRINGING ME THAT LITTLE BABY GIRL. Philadelphia, J. B. Lippincott Co., 1974.

A young boy overcomes his disappointment and ambivalent feelings about his new sister.

3–7   Minarek, E. H.: LITTLE BEAR'S FRIEND. New York, Harper & Row, 1960.

One of the four vignettes concerns a doll whose arm needs repair.

3–7+   Rockwell, H.: MY DOCTOR. New York, Macmillan Publishing Co., Inc., 1973.

A young boy has a physical checkup by a woman pediatrician. Step-by-step account reassuringly described with detailed drawings.

3–7   Skorpen, L. M.: THAT MEAN MAN. New York, Harper & Row, 1968.

An unsavory character gets his comeuppance, but not before he tries a lot of things that children are told not to do.

3–7   Stein, S. B.: ABOUT HANDICAPS. New York, Walker and Co., 1974.

A young boy is afraid of a child with cerebral palsy until his father helps him resolve his fears.

3–7+   Viorst, J.: ALEXANDER AND THE TERRIBLE, HORRIBLE, NO GOOD, VERY BAD DAY. New York, Atheneum, 1977.

Nothing was right, including lima beans for supper and kissing on TV. Alexander learns that some days are like that for everyone.

3–8   Viorst, J.: ALEXANDER, WHO USED TO BE RICH LAST SUNDAY. New York, Atheneum, 1978.

Alexander discovers how hard it is to save money when too many temptations get in the way.

4–10   Bartoli, J.: NONNA. New York, Harvey House, 1975.

A strong, natural and realistic story of two youngsters who participate fully in all events surrounding the death of their grandmother. Focuses on feelings, customs regarding funeral, burial and family unity.

4–6   Brenner, B.: BODIES. New York, E. P. Dutton, 1973.

Body types and functions.

4–8   Brown, M. W.: THE DEAD BIRD. Reading, Mass., Addison-Wesley, 1958.

This longtime classic concerns a dead bird found by children playing in the park. It is buried with funeral rites. The children are appropriately sad over a period of time but eventually return to their everyday routines.

4–8   Kroll, S.: IS MILTON MISSING? New York, Holiday, 1975.

The reader accompanies a young boy on a suspenseful search for his missing Great Dane.

4–8   Perry, P., and Lynch, M.: MOMMY AND DADDY ARE DIVORCED. New York, Dial, 1978.

Learning to cope with feelings and changes in the family. Straightforward and compassionate introduction.

4–8   Raskin, E.: MOOSE, GOOSE AND LITTLE NOBODY. New York, Parents' Magazine Press, 1974.

Separated from his mother, a mouse is befriended by a moose and a goose. Together they visit various animate and inanimate objects in an effort to establish the mouse's identity. Humorously told.

4–8+   Rogers, H.: MORRIS AND HIS BRAVE LION. New York, McGraw-Hill, 1975.

On the occasion of his parents' divorce, Morris is given a stuffed lion to help him remember his father's request to remain brave despite his feelings of despair. When the father abandons his son because of his own emotional turmoil, Morris arranges a reunion by sending his father the lion.

4–7   Stein, S. B.: ABOUT DYING: An Open Family Book for Parents and Children Together. New York, Walker, 1974.

One of a series of read-together books designed to help the child through parent education. Parallel narratives accompany the photographs: for the parent, explanations on the psychodynamics of loss and children's concepts of death; for the child, the story of one youngster's reactions to the death of a pet and then to the death of his grandfather. Written in consultation with the Center for Preventive Psychiatry, White Plains, New York.

4–8   Schick, E.: KATIE GOES TO CAMP. New York, Macmillan, 1968.

A child projects her feelings of anxiety and excitement about her first separation from home to her doll. Deals with the sense of loss and adjustment to an unfamiliar environment.

4–10   Viorst, J.: THE TENTH GOOD THING ABOUT BARNEY. New York, Atheneum, 1971.

A young boy is distraught over the death of his cat. To help him resolve his loss, his mother suggests that he prepare a eulogy for Barney's funeral, including ten good things about his beloved pet. This and the support of parents and friends lead to open discussion that helps him to accept the death. Realistically and sensitively done.

4–8   Waber, B.: IRA SLEEPS OVER. Boston, Houghton Mifflin Co., 1972.

Ira accepts an invitation to sleep over and then worries about what his friend will say if he takes along his teddy bear.

4–10   Weber, A.: ELIZABETH GETS WELL. New York, T. Y. Crowell, 1970.

A girl has surgery, after which she gets well.

5+   Bernstein, J. E., and Gullo, S. V.: WHEN PEOPLE DIE. New York, Dutton, 1977.

A nonfiction book that investigates major issues surrounding life, death and loss by focusing on one woman's death. Some of the areas covered include the aging process, efforts to stay healthy, death and medical checking for signs of life. Also deals with the universality of death, cross-cultural and religious customs, and common grief reactions as a normal process.

5–8   Carrick, C.: LOST IN THE STORM. New York, Seabury, 1974.

Distressed children must wait for a storm to pass before they can search for their lost dog.

5–10   Lasker, J.: HE'S MY BORTHER. Toronto, G. J. McLeod Ltd., 1975.

Deals with ambivalent feelings about a sibling with a learning disability.

5–10   Shecter, B.: ACROSS THE MEADOW. Garden City, N.Y., Doubleday, 1973.

The story of Alfred, a worn-out cat in need of a vacation. In preparation, he bids farewell to animal friends and savors the pleasures of his old environment before departure. Told on two levels, for the very young and for older readers who will understand the allegory: orderly preparation for death as the natural conclusion to a full, rich life.

5–10   Showers, P.: HEAR YOUR HEART. Toronto, Fitzhenry and Whiteside, Ltd., 1968.

Accurate description of the heart and its work, which will hold the attention and interest of latency-age children.

5+   Smith, G.: THE HOSPITAL IS WHERE. 1417 Ocean Drive, Manhattan Beach, California, 1975.

An open-ended book that encourages children to discuss their own experiences and feelings as a way of coping with hospitalization.

5–8   Stanek, M.: I WON'T GO WITHOUT A FATHER. Chicago, Whitman, 1972.

Steve thinks that his problem is unique until he meets other single-parent families at his school's Open House.

5–8   Welber, R.: THE TRAIN. New York, Pantheon, 1972.

Elizabeth slowly builds her courage to face separation from home and shows additional maturity and pride in accomplishment when she is able to help a younger sister make the same trip.

5–8   Zolotow, C.: MY GRANDSON LEW. New York, Harper, 1974.

Assuming that he was unable to understand at age two, Lewis was not told of his grandfather's death. Years later, Lewis tells his mother that he has waited longingly for the old man's return. Together they reminisce and conclude that sharing the loss makes each of them less lonely.

6+   Sendak, M.: HIGGLETY PIGGLETY POP! OR THERE MUST BE MORE TO LIFE. New York, Harper, 1967.

A sophisticated dog, Jennie, concludes that there must be more to life than the accumulation of material possessions. She sets out to gain experience that eventually prepares her for being an actor. Can be read on several age levels.

6–8   Viorst, J.: ROSIE AND MICHAEL. New York, Atheneum, 1974.

All problems are overcome for the best of friends.

8–12   Agle, N. H. SUSAN'S MAGIC. New York, Seabury, 1973.

Susan works out feelings over her parents' divorce through a painful series of small losses. In the process she learns that magical thinking is nonproductive in setting things right.

8–12   La Farge, P.: ABBY TAKES OVER. Philadephia, J. B. Lippincott, 1974.

Helping to care for the family during her mother's absence contributes to the maturity of a preadolescent girl.

8–12   Le Shan, E.: WHAT MAKES ME FEEL THIS WAY? GROWING UP WITH HUMAN EMOTIONS. New York, Macmillan, 1972.

Concerns feelings common to all and gives an overview of psychological thought regarding each.

8–12+   Smith, D. B.: A TASTE OF BLACKBERRIES. New York, Crowell, 1973.

A classic on the topic of grief responses, told in the first person. Concerns Jamie, who dies from a bee sting, and his friend's effort to cope with tragic loss.

10+   Bernstein, J. E.: LOSS AND HOW TO COPE WITH IT. New York, Seabury, 1977.

A comprehensive nonfiction work designed to help children deal with the death of a significant person. Some of the areas covered include what happens when someone dies; children's concepts of death; bereavement; management of feelings; practical issues that must be faced.

10–14   Blume, J.: DENNIE. Scarsdale, New York, Bradbury Press, 1973.

Dennie's bad posture is diagnosed as scoliosis, a congenital deformity for which wearing a brace is prescribed. The event precipitates a maturational crisis for this young teenager.

10–13   Burch, R.: QUEENIE PEARL. New York, Viking, 1966.

A study of maladaptive defenses in a young girl who feels humiliation and loss as the result of her father's imprisonment. She is befriended by a local doctor whose support is influential in helping her cope constructively.

10+   Gardner, R. A.: BOYS AND GIRLS BOOK ABOUT DIVORCE. New York, J. Aronson, 1970.

A comprehensive self-help book meant specifically for children, but helpful as well to parents. Includes universal reactions in children after divorce, including guilt and blame, anger, fear of abandonment, and depression, with an emphasis on a problem-solving approach.

10–14   Greene, C. C.: A GIRL CALLED AL. New York, Viking, 1969.

A story of two preteen girls and their great friendship with Mr. Richards, superintendent of their building. Mr. Richards' sudden death precipitates a crisis in the lives of both girls, who lose his supportive influence.

11+   Hyde, M. O., and Forsyth, E. H.: KNOW YOUR FEELINGS. New York, Watts, 1975.

The importance of recognizing and dealing with feelings as a basis for good mental health is documented in case histories and the work of mental health professionals. A positive, caring approach for young readers.

12–16   Degens, T.: TRANSPORT 7–41–R. New York, Viking, 1974.

Suspenseful tale of displaced persons being evacuated from the Russian-occupied sector of Germany after World War II. Prominently featured are a young adolescent girl and the old couple who befriend her in their flight for survival. Humorous incidents offer the reader moments of relief from the acute tension surrounding the dangerous journey.

12–16   Holland, I.: HEADS YOU WIN, TAILS I LOSE. Philadelphia, J. B. Lippincott, 1973.

An unhappy adolescent girl is entangled in the marital problems of her parents. Family disorganization and misdirected efforts to cope finally lead her and mother to appropriate help and new insights. The fast pace and language hold the reader's interest.

12–16   Klein, N.: IT'S NOT WHAT YOU EXPECT. New York, Pantheon, 1973.

Parental separation teaches a 14-year-old girl and her adolescent siblings that they are capable survivors. Before their parent's eventual reunion, the children get a taste of life in the outside world, including working for a living, pregnancy, abortion, mental illness, etc., all resulting in positive, maturing experiences.

12+   Shanks, A. Z.: OLD IS WHAT YOU GET: DIALOGUES ON AGING BY THE OLD AND THE YOUNG. New York, Viking, 1976.

Fascinating collection of interviews between 17 old persons and 9 adolescents who are involved in projects to help the aged. Discussions on loneliness, retirement, work, marriage, sex, death, etc., contribute to greater understanding of the aging process. Enhanced by quality of photos.

12–16   Sherburne, Z.: STRANGER IN THE HOUSE. New York, Morrow, 1963.

Family relationships change after the return of Kathleen's mother, who was hospitalized several years for mental illness. Story describes the process of reentry and the eventual acceptance of the mother as a capable woman.

14–16   Childress, A.: A HERO AIN'T NOTHIN' BUT A SAND-WICH. New York, Coward, 1973.

A 13-year-old black boy, on the brink of self-destruction from drug abuse, is placed in a rehabilitation program. At first, overcome with bitterness from early-life experiences, he resists the genuine efforts of his stepfather to be supportive. Each chapter relates the story of Benjie through the eyes of significant others. Hard-hitting, explicit and potentially shocking to some readers.

14–adults   Lund, D.: ERIC. Philadelphia, J. B. Lippincott, 1974.

Strong, realistic, moving account of an adolescent's attempts to live a full life despite being afflicted with leukemia. The effects of fatal illness on the family are poignantly described by the author, his mother.

IX
The Pediatric Bill of Rights

Reprinted with the permission of The National Association of Children's Hospitals and Related Institutions, Inc.

"Moved that the Board of Trustees of the National Association of Children's Hospitals and Related Institutions, Inc., endorse the February 25, 1974 proposed Pediatric Bill of Rights as a guideline to be used by agencies and organizations in the development of the mechanics to assure that the children and young adults of our nation are protected in their rights to receive appropriate medical care and treatment where there is conflict between the parents and the child. It is the feeling of the Board that these guidelines shall not be constructed to bypass the rights of parents unless they are in direct conflict with and not in the best interest of the child; and that provisions be made for adequate counseling as to the child's right both to receive and to deny medical care."

Action of
The Board of Trustees
February 25, 1974

PREAMBLE

Every child, regardless of race, religion, ethnic background or economic standing, has the right to be regarded as a person and shall have the right to receive appropriate medical care and treatment. The Pediatric Bill of Rights shall not be construed as a by-passing of the family's right to personal privacy, but shall become operative when parental rights and the child's rights are in direct conflict and it becomes necessary to act in the best interests of the child. Provision shall be made for adequate counseling of the child as to his right to receive and to deny medical care. To the extent that a child cannot demand his rights as a person, those involved in his health care shall move to protect that child's medical interests to the best of their ability.

Canon I.

Every person, regardless of age, shall have the right of timely

425

access to continuing and competent health care.

Canon II.

Every person, regardless of age, shall have the right to seek out and to receive information concerning medically-accepted contraceptive devices and birth-control services in doctor-patient confidentiality. Every person, regardless of age, shall have the right to receive medically-prescribed contraceptive devices in doctor-patient confidentiality.

Canon III.

Every person, regardless of age, shall have the right to seek out and to receive information concerning venereal disease; and every person, regardless of age, shall have the right to consent to and receive any medically-accepted treatment necessary to combat venereal disease in doctor-patient confidentiality.

Canon IV.

Every person, regardless of age, shall have the right to seek out and to accept in doctor-patient confidentiality, the diagnosis and treatment of any medical condition related to pregnancy. Every person, regardless of age, shall have the right to adequate and objective counseling relating to pregnancy and abortion in doctor-patient confidentiality; and every person, regardless of age, shall have the right to request and to receive medically accepted treatment which will result in abortion in doctor-patient confidentiality.

Canon V.

Every person, regardless of age, shall have the right to seek out and to receive psychiatric care and counseling in doctor-patient confidentiality.

Canon VI.

Every person, regardless of age, shall have the right to seek out and to receive medically-accepted counseling and treatment for drug or alcohol dependency in doctor-patient confidentiality.

Canon VII.

Every person, regardless of age, shall have the right to immediate medical care when the life of such person is in imminent danger. The decision of imminent danger to the life of such person is a decision to be made solely by the attending physician; and the attending physician shall decide what treatment is medically indicated under the circumstances.

Canon VIII.

Any person, regardless of age, who is of sufficient intelligence to appreciate the nature and the consequences of the proposed medical care, and if such medical care is for his own benefit, may effectively consent to such medical care in doctor-patient confidentiality. The same shall not apply to Canons II through VII which are deemed to be absolute rights.

Canon IX.

In every case in which a child is being examined by, being treated by or under the medical care of a qualified medical practitioner, and where, in the opinion of that qualified medical practitioner, the child is in need of immediate medical care and where the parent or the legal guardian of said child refuses to consent to such needed, immediate medical treatment, said medical practitioner shall notify the juvenile court or the district court with juvenile jurisdiction immediately. The juvenile court or the district court with juvenile jurisdiction shall immediately appoint a guardian ad litem who shall represent the child's interests in all subsequent legal proceedings. The juvenile court or the district court with juvenile jurisdiction shall immediately set a date for hearing, not to exceed 96 hours from the receipt of the initial report.

The court shall determine at the hearing, based upon medical and other relevant testimony and the best interests of the child, whether or not said medical treatment should be so ordered by the court.

Canon X.

Every person, regardless of age, shall have the right to considered and respectful care. During examinations, every attempt shall be made to insure the privacy of every patient, regardless of age; and every person, regardless of age, has the right to know if observers are present, what role the observer may have in regard to the patient's treatment and shall have the right to request that observers remove themselves from the immediate examining area.

Canon XI.

Every person, regardless of age, shall have the right to know which physician is responsible for his care. Every person, regardless of age, shall have the right to be informed concerning his diagnosis, his treatment and his prognosis in language that is readily understandable to him. Every person, regardless of age, shall have the right to ask pertinent questions concerning the diagnosis, the treatment, tests and surgery done, on a day-to-day basis in a hospital setting; and every person, regardless of age, shall have the right to immediate response to the best of the attending physician's knowledge and in language that the patient clearly understands.

The National Association of Children's Hospitals and Related Institutions is organized in recognition of the importance of child health care. Furthermore, it is organized for the exclusive purpose of creating an organization of hospitals and related institutions which specialize in the health care of children. The main objective of the Association is to promote the quality of health care through the dissemination of information, the promotion of research and education programs related to care, and to participate in such related charitable, scientific, or educational endeavors as determined by the Board of Trustees.

Statements of Policy for the Care of Children and Families in Health Care Settings

PREAMBLE

Advancement of technology and medical science has permitted more children to live, to live longer and in most cases, to live more fully. In the process, other dangers to children's healthy development have arisen or come to light. These problems have in turn stimulated the current progress in the behavioral sciences.

Threats posed to the emotional security and development of many children and their families by serious illness, disability, disfigurement, treatment, interrupted human relationships and nonsupportive environments have been clearly demonstrated by worldwide research studies. The outcomes can range from temporary but frequently overwhelming anxiety and emotional suffering to long-standing or permanent developmental handicaps. Such interference with the fullest possible development and

Date of endorsement July 31, 1977

expression of individual potential is an unacceptable price to pay.

Closer contact with the emotional life of children, increased parent involvement and communication amongst professionals have also contributed to greater understanding as well as to improvements of care. Whereas there is still much to learn regarding the inter-relatedness of such factors as age, type of illness, length of hospitalization, critical developmental periods and vulnerability, sufficient knowledge now exists to direct action toward both minimizing and preventing such harm.

The Association for the Care of Children in Hospitals endorses the following policies:

ALL PEDIATRIC HEALTH CARE SETTINGS SHOULD:

1. Have a stated philosophy of care which is specific, easily understood by, and made available to patients and families,

429

and which applies in a coordinated manner to all disciplines and departments.

2. Assist or provide programs of prevention and restorative care which respond to emotional, social and environmental causal factors of accidents and illness.

3. Create and maintain a social and physical environment which is as welcoming, unthreatening and supportive as possible, and which fosters open communication, encourages human relationships, and invites involvement of children, their families and the community in decisions affecting their care.

4. Avoid hospitalizing children whenever possible through the development of alternatives.

5. Develop and utilize ambulatory, day and home care programs which are financially and geographically accessible.

6. Minimize the duration of unavoidable hospital stays, while recognizing discharge planning needs.

7. Provide for and encourage the presence and participation in the hospital of persons most significant to the child, to approximate supportive home patterns of interactions and routines.

8. Provide consistent, emotionally supportive nurturing care for young children during the absence of their parents.

9. Respect the unique care-taking role of parents as well as their individual responses, and provide ongoing understandable information and support which will enable them to utilize their strengths in supporting their child.

10. Provide a milieu which is responsive to the uniqueness of each child and adolescent, their ethnic and cultural backgrounds and developmental needs.

11. Provide readily accessible, well designed space, equipment and programs for the wide range of play, educational and social activities which are essential to all children and adolescents, particularly those who have been deprived of normal opportunities for development.

12. Provide child care professionals who are skilled at assessing emotional, developmental and academic needs, communicating with and fostering the involvement of patients and their families in activities appropriate to their needs.

13. Ensure that children and their parents are informed, understand and are supported prior to, during, and following experiences which are potentially distressing.

14. Carefully select all staff and volunteers according to their commitment to the foregoing policies. Those in direct contact, however limited, with

children, youth, and families should be sensitive, perceptive and compassionate. Professionals involved in more extended, intimate and responsible positions of child care should have special training in child development, family dynamics and the unique psychological needs of children when ill and under stress.

15. Facilitate orientation, continued learning, and consultation in relation to all of the above, and provide support which recognizes the emotional demands on staff.

16. Encourage and foster the inclusion of the above educational focus in the basic curriculum and field experiences of the various professional and technical personnel preparing for careers in pediatric settings.

17. Support the evolvement of resources for early detection, and of attitudes and facilities for ongoing care of children with health and/or developmental problems.

18. Provide for ongoing evaluation of policies and programs by the recipients of care and staff at all levels.

19. Support and disseminate research which clarifies and pertains to the above.

20. Promote education within the community about the health and developmental needs of children.

XI

Publications of the Association for the Care of Children in Hospitals

ACCH
3615 Wisconsin Avenue N.W.
Washington, D.C. 20016
(202) 244-1801

Available at Nominal Cost:

1. The Hospitalized Child Bibliography.
2. Directory of Child Life Activity Programs in North America.
3. Survey of Activity Programs for Hospitalized Adolescents and an Annotated Bibliography.
4. Guidelines for the Development of Hospital Programs and for the Personnel Conducting Programs of Therapeutic Play for Pediatric Patients.
5. Ideas for Activities with Hospitalized Children.
6. Directory of Child Life Activity Practicum Experiences in North America.
7. Journal of the Association for the Care of Children in Hospitals.

XII

Colleges Preparing Child Life Personnel

Utica College of Syracuse University

A four-year major in Psychology-Child Life leads to the Bachelor of Science degree and certification as a Child Life Specialist. Special emphases include working with adolescents as well as young children, responding to death-related concerns, and establishing child life programs in hospitals where none previously existed. Field experiences begin in the first year, continue during each subsequent year, and culminate in an internship in one of many outstanding child life programs throughout the United States and Canada. For information contact: Director, Child Life Specialist Program, Utica College of Syracuse University, Burrstone Road, Utica, NY 13502.

Northeastern Illinois University

A four-year undergraduate program leads to a degree in Child Development-Hospital Play Specialist. Combining both practical experience and classroom work, the program starts field experiences as early as the sophomore year and culminates with a two-semester practicum and internship in major hospital facilities in the Chicago area. For further information contact: Director, Hospital Program, Department of Early Childhood Education, Northeastern Illinois University, Chicago, IL 60625.

Mills College

Undergraduate students may major in Child Development, with a special emphasis on Child Life in Hospitals. Five hundred clock hours of

435

supervised work with children is required, including work with healthy children as well as children in hospitals. On completion of the undergraduate program, students receive certificates as Child Life Workers. A similar graduate program leads to a master's degree in education and a certificate as a Child Life Specialist. Supervised field placements are made in children's hospitals and pediatric units in the San Francisco Bay Area. For information contact: Coordinator, Child Life in Hospitals Program, Mills College, Oakland, CA 94613.

Wheelock College

A four-year major in The Hospitalized Child leads to the Bachelor of Science in Education degree. Graduate programs in Advanced Study in Early Childhood Education and Leadership in Early Childhood Education, which can focus on the hospitalized child, lead to the Master of Science in Education degree. Field experiences with both well and hospitalized children are included, with placements made in hospitals in the Greater Boston area. For information contact: Coordinator, Hospitalized Child Program, Wheelock College, 200·The Riverway, Boston, MA 02215.

Index